Arrhythmias
Case Studies

50 Case Histories Related To Arrhythmias

By

LESTER B. JACOBSON. M.D.. F.A.C.C., F.A.C.P.
Attending Physician and Staff Cardiologist
Pacific Medical Center
Attending Physician
Ralph K. Davies Medical Center
San Francisco, California

and

NORA GOLDSCHLAGER, M.D., F.A.C.C., F.A.C.P., F.C.C.P.
Director, Coronary Care Unit
Pacific Medical Center
San Francisco, California

MEDICAL EXAMINATION PUBLISHING Co., INC.
969 STEWART AVENUE   GARDEN CITY, N.Y. 11530

Copyright © 1978 by
MEDICAL EXAMINATION
PUBLISHING CO., INC.

Library of Congress Card Number
78-53586

ISBN 0-87488-070-X

August, 1978

Printed in the United States of America

INTRODUCTION

Advances in technology, electrophysiology, pharmacology, and histopathology have made possible detection and elucidation of the mechanism of many cardiac rhythm disturbances encountered clinically. Accurate analysis of the cardiac rhythm is essential for the optimum management of patients with arrhythmias. This book, presenting the actual case histories and electrocardiographic tracings of fifty patients who have at some time in their course been cared for personally by the authors, offers the reader an opportunity to broaden his experience in the important areas of arrhythmia analysis and patient management. In many cases, electrocardiographic tracings and clinical information accumulated over periods of several years demonstrate the clinical course of the arrhythmia, and allow evaluation of the effects of specific therapeutic interventions.

The case histories have been grouped into three categories on the basis of the complexity of the arrhythmias illustrated. The first twenty case histories demonstrate "simple" arrhythmias, aimed both at the beginning electrocardiographic reader and at the more experienced reader who wishes to review basic principles. The middle eighteen case histories illustrate arrhythmias of intermediate complexity, and the last twelve cases illustrate complex arrhythmias aimed at the sophisticated reader. Emphasis is placed upon systematic analysis of the tracings in which the ventricular and the atrial rhythms are individually defined, and then the relationships between them deduced. Ladder diagrams, which greatly facilitate arrhythmia analysis, accompany several of the more complex tracings. In tracings in which the diagnosis or mechanism of an arrhythmia seems impossible to establish with certainty, the adjective "likely" is used to emphasize the uncertainty; and, in recognition that multiple therapeutic approaches to a patient with an arrhythmia may result in a similar outcome, the adjective "reasonable," rather than "correct" or "incorrect," is used in discussions of patient management.

L.B.J.
N.G.

ACKNOWLEDGMENTS

A book of this type could not have been written without a large number of original electrocardiographic tracings of excellent technical quality. The recording of these tracings required the time and energy of many people, to whom I am indebted. The staff in the Coronary Care Unit, the Cardiac Surgical Intensive Care Unit, and the Heart Station, at the University Hospital of San Diego County; the staff in the Coronary Care Unit and Electrocardiographic Laboratory at Moffitt Hospital, of the University of California, San Francisco; and the staff in the Cardiac Catheterization Laboratory, at Pacific Medical Center, San Francisco, were most helpful in this regard.

Special mention is given to Ms. Lynne Gorum, at the University Hospital of San Diego County, and to the Coronary Care Unit nurses at the Ralph K. Davies Medical Center, San Francisco, for their initiative and kindness in carefully collecting many of the tracings and in calling to my attention the arrhythmias of many of the patients presented in this book. Finally, I gratefully acknowledge the superior secretarial assistance provided by my co-author.

L.B.J.
San Francisco, 1978

To the Memory of

Reuben E. Thalberg, M.D.

and

Theodore T. Fox, M.D.

And to Norma and Lou

ARRHYTHMIAS CASE STUDIES

CONTENTS

THE LADDER DIAGRAM

Analysis of complex arrhythmias is greatly facilitated by use of the ladder diagram, which is usually constructed just below an electrocardiographic tracing. The ladder diagram is composed of a skeleton representing regions of the heart in which impulse formation and/or impulse conduction occur. The typical ladder diagram, shown at the upper lefthand portion of the accompanying Figure, consists of equally spaced areas depicting the atria (A), the AV junction (AV) which includes the AV node and His bundle, and the ventricles (V). The height of each area is usually equal. In those instances in which it is important to depict the sinus node (SN) and sinoatrial junction (SA), two rows are added above the A level, as shown in the upper righthand portion of Figure 1.1.

The ladder is constructed upon the skeleton by drawing vertical lines in the A level directly under the P waves inscribed in the electrocardiogram, and vertical lines in the V level directly under the QRS complexes inscribed in the electrocardiogram. The time intervals (in hundredths of a second) are then written between consecutive atrial and/or ventricular deflections. The focus of origin of an impulse is designated by a solid circle. Solid circles representing impulses arising in the sinus node are located at the top of the atrial level, those representing impulses arising within the atria (but not in the sinus node) are located in the middle of the A level, those representing impulses arising in the AV junction are located in the middle of the AV level, and those representing impulses originating in the ventricles are located at the bottom of the V level. Block of an impulse within the cardiac conduction system is designated by a small straight line at right angles to the impulse at the hypothesized area of block. Fusion complexes, i.e., P waves or QRS complexes that occur when atrial or ventricular activation is contributed to by impulses arising in two foci, are detected by closely spaced vertical lines within the A or V levels. When intraventricular conduction occurs with delay or block in either the right or left bundle branch, the bundle branches may be depicted as lines diverging from a common origin at the junction of AV and V levels. These constructs are illustrated in Tracings 1 through 4 of the accompanying Figure.

In Tracing 1, each of two sinus impulses occurring 0.72 seconds apart traverses the atrium and the AV conduction system (which includes the AV node and His-Purkinje system) to stimulate normal-appearing QRS complexes. The PR interval of each PQRST complex is 0.20 seconds.

In Tracing 2 four consecutive sinus impulses are conducted to the ventricles with intraventricular conduction pattern that alternates between normal and left bundle branch block (LBBB).

9

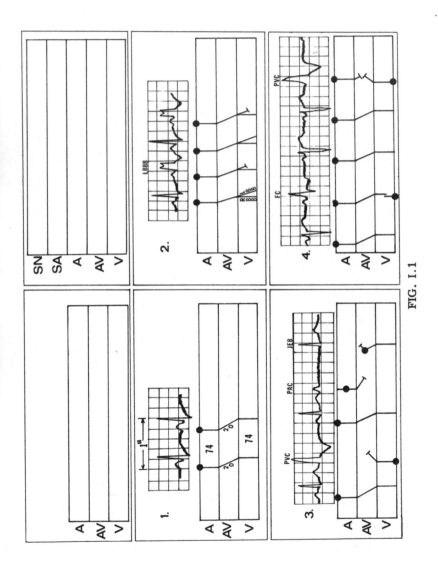

FIG. I.1

In Tracing 3, a sinus-stimulated QRS complex is followed by a premature ventricular complex (PVC) whose retrograde transmission is blocked in the AV junction. The pause occasioned by the PVC is terminated by a sinus impulse which stimulates a normal QRS complex which is followed by a premature atrial complex (PAC) which is blocked within the AV junction. The pause occasioned by the PAC is terminated by a normal-appearing QRS complex which, not preceded by a P wave, is a junctional complex. The occurrence of the junctional complex after a pause of about 1.34 seconds makes it a junctional escape beat (JEB). Retrograde transmission of the junctional impulse has presumably been blocked within the AV junction, since atrial activity does not occur following the junctional complex.

In Tracing 4 the atrial rhythm is sinus, and the first, third and fourth QRS complexes are stimulated by the P waves which precede them. The last QRS complex is a premature ventricular complex. Retrograde transmission of this premature ventricular complex into the atrium, and antegrade transmission of the on-time sinus impulse into the ventricles, are precluded by collision of the two impulses within the AV junction. The second QRS complex, whose initial portion resembles the initial portion of the premature ventricular complex and whose terminal portion resembles the terminal portion of the sinus-stimulated QRS complex is a fusion complex (FC) in which both sinus and ventricular impulses have contributed to ventricular activation.

I: SIMPLE ARRHYTHMIAS

CASE 1: Congestive heart failure precipitated by an arrhythmia,
the treatment of which causes syncope.

A 70-year-old man with no past history of heart disease comes to
the Emergency Room complaining of shortness of breath, orthopnea,
and paroxysmal nocturnal dyspnea, which have progressed over a
period of six weeks. He denies ever having had chest pain, syncope,
or awareness of rapid or irregular heart action. Physical examination suggests generalized cardiomegaly, pulmonary and systemic
venous hypertension, and no valvular dysfunction. An ECG recorded
after the physical examination is shown in Fig. 1.1.

1. What is the cardiac rhythm?
    a) ectopic atrial tachycardia
    b) atrial flutter with 2:1 AV conduction
    c) sinus tachycardia
    d) supraventricular tachycardia (SVT)
    e) atrial fibrillation with rapid ventricular response

ANSWER: (b) QRS complexes occur with perfect regularity at a rate
of about 150/minute. Their normal contour and duration indicate
that ventricular activation occurs normally via the AV junction-His-
Purkinje system. Atrial activity, seen most distinctly in Lead V1,
occurs with regularity at a rate of about 300/minute. The constant
temporal relationship between atrial activity and QRS complexes
suggests that the atrial rhythm is stimulating the ventricular rhythm,
but that only alternate atrial impulses are conducted to the ventricles.
Lead II shows best the sawtooth contour of the atrial activity and the
absence of isoelectric periods in the baseline, indicating that the
atrial rhythm is flutter.

In ectopic atrial tachycardia the atrial rate is usually slower, ranging from about 180 to 220/minute, and discrete P waves are usually
seen between isoelectric segments in Lead II. In sinus tachycardia
clearly defined P waves of normal contour and axis and an isoelectric baseline would be seen. In atrial fibrillation the baseline would
be disorganized and the ventricular rhythm would be irregular. In
SVT, which until recently had been called "PAT", the atrial rate
almost never exceeds 240/minute, and atrial and ventricular rates
are almost invariably identical.

2. The initial use of which of the following therapeutic modalities
    might be expected to be of benefit in this patient who has con-
    gestive heart failure?
    a) quinidine preparation   d) DC cardioversion
    b) digoxin   e) diuretic agents
    c) propranolol

12

ANSWER: (d, e) Congestive heart failure in this patient is most likely the result of atrial flutter with rapid ventricular rate that has been sustained over a period of several weeks. DC cardioversion of the atrial flutter to sinus rhythm, which can usually be achieved with very low energy levels (10-30 watt-seconds), is a useful first-line maneuver with negligible risk; the flutter would be less likely to recur, however, if the rhythm is converted after the congestive failure has resolved.

Diuretic agents would be useful in relieving the circulatory congestion, and digoxin might also be helpful in this regard if it effectively slowed ventricular rate. However, since digitalis preparations are not nearly as effective in decreasing the ventricular response in atrial flutter as they are in atrial fibrillation, significant clinical improvement is not likely to follow the administration of digoxin at this time. Quinidine preparations might convert the flutter to sinus rhythm, but prior to achieving this the atrial rate might be slowed to a point at which the AV node could transmit every impulse, resulting in 1:1 AV conduction and an extremely rapid ventricular rate. The pure vagolytic effect of quinidine, independent of slowing of atrial rate, is rarely seen in clinical dosages used. Propranolol might slow the ventricular response, and in so doing relieve the congestive failure, but this medication is relatively contraindicated as a first-line agent in this patient, as the effects of beta-blockade might produce further myocardial depression and a worsening of the pulmonary congestion.

The patient is treated with oral diuretic agents which clear his congestion, and oral digoxin in doses which achieve a serum digoxin level of 2.2 ng/ml but alter neither AV conduction nor atrial rate. Oral quinidine sulfate is then administered in doses which achieve therapeutic serum levels of 5.0 mg/L, and results in slowing of the atrial rate from 300/minute to about 240/minute but no change in the 2:1 AV conduction of the flutter impulses.

3. At this point the patient is clinically improved. What therapeutic maneuver is most likely to result in restoration of sinus rhythm?
a) adding propranolol
b) stopping digoxin
c) increasing quinidine
d) continuing digoxin
e) performing DC cardioversion

ANSWER: (e) DC cardioversion is the procedure most likely to restore sinus rhythm. Discontinuation of digitalis preparations one to two days prior to DC cardioversion is advocated by some in order to prevent digitalis-induced post-cardioversion arrhythmias. At the low energy levels required to convert atrial flutter to sinus rhythm, however, digitalis preparations need not be withheld unless the patient is obviously digitalis intoxicated. The atrial flutter is treated with DC cardioversion using 10 watt-seconds, and the rhythm shown in Figure 1.2 is then recorded.

4. What is the rhythm?
a) junctional rhythm with 1:1 retrograde conduction
b) sinus rhythm
c) junctional rhythm with atrioventricular dissociation

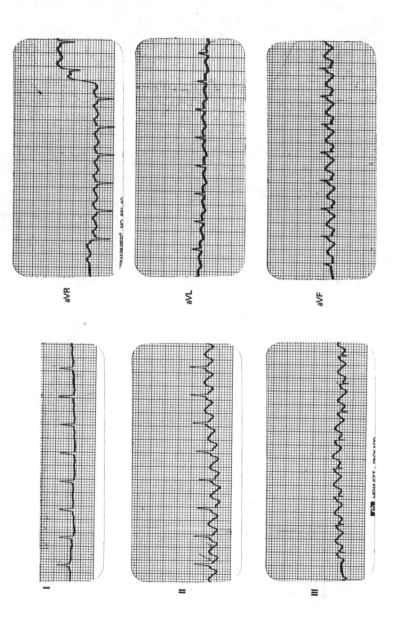

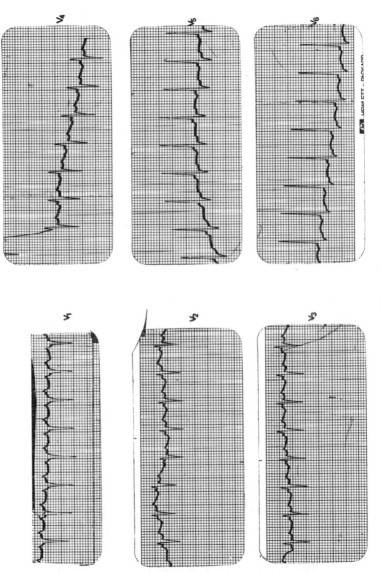

FIG. 1.1

ANSWER: (b) The P waves have a normal axis of +80 degrees, and
precede each QRS complex by identical intervals of about 0.13
seconds. These features establish the diagnosis of sinus rhythm.

5. To which of the following conditions are the ST segment and T
wave abnormalities best attributed in this patient?
   a) left ventricular hypertrophy   e) anterior wall myocardial
   b) digitalis   ischemia
   c) quinidine   f) prolonged period of
   d) hypokalemia   tachycardia

ANSWER: (b, c) Quinidine commonly produces prolongation of the
QT interval and increases U wave amplitude, presumably because
it prolongs His-Purkinje system repolarization time. QT interval prolongation occurs prior to prolongation of either P wave or QRS
duration, but is not absolutely related to the serum quinidine level.
ST segment displacement from the baseline is not a feature of
quinidine effect.

Pronounced U waves are found in about one-fourth of patients with
hypokalemia, but the QT interval itself is usually normal in such
individuals, and the ST segment is not displaced. In this patient,
the ST segment displacement is most likely due to recent digitalis
therapy, but left ventricular hypertrophy, myocardial ischemia,
and recent sustained tachycardia may all be contributing factors.

The patient remains in sinus rhythm and no longer has symptoms
and signs of congestive heart failure. He is discharged home taking
digoxin 0.25 mg orally daily, and oral quinidine sulfate in doses
which achieve therapeutic serum levels. Thirty-six hours after discharge he loses consciousness and falls to the ground, awakening a
few minutes later. Over the ensuing four hours he has three more
such episodes of loss of consciousness. Upon presentation to the
Emergency Room the ECG is identical to that shown in Fig. 1.2.

6. What are likely causes of the patient's episodes of loss of consciousness?
   a) paroxysmal atrial flutter
   b) high grade atrioventricular block
   c) paroxysmal ventricular tachycardia
   d) paroxysmal atrial fibrillation
   e) periods of sinus arrest

ANSWER: (c) Syncope in patients taking quinidine should be presumed to be due to quinidine-induced or-facilitated ventricular tachycardia or ventricular fibrillation until proved otherwise, even though
the estimated incidence is in the range of only one percent. In the
presence of marked QTU interval prolongation, which reflects in-
homogeneity of recovery times of specialized intraventricular conduction tissue produced by quinidine, a premature ventricular impulse may well fall in the "vulnerable period" of ventricular tissue,
leading to repetitive ventricular beating, that is, ventricular tachycardia and/or fibrillation.

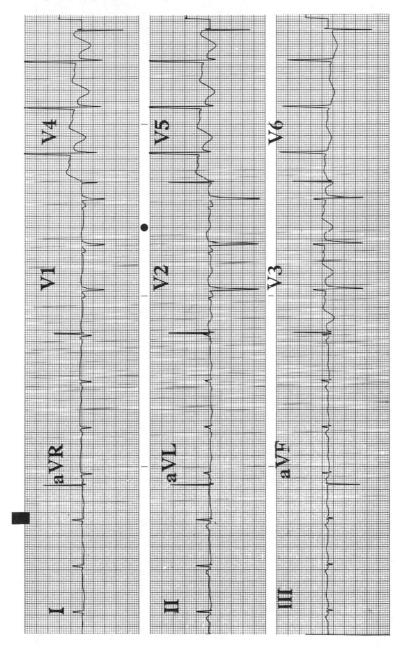

FIG. 1.2

Paroxysmal atrial flutter would not be expected to result in syncope
unless the flutter impulses were being conducted to the ventricles in
a 1:1 ratio, an unlikely possibility in this patient taking digoxin.
Paroxysmal atrial fibrillation could result in syncope if the ventricular response were unusually rapid, but again the patient's digoxin
therapy should be expected to preclude this possibility. Sinus arrest
could conceivably be causing the syncopal episodes in this setting if
it had been demonstrated that prolonged atrial standstill occurred
following the termination of tachycardia, an event that was not observed at the time of conversion of the patient's atrial flutter to
sinus rhythm. High grade AV block would be unlikely to occur in
this man who, while taking digoxin, had nevertheless been able to
conduct 150 flutter impulses per minute to the ventricles.

The patient is admitted to the Coronary Care Unit and his cardiac
rhythm monitored. He has a syncopal episode at a time when the
MCL_1 rhythm strip shown in Fig. 1.3 is recorded.

7. What is the rhythm?
   a) sinus rhythm with a paroxysm of atrial fibrillation and
      aberrant intraventricular conduction
   b) sinus rhythm with a paroxysm of atrial flutter with aberrant
      intraventricular conduction
   c) sinus rhythm with a run of ventricular tachycardia
   d) artifact

ANSWER: (c) Sinus rhythm is present in the beginning of the MCL_1
rhythm strip. The prolonged QTU interval measures about 0.56
seconds. The first premature beat is wide, bizarre, and purely
upright in configuration, and falls on the downslope of the U wave,
but the P wave rhythm and rate are not disturbed. These features
suggest that the premature beat originates in ventricular tissue.
The expected sinus P wave is seen in the early portion of the ST segment of the premature ventricular beat. The pause following the
premature ventricular beat is terminated by a sinus P wave which
is in turn followed by a wide bizarre QRS complex suggesting another premature ventricular beat. The expected sinus P wave falls
on the ST segment of this ventricular beat. Following this, four
wide bizarre QRS complexes occur at intervals of 0.36, 0.33, 0.29
and 0.26 seconds, corresponding to rates of up to about 230/minute.
Since the sinus rate is not altered by these QRS complexes (that is,
there is AV dissociation), it seems most likely that the QRS complexes are stimulated by impulses originating below the bundle of
His, that is, in ventricular tissue, and that the QRS rhythm represents ventricular tachycardia.

8. What is appropriate therapy at this point?
   a) isoproterenol
   b) lidocaine
   c) electrical conversion
   d) discontinuation of the quinidine sulfate

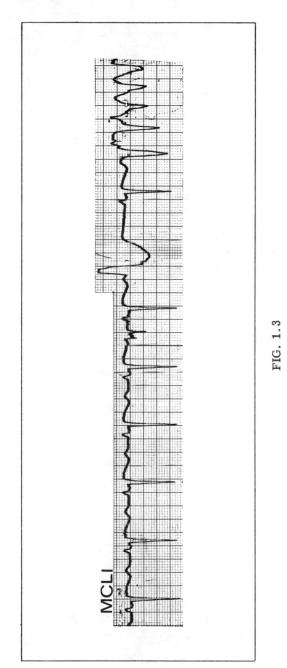

FIG. 1.3

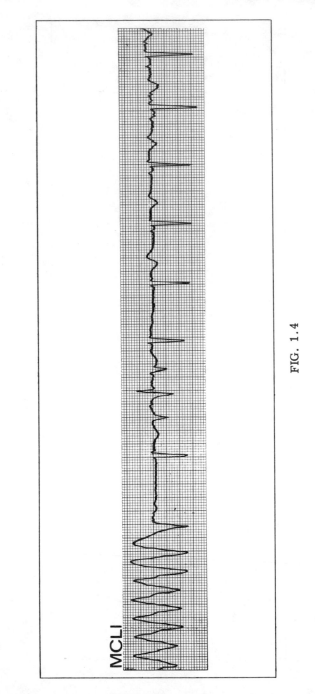

FIG. 1.4

ANSWER: (c, d) This patient's paroxysms of ventricular tachycardia documented to occur in the Coronary Care Unit (this episode subsided spontaneously after about thirty seconds) are most likely related to the quinidine sulfate administration, and represent episodes of "quinidine syncope"; similar paroxysms of ventricular tachycardia were probably responsible for the patient's syncopal episodes at home. The phenomenon of "quinidine syncope" is not clearly dose-related, and in fact occurred in this patient when the serum quinidine level was below the therapeutic range. Quinidine syncope appears to represent an idiosyncratic phenomenon related to prolongation of the QTU interval such that premature ventricular beats occur at a time when repetitive ventricular beating is facilitated.

Although the electrophysiologic properties of isoproterenol seem to be opposite to those of quinidine, intravenous isoproterenol in this clinical setting usually has no effect on preventing quinidine-induced ventricular tachycardia or fibrillation. Repeated electrical conversions and closed-chest cardiac massage seem to be the only modalities useful in the therapy of this problem, and should be performed whenever warranted by the hemodynamic situation. When quinidine is metabolized and excreted from the body these rhythms no longer occur. Acidification of the urine has been reported to increase the renal clearance and therefore the rate of disappearance of quinidine but the clinical effectiveness of this therapy remains conjectural. Fig. 1.4 displays the spontaneous termination of an episode of ventricular tachycardia which lasted about thirty seconds.

The quinidine sulfate is discontinued, the digoxin continued, and the episodes of ventricular tachycardia disappear over a twelve-hour period. The patient is discharged and when last seen five months later remains in sinus rhythm, reports no symptoms of congestive failure, syncope or presyncope, and has no signs of heart failure.

BIBLIOGRAPHY

Selzer A, Wray HW: Quinidine syncope: paroxysmal ventricular fibrillation occurring during treatment of chronic atrial arrhythmias. Circulation 30:17, 1964.

Kassebaum DG, Van Dyke AR: Electrophysiological effects of isoproterenol on Purkinje fibers of the heart. Circulation Res. 19:940, 1966.

Dreifus LS, de Azevedo IM, Watanabe Y: Electrolyte and antiarrhythmic drug interaction. Amer Heart J. 88:95, 1974.

Gerhardt RE: Quinidine excretion in aciduria and alkaluria. Ann Int Med 71:927, 1969.

Kaplinsky E: Quinidine syncope: report of a case successfully treated with lidocaine. Chest 62:764, 1972.

Surawicz B, Lasseter KC: Effect of drugs on the electrocardiogram.
Prog Cardiovasc Dis 13:26, 1970.

Rainer-Pope CR, Schrire V, et al.: The treatment of quinidine induced ventricular fibrillation by closed chest resuscitation and external defibrillation. Amer Heart J 63:582, 1962.

Wallace AG, Cline RE, et al.: Electrophysiologic effects of quinidine:
studies using chronically implanted electrodes in awake dogs with and
without cardiac denervation. Circulation Res 19:960, 1966.

Sokolow M: The present status of therapy of the cardiac arrhythmias
with quinidine. Amer Heart J 42:771, 1951.

Watanabe Y: Purkinje repolarization as a possible cause of the U
wave in the electrocardiogram. Circulation 51:1030, 1975.

Paulk EA Jr, Hurst JW: Clinical problems of cardioversion. Amer
Heart J 70:248, 1965.

Wagner GS, McIntosh HD: The use of drugs in achieving successful
DC cardioversion. Prog Cardiovasc Dis 11:431, 1969.

CASE 2: Hip fracture following syncope in a patient with dizzy spells.

A 72-year-old woman with hypertension and chronic stable angina and occasional dizzy spells is admitted to the hospital for treatment of a hip fracture which resulted from a fall suffered during a dizzy spell. She has never had syncope, symptoms of congestive heart failure, or myocardial infarction. Her only medication is hydrochlorothiazide, which she takes once daily. Her 12-Lead ECG is shown in Fig. 2.1A. The basic rhythm is sinus at a rate of about 58/minute. In Leads aVF, V1, and V4 premature, wide QRS complexes occur at constant coupling intervals of about 0.47 seconds, suggesting that these are ventricular premature beats. The PR interval of about 0.21 seconds is mildly prolonged. The mean frontal plane QRS axis and the QRS duration are normal. The QRS voltage is somewhat increased, raising the possibility of left ventricular hypertrophy. There are non-diagnostic ST and T wave abnormalities, prominent U waves, and a prolonged QTU interval.

Reduction of the hip fracture is performed under general anesthesia without incident. After discharge from the hospital, the patient again experiences dizzy spells that last for several seconds, so the 12-Lead ECG shown in Fig. 2.1B is recorded. All QRS complexes are narrow, suggesting a supraventricular origin. The RR intervals range from 1.18 seconds (corresponding rate about 51/minute) in Lead I, to 1.62 seconds (corresponding rate about 37/minute) in Lead V4. While P waves are clearly identifiable in some Leads (II, aVR, aVL, and V3-V6), they are not so obvious in others (I, III, aVF, V1-V2), suggesting that some QRS complexes are stimulated by sinus impulses and others by junctional impulses. Dissociation of atrial and ventricular complexes is suggested by the variability in PR intervals (shorter in Lead V6 than in Leads V3 and V5), and by the superimposition of a P wave on the early portion of the first QRS complexes in Leads I and V6. The PP intervals range from 1.24 seconds in Lead V5 to 1.64 seconds in Lead aVL.

1. In view of these two tracings, what are the likely rhythm disturbances that might be causing this patient's dizzy spells which are probably due to inadequate cerebral blood flow?
   a) marked bradycardia with periods of sinus pauses
   b) ventricular tachycardia
   c) paroxysmal complete AV block
   d) pauses occasioned by AV Wenckebach periods
   e) marked bradycardia with periods of sinoatrial block

ANSWER: (a, b, e)   While slow sinus rhythm of the degree seen in Fig. 2.1A is not unusual in a patient of this age, the profound sinus bradycardia seen in Fig. 2.1B makes sinus arrest and/or sinoatrial exit block likely causes of the patient's dizzy spells. The ventricular premature beats in Fig. 2.1A suggest that paroxysmal ventricular tachycardia may also be causing dizzy spells, especially in this patient

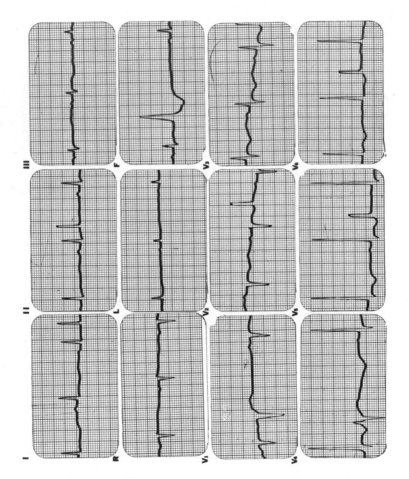

FIG. 2.1A

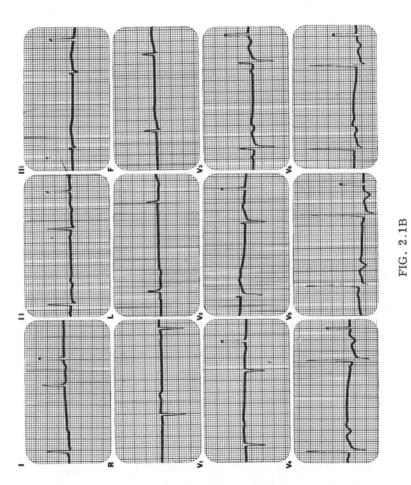

FIG. 2.1B

with symptomatic ischemic heart disease. Since the intraventricular conduction time is normal, it is unlikely that transient complete AV block is occurring. While pauses occasioned by AV
Wenckebach periods are generally not long enough to cause symptoms of inadequate cerebral perfusion, such symptoms might
occur if the patient's sinus rate is very slow and the AV Wenckebach periods are high-grade (e.g., 3:2 and 2:1).

After discharge from the hospital, the patient continues to have
intermittent dizzy spells, but no angina, no symptoms of congestive heart failure, and no syncope. Two years later, she begins
to notice episodes of rapid heart action, during one of which the
12-lead ECG shown in Fig. 2.2 is recorded.

2. What is the rhythm?
    a) atrial fibrillation
    b) atrial flutter with variable AV conduction
    c) multifocal atrial tachycardia
    d) sinus rhythm with paroxysms of atrial tachycardia

ANSWER: (a) The irregularly irregular narrow QRS rhythm and
the irregular baseline suggesting irregular atrial activity indicate
that the atrial rhythm is fibrillation.

3. What are likely pathologic processes that predispose to the de-
    velopment of atrial fibrillation in this patient?
    a) sinus node disease
    b) atrial conduction pathway disease
    c) AV nodal disease
    d) His bundle and bundle branch disease

ANSWER: (a, b) The dramatically slow sinus rates in this patient's
previous ECGs indicate abnormalities of impulse formation and/or
impulse conduction in the area of the sinus node. The slow and
variable rates of the junctional escape rhythm suggest abnormalities
in automaticity and/or conductivity in the area of the AV node and
His bundle. In patients with such rhythm disturbances, histopatho-
logic studies demonstrate fibrosis in pacemaking and conduction
tissue. These pathologic processes result in electrical instability
by causing disparities in rates of impulse formation, and in refractory periods and conduction velocities, thus enhancing the proclivity
to reentrant arrhythmias. Fibrosis of the AV node, His bundle, and
bundle branches, while not uncommon in these patients, is not a
direct cause of atrial arrhythmias.

The patient is treated with oral digoxin and oral quinidine sulfate,
which result in conversion of the atrial fibrillation to sinus bradycardia at a rate of about 50/minute. She is instructed to take digoxin
0.25 mg orally daily, and quinidine sulfate, 200 mg orally every six
hours. Six months later, during a routine office visit, with the patient's only complaint being that of occasional dizzy spells lasting a
few seconds, the 12-lead ECG in Fig. 2-3 is recorded.

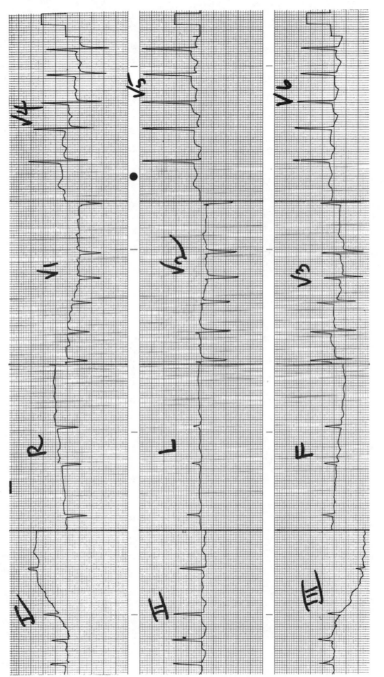

FIG. 2.2

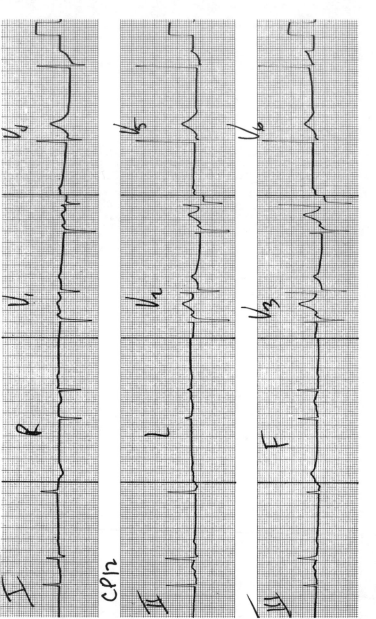

FIG. 2.3

4. What are the possible rhythms?
   a) junctional, with and without retrograde conduction and echo beats
   b) slow sinus rhythm
   c) sinus pauses terminated by junctional escape beats
   d) atrial bigeminy
   e) ventricular bigeminy

ANSWER: (a, b, c) All QRS complexes are narrow (0.06-0.09 seconds duration), indicating their supraventricular origin. Except in Leads V4-V6, QRS complexes occur in a bigeminal pattern with reasonably constant coupling intervals of about 0.40 seconds. The second QRS complex of each pair is a bit wider and of different contour from the first, possibly because of rate-dependent aberrant intraventricular conduction. P waves do not precede the QRS complexes in Leads V4-V6, or the first of each pair of QRS complexes in the other Leads, indicating that these complexes are probably junctional in origin. During the periods of bigeminal rhythm, the ST-T waves of the first QRST complexes are deformed, suggesting that P waves are superimposed. These P waves might represent retrograde atrial capture by the preceding junctional beats. The second QRS complex of each pair might then be stimulated by either antegrade conduction of this atrial impulse (echo beat) or by AV nodal reentry of the original junctional impulse. It is also possible that the junctional escape beat somehow triggers sinus node discharge, with the resulting P wave stimulating the second QRS complex. The origin of the P waves cannot be discerned from this ECG, as P wave contour and therefore P wave axis cannot be precisely determined.

Although the patient is asymptomatic, she is admitted to the Coronary Care Unit for further observation of her rhythm disturbance. Serum potassium, blood urea nitrogen, serum digoxin, and serum quinidine levels are measured; the serum potassium and blood urea nitrogen are normal. Shortly after admission the two continuous strips shown in Fig. 2.4A are recorded. A probable sinus impulse, conducted to the ventricles with first degree AV block, is followed by a pause of 4.90 seconds, which is terminated by a junctional escape beat. The ensuing pause of 2.04 seconds is terminated by another junctional escape beat. A P wave, seen in the T wave of the second junctional escape beat, stimulates the next QRS complex. The remainder of the strip is characterized by a junctional escape beat, followed by two sinus beats, two long pauses terminated by junctional escape beats, and finally, two sinus beats. All atrial impulses are conducted to the ventricles with first degree AV block.

5. How might this rhythm reasonably be managed in this asymptomatic patient?
   a) withhold digoxin
   b) withhold quinidine
   c) administer intravenous atropine
   d) administer intravenous propranolol
   e) insert a temporary pacemaker

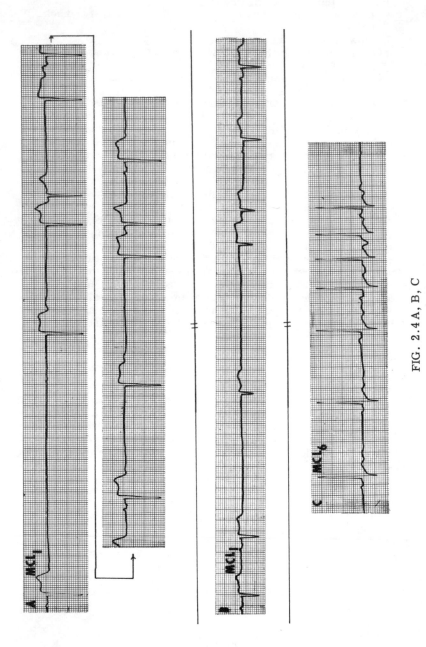

FIG. 2.4 A, B, C

ANSWER: (a, b, c, e) Digoxin and/or quinidine administration might
be playing a role in the rhythm disturbance in this patient at this
time, and should be withheld. Intravenous atropine might improve
sinus node and AV junction automaticity and sinoatrial and AV nodal
conductivity, thereby increasing the ventricular rate. Isoproterenol
might achieve the same effect, but could cause troublesome tachyarrhythmias and even angina pectoris in this patient with coronary
artery disease. Temporary pacing from the right atrium or right
ventricle would, of course, prevent the bradycardia.

Digoxin and quinidine are withheld. The serum digoxin level on admission is reported to be elevated at 3.1 ng/ml (normal therapeutic
range = 0.5-2.0 ng/ml), and the serum quinidine level well below
the therapeutic range at 0.4 mg/L. Digoxin might therefore be
playing at least some role in the rhythm disturbance. Intravenous
atropine, administered periodically in 1-2 mg doses, results in a
greater number of atrial impulses, fewer junctional escape beats,
and shorter pauses. Five days later, when the serum digoxin and
serum quinidine levels are reported to be "zero", the rhythm strips
in Figs. 2.4B and 2.4C are recorded. In Fig. 2.4B, two sinus
beats conducted to the ventricles with first degree AV block and
occurring at intersinus intervals of about 1.10 seconds (corresponding rate about 55/minute) are followed by a pause of 2.68 seconds,
which is terminated by a junctional escape beat. A pause of 2.80
seconds follows, which is terminated by a second junctional escape
beat. A P wave falling on the T wave of this second junctional escape beat stimulates the next QRS complex. The final two beats in
this strip are conducted from the atria, and the different contour
of the P waves suggests that they originate from different atrial
foci. In Fig. 2.4C, two beats which are probably sinus in origin
are followed by a somewhat early ectopic atrial beat, after which a
brief burst of probable atrial tachycardia occurs. So, while the
digoxin may have contributed to the slow heart rate and sinus pauses,
it clearly is not the primary cause.

6. At this time, reasonable management might include:
   a) permanent ventricular pacing
   b) quinidine administration
   c) digoxin administration
   d) no treatment
   e) propranolol administration

ANSWER: (a, b, c) This patient manifests the typical rhythm disturbances seen in the bradycardia-tachycardia syndrome (so-called
"sick sinus syndrome"). The dizzy spells, if due to bradycardia,
can effectively be prevented only by permanent ventricular pacing.
However, ventricular pacing may not prevent the occurrence of
atrial tachyarrhythmias, the development of which is related to abnormal impulse formation and conduction in the sinus node, atria,
and AV junction. Prevention of atrial tachyarrhythmias will require
prevention of atrial premature beats for which quinidine is usually

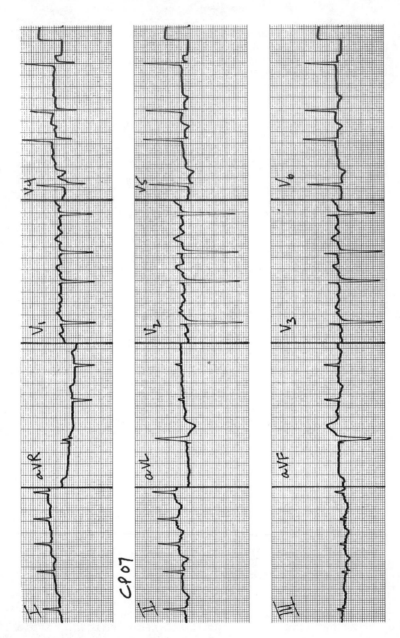

FIG. 2.5

administered. Control of the ventricular rate during atrial flutter
or fibrillation will generally require digoxin and/or propranolol administration. It is unlikely that the patient would do well with no
treatment.

Digoxin and quinidine are withheld until a permanent right ventricular endocardial demand pacemaker, set at a rate of 72 beats per
minute, is implanted. On the second postoperative day digoxin,
0.25 mg orally daily, is restarted. For the first three days postoperatively, the QRS complexes are stimulated almost entirely by
the pacemaker. Only rare P waves are seen, but most of these
are conducted into the ventricles. On the fourth postoperative day
the patient complains of rapid heart action, and the 12-lead ECG
shown in Fig. 2.5 is recorded. The rhythm is atrial fibrillation,
with an average ventricular rate of about 100/minute. The first
QRS complex in the second panel is a paced beat which terminates
a pause which, while not accurately measurable because of the
change in Leads, is at least 0.78 seconds long. Thus, while preventing bradycardia, the pacemaker has not prevented the onset of
atrial fibrillation. Oral quinidine sulfate is then administered in a
dosage which achieves a therapeutic serum level of 4.4 mg/L, and
the atrial fibrillation converts to slow sinus rhythm, with the pacemaker stimulating most QRS complexes. The patient is discharged
from the hospital on digoxin 0.125 mg daily, and quinidine sulfate
in the dose which had achieved therapeutic serum levels. When
last seen 16 months after pacemaker implantation, she feels well,
has no further dizzy spells, and is aware of only brief episodes of
rapid heart action occurring every few days.

BIBLIOGRAPHY

Aroesty JM, Cohen SI, Morkin E: Bradycardia-tachycardia syndrome: Results in 28 patients treated by combined pharmacologic
therapy and pacemaker implantation. Chest 66:257, 1974.

Bharati S, Lev M, et al.: Pathologic correlations in three cases of
bilateral bundle branch disease with unusual electrophysiologic
manifestations in 2 cases. Amer J Cardiol 38:508, 1976.

Bigger JR Jr, Reiffel JA, Cramer M: Effects of digoxin in patients
with sinus bradycardia before and after vagal blockade. Circulation
54: II-187 (Abstr.), 1976.

Cheng TO: Transvenous ventricular pacing in the treatment of
paroxysmal atrial tachyarrhythmias alternating with sinus bradycardia and standstill. Amer J Cardiol 22:874, 1968.

Cohn AE, Lewis T: Auricular fibrillation and complete heart block.
A description of a case of Adams-Stokes syndrome, including the
post-mortem examination. Heart 4:15, 1912-1913.

Ferrer MI: The Sick Sinus Syndrome, Futura Publishing Company, Inc., Mount Kisco, New York, 1974.

Kaplan BM: The tachycardia-bradycardia syndrome. Med Clin No Amer 60: I-81, 1976.

Kaplan BM, Langendorf R, et al.: Tachycardia-bradycardia syndrome (So-called "sick sinus syndrome") Amer J Cardiol 31: 497, 1973.

Kulbertus HE, de Leval-Rutten F, et al.: Sinus node recovery time in the elderly. Brit Heart J 37:420, 1975.

Obel IWP, Cohen E, Millar RNS: Chronic symptomatic sino-atrial block: A review of 34 patients and their treatment. Chest 65: 397, 1974.

Rosen KM, Rahimtoola SH, et al.: Bundle branch block with intact atrioventricular conduction. Electrophysiologic and pathologic correlations in 3 cases. Amer J Cardiol 32:783, 1973.

CASE 3:   Anorexia and malaise two years after beginning therapy
           for an asymptomatic arrhythmia.

A 69-year-old man complains of occasional episodes of exertional
chest discomfort which is felt to be angina pectoris. His resting ECG
(Fig. 3. 1) shows sinus arrhythmia at an average rate of about 65/
minute, and probable atrial premature beats conducted with aberrant intraventricular conduction in Lead I and with no change in intraventricular conduction in Lead aVR. The P waves are normal,
the PR intervals are 0. 13-1. 04 seconds, and the QRS duration is
about 0. 11 seconds. The rSR' configuration in Lead V1 suggests a
mild right bundle branch conduction delay. The mean frontal plane
QRS axis is normal at about -25 degrees. The ST segments and T
waves are normal. The patient is advised to use nitroglycerin, gr.
1/150 sublingually for his chest discomfort. At a routine follow-up
visit two years later his only complaint is of infrequent episodes of
angina pectoris. His ECG now (Fig. 3. 2) shows an increase in QRS
duration from 0. 11 to about 0. 12 seconds, and a change in the rhythm.
The irregular baseline suggests that the atrial rhythm is fibrillation.
The irregularly irregular QRS rhythm, occurring at an average rate
of about 100/minute, is most likely stimulated by the atrial fibrillatory impulses. The patient has no evidence of congestive heart
failure, and his levels of blood urea nitrogen and serum potassium are
normal. Digoxin, 0. 25 mg orally daily, is prescribed.

1. For this patient, this digoxin dosage is probably:
    a) inadequate
    b) appropriate
    c) excessive

ANSWER: (c) Administration of digoxin to patients with atrial fibrillation is aimed at maintaining the ventricular rate at levels that permit adequate cardiovascular performance at rest and during activity.
The AV node, which has the slowest conduction velocity of all cardiac
conduction tissue and often the longest refractory period almost always
determines the ventricular rate in atrial fibrillation. The number of
fibrillatory impulses conducted through the AV node and into the His-
Purkinje system per minute is dependent upon the AV nodal refractory period and the number of impulses which penetrate into but not
through the AV node. These impulses, by depolarizing AV nodal cells
to varying depths, slow the transmission of subsequent impulses. The
phenomenon by which impulses that are not themselves electrocardiographically manifest but make their presence known by affecting subsequent electrocardiographic events, is called "concealed conduction".

The usual ventricular response to atrial fibrillation in an individual
who is euthyroid, has no medical problems, receives no medication,
and has normal AV nodal function is in the range of 150-170 beats
per minute. Medications and autonomic nervous system traffic can
alter the ventricular response by their effects on AV nodal function.

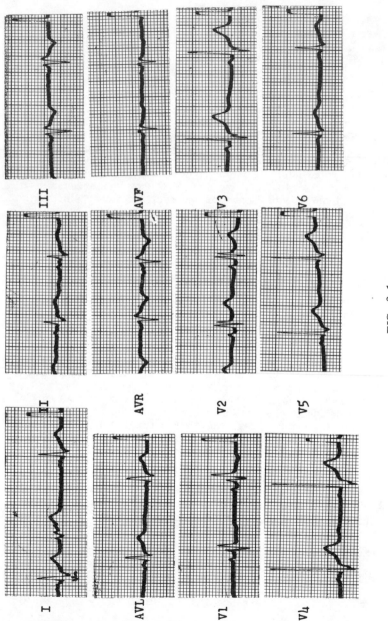

FIG. 3.1

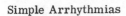

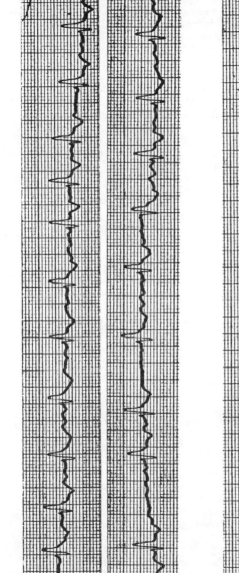

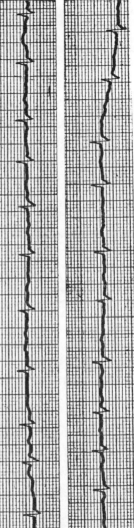

FIG. 3.2

V_1

$=$

Sympathetic stimulation, beta-adrenergic agents, and parasympatholytic agents tend to increase the ventricular response while parasympathetic stimulation, beta-adrenergic blocking agents, and para-
sympathomimetic agents tend to decrease it. Digoxin, which slows
AV nodal conduction velocity and prolongs AV nodal refractory
period does so predominantly by modification of autonomic nervous
system traffic into the AV node.

In this patient who takes no medications and has no complicating
medical problems, the ventricular rate of about 100/minute suggests
abnormally depressed AV nodal function. Digoxin, if administered
in doses usually prescribed for patients with normal AV nodal function, may cause undue slowing of the ventricular rate. Rather than
administer the "usual" daily dose of digoxin to this patient, it would
be preferable to prescribe a lower starting dose and evaluate the
patient frequently to ensure that his ventricular rate at rest and with
activity remains in a range which optimizes his cardiovascular performance. Since this patient is asymptomatic and unaware of the
atrial fibrillation, consideration should be given to administering
no digoxin at all.

The patient does well for a period of about two years, until he begins
to feel generally unwell and has a poor appetite. He reports no
symptoms of congestive heart failure and has had no angina pectoris for
the past several months. His radial pulse is irregularly irregular
at a rate of about 40/minute, and his apical pulse is counted at a
rate of 60/minute. The ECG recorded at this time is shown in
Fig. 3.3.

2. What rhythms are present in this tracing?
    a) atrial fibrillation
    b) ventricular parasystole
    c) ventricular extrasystoles
    d) ventricular bigeminy
    e) AV dissociation with AV junctional rhythm

ANSWER: (a, c, d) The atrial rhythm is fibrillation. The irregularly irregular ventricular rhythm in Leads I, II, III and V1 indicates that the QRS complexes in these Leads are stimulated by the
atrial fibrillatory impulses. As in the previous electrocardiogram,
intraventricular conduction shows right bundle branch conduction
delay. In Leads I, II, and III wider QRS complexes, occurring at
coupling intervals of 0.49-0.53 seconds, are interposed between
narrower QRS complexes, resulting in a bigeminal rhythm. The
duration of these wider QRS complexes suggests that they originate
below the His bundle, and their left bundle branch block contour
suggests that they initiate ventricular activation in the area of the
right bundle branch. Their essentially fixed coupling intervals to
preceding QRS complexes suggests that they are extrasystolic. The
diagnosis of ventricular parasystole is excluded by the absence of
variable coupling intervals, by the marked variability in interectopic

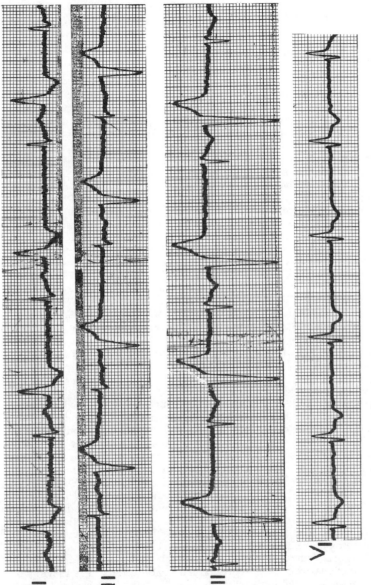

FIG. 3.3

intervals, and by the absence of fusion beats. AV dissociation with atrial fibrillation and independent AV junctional rhythm would be characterized by a regular QRS rhythm which, in this patient, would probably have a right bundle branch block pattern.

3. Reasonáble management at this time might include:
   a) quinidine administration
   b) potassium administration
   c) lidocaine administration
   d) procainamide administration
   e) withholding digoxin
   f) evaluation of creatinine clearance
   g) measurement of serum digoxin level

ANSWER: (e, f, g) The patient's loss of appetite and the ventricular bigeminal rhythm strongly suggest the possibility of digitalis intoxication, primary therapy of which includes withholding further digoxin and maintaining normal serum potassium levels. Potassium, which may itself depress AV nodal conduction, should be administered to patients with depressed AV nodal function only if serious ventricular arrhythmias occur in the presence of hypokalemia. If the ventricular extrasystolic beats should have an adverse hemodynamic effect and/or lead to ventricular tachycardia, suppressant medication such as lidocaine, quinidine, or procainamide could be prescribed. Creatinine clearance, a major determinant of digoxin excretion, should be measured to help explain the appearance of digoxin intoxication at this particular time, and to estimate appropriate digoxin dosage for the future. Measurement of serum digoxin level might help support the diagnosis of digitalis intoxication (this rhythm occurred in 1968, before widespread availability of serum digoxin assays).

Digoxin is withheld, the measured serum potassium level is normal, and the measured creatinine clearance is moderately reduced at 50 ml/min. Over a four-day period, the anorexia and runs of ventricular bigeminy disappear, suggesting that digoxin administration was indeed responsible for these problems. Three days later, at the time of discharge, the patient feels well, the resting ventricular rate has increased from about 55/minute to about 90/minute, and only rare ventricular premature beats are occurring. Since the patient is feeling well without digoxin, and since he has AV nodal dysfunction and somewhat impaired renal function, the decision is made to prescribe no further digoxin until the patient is reevaluated one month later. At the time of this visit he looks and feels well, has no symptoms or signs of congestive heart failure and is having no angina. His ventricular rate is about 90/minute at rest and there are occasional ventricular premature beats. Digoxin is therefore not prescribed, and the patient does well over the next five years.

It is unclear why this man, who tolerated digoxin for almost two years without problems, should suddenly develop manifestations of digitalis intoxication. This phenomenon is seen most commonly in the aged, usually in the setting of an acute illness complicated by fluid and electrolyte disturbances. In this man it may have been due to interval asymptomatic deterioration in renal function, but since creatinine clearances had not been measured before, this possibility remains conjectural.

BIBLIOGRAPHY

Childers R: Concealed Conduction, Med Clin No Amer 60: I-149, 1976.

Cohen SI, Lau SH, et al.: Concealed conduction during atrial fibrillation. Amer J Cardiol 25:416, 1970.

Goodman DJ, Rossen RM, et al.: Effect of digoxin on atrioventricular conduction. Studies in patients with and without cardiac autonomic innervation. Circulation 51:251, 1975.

Haft JI, Levites R, Gupta PK: Effects of ventricular premature contractions on atrioventricular conduction. Amer J Cardiol 32:794, 1973.

Langendorf R, Pick A, Katz LN: Ventricular response in atrial fibrillation. Role of concealed conduction in the AV junction. Circulation 32:69, 1965.

Lau SH, Damato AN, et al.: A study of atrioventricular conduction in atrial fibrillation and flutter in man using His bundle recordings. Circulation 40:71, 1969.

Langendorf R: Concealed A-V conduction: The effect of blocked impulses on the formation and conduction of subsequent impulses. Amer Heart J 35:542, 1948.

Przybyla AC, Paulay KL, et al.: Effects of digoxin on atrioventricular conduction patterns in man. Amer J Cardiol 33:344, 1974.

Mendez C, Han J, Moe GK: Comparison of the effects of epinephrine and vagal stimulation upon the refractory periods of the A-V node and the bundle of His. Arch Exp Pathol Pharmacol 248:99, 1964.

CASE 4: Arrhythmias following surgical closure of an atrial septal defect.

A 54-year-old woman with an atrial septal defect has had episodes of supraventricular tachycardia for the past five years. Despite taking digoxin 0.25 mg daily, her episodes have been occurring with increasing frequency, but they can be converted to sinus rhythm with vigorous carotid sinus massage. Cardiac catheterization reveals a 2:1 left-to-right shunt at the atrial level, moderate pulmonary hypertension, and moderately elevated pulmonary vascular resistance; surgical closure is recommended. At surgery a prosthetic patch is used to close a large secundum defect. When cardiopulmonary bypass is discontinued there is no visible atrial activity, and the cardiac rhythm is junctional at a rate of about 60/minute. Pairs of bipolar pacing electrodes are sewn onto the right atrium and right ventricle for use in the event that this rhythm is unstable, and bipolar right atrial pacing at a rate of about 80/minute is instituted. The operation is completed, and the patient transferred to the Intensive Care Unit. Digoxin 0.25 mg daily is continued, and is administered intravenously during the perioperative period.

In order to assess spontaneous atrial activity the current output of the pacemaker is decreased below the bipolar atrial pacing threshhold level every twelve hours, as shown in Fig. 4.1 (two continuous Lead II rhythm strips). The top strip shows a regular QRS rhythm at intervals of about 0.94 seconds (rate about 64/minute), which is unrelated to the atrial pacing artifacts that are seen at intervals of about 0.74 seconds (rate about 81/minute). In the lower strip the current output of the pacemaker is increased with the result that, beginning with the fifth (●) QRS complex, the RR intervals shorten, becoming essentially equal to the interstimulus interval of the pacemaker, and the stimulus-to-R interval becomes constant at about 0.22 seconds. Even though P waves are not clearly seen, the constant 0.22 second stimulus-to-R interval suggests that the atrial pacemaker is stimulating these QRS complexes. P waves are clearly seen in Lead aVF of Fig. 4.2, recorded during constant atrial pacing a few minutes later.

For four days there is no evidence of spontaneous atrial activity. On the fifth postoperative day the pacemaker is transiently turned off while the two continuous Lead V₆ rhythm strips in Fig. 4.3 are recorded. The first four QRS complexes in the top strip are stimulated by the atrial pacemaker.   The pause following cessation of atrial pacing is terminated by the first of a series of spontaneously occurring P waves which precede, at intervals of 0.24 seconds, QRS complexes which have contours identical to QRS complexes stimulated during atrial pacing. The atrial rhythm is probably sinus, and the progressively shortening PP intervals indicate a rhythm of development, or "warmup" phenomenon. Effective sinus node function has returned for the first time since the operation, but atrial pacing is continued for another 24 hours. About two hours after

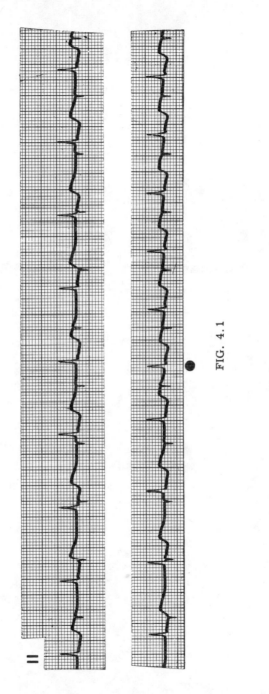

FIG. 4.1

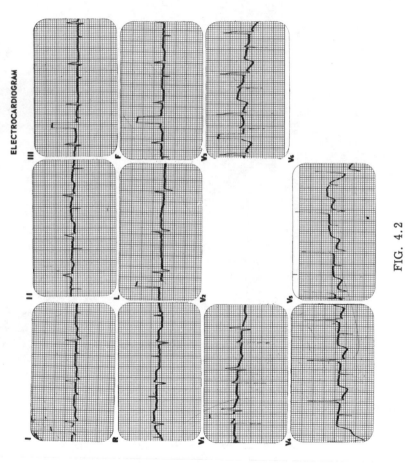

FIG. 4.2

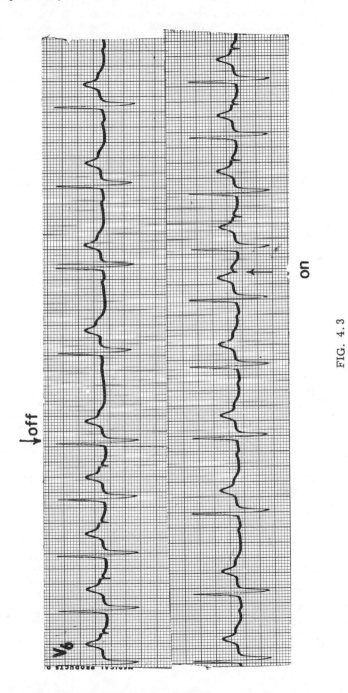

FIG. 4.3

cessation of atrial pacing the rhythm is noted to have changed from
sinus to atrial flutter with 2:1 AV conduction. The ventricular rate
is about 130/minute, but there is no change in the adequate hemodynamic state.

1. Reasonable management of this patient at this time might include:
   a) slowing the ventricular rate with propranolol and/or additional
      digoxin
   b) DC cardioversion
   c) quinidine administration

ANSWER: (a) Atrial arrhythmias are common in the first few days
following surgical closure of defects of the interatrial septum, especially in adult patients. They are presumably due, at least in
part, to irritation of the atrium and sinus node area from manipu-
lation of the atrium during the surgical procedure itself; the commonly seen postoperative pericarditis and increased sympathetic
nervous system traffic may facilitate their appearance. In this
setting, stable sinus rhythm usually cannot be maintained until
several days to weeks postoperatively. Therefore, while DC cardioversion might achieve sinus rhythm, recurrence of atrial arrhythmias would be expected. Propranolol and/or digoxin administration
in order to slow the ventricular response would seem to be the most
reasonable therapy. If restoration of sinus rhythm is felt to be advisable at this time and is achieved with DC cardioversion, a quinidine preparation might help prevent the recurrence of atrial arrhythmias.

The decision is made to slow the ventricular rate by the intravenous
administration of additional digoxin, 0.25 mg every four hours, until alternating 4:1 and 2:1 AV conduction of the atrial flutter occurs.
The amount of digoxin required to slow the ventricular response to
atrial flutter is usually much greater than that required to slow the
ventricular response to atrial fibrillation. Despite the fact that
serum digoxin levels are often above the "therapeutic range" when
alternating 4:1 and 2:1, or consistent 4:1 AV conduction is achieved
in atrial flutter, digoxin-induced arrhythmias are rarely seen at
such times. Propranolol might be used to slow the ventricular
response, and usually does so more rapidly and more consistently
than digoxin in this clinical setting.

The patient's rhythm continues to be atrial flutter with 4:1 and 2:1
AV conduction for the next three days, at which time the atrial and
ventricular pacing wires are removed. Ten days later quinidine sulfate is administered in doses which achieve a therapeutic serum
level, and DC cardioversion of the atrial flutter is attempted with a
10 watt-second discharge. The continuous Lead II rhythm strips
shown in Fig. 4.4 record the events surrounding the electrical discharge.

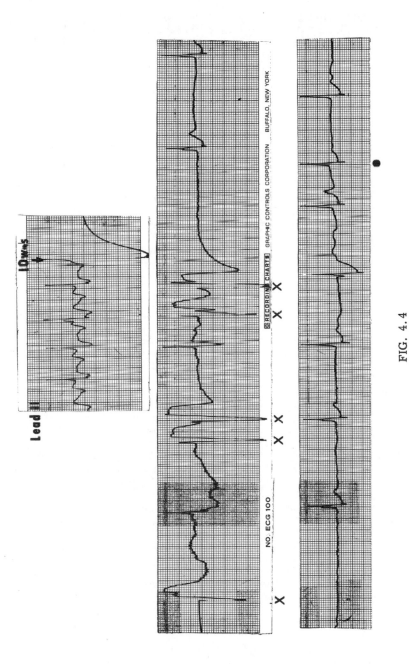

FIG. 4. 4

In the top strip the atrial rhythm is flutter at a rate of about 220/
minute, and the RR intervals vary, with the ventricular response
averaging 110/minute. At the arrow, a 10 watt-second discharge,
synchronized to the R wave, is introduced, and is followed by a
1.4 second period during which the ECG machine is not recording.

2. Which terms characterize the rhythm emerging after the electrical discharge?
   a) junctional rhythm   e) "warmup" phenomenon
   b) ventricular ectopic beats   f) escape beats
   c) atrial standstill   g) atrial fibrillation
   d) complete AV block

ANSWER: (a, b, c, e, f) The QRS complexes are of two types.
Those labeled "X" are wide, bizarre, predominantly negative, and
different from the QRS complexes during atrial flutter; the other
QRS complexes are narrow, and identical to the QRS complexes
during atrial flutter. The wide bizarre QRS complexes are probably ventricular in origin. Since the first and second of these wide
QRS complexes terminate long pauses they are ventricular escape
beats; and the remainder of them, which occur at short cycle length,
are ventricular premature beats.

The resemblance of the narrow QRS complexes occuring after the
electrical discharge to those that occurred during atrial flutter indicates that these QRS complexes are conducted to the ventricles
from the AV junction, but does not establish whether they are stimulated by junctional or by atrial impulses. However, their appearance
following long pauses suggests that they are junctional escape beats,
and their generally shortening cycle length, which demonstrates a
rhythm of development or "warmup" phenomenon, supports the diagnosis of junctional rhythm. The next-to-last QRS complex (●) in
the bottom strip occurs at an unexpectedly short cycle length, and
follows an identical QRS complex whose T wave is taller and sharper
than those of the remaining narrow QRS complexes. This suggests
that there is, superimposed on this T wave, a P wave which stimulates
the prematurely occurring QRS complex. If indeed this is a P wave,
the atrial rhythm could not be fibrillation. Since atrial activity has
not been apparent until this P wave occurs 22 seconds after the
electrical discharge, "atrial standstill" may be said to have been
present up to this time. Atrial standstill may be due to sinus arrest
and/or to sinoatrial exit block, but currently available techniques
do not allow this differential diagnosis to be established in man.
Since the solitary P wave stimulates a QRS complex, there is no
evidence of complete AV block, although, because the P wave occurs
shortly after the junctional beat, it is conducted with a markedly prolonged PR interval (first degree AV block). A 12-Lead ECG recorded
during the junctional rhythm is shown in Fig. 4.5.

Since a serum digoxin level is in the therapeutic range at this time,
digoxin 0.25 mg daily is continued. For three days the patient's
rhythm remains junctional until atrial flutter with alternating 2:1 and

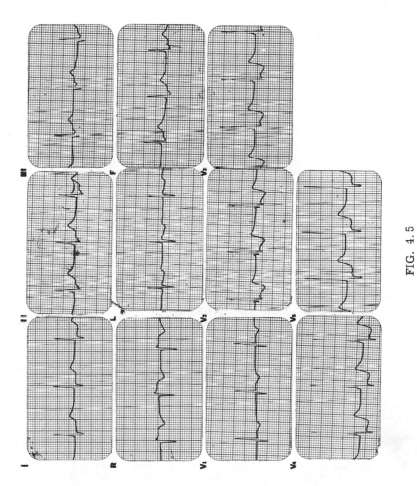

FIG. 4.5

4:1 AV conduction recurs. As the atrial flutter causes no hemodynamic deterioration and the patient does not feel uncomfortable
with the irregular rhythm, the decision is made to postpone electrical conversion for about six weeks. This delay may allow further
recovery of sinus node and atrial conduction system function which
would optimize the chances of achieving and maintaining sinus
rhythm.

3. Reasonable management prior to the second attempt at DC
   cardioversion of this patient might include:
   a) temporary transvenous pacemaker insertion
   b) propranolol administration
   c) atropine administration
   d) quinidine administration

ANSWER: (a, d) In this patient, whose course after her first DC
cardioversion was characterized by long pauses and ventricular
ectopic beats, recurrence of similar events, although less likely
at this time, must be anticipated and prepared for. A temporary
transvenous pacemaker, located in the right atrium or right ventricle could be used to prevent long periods of cardiac standstill
which might be terminated by serious ventricular arrhythmias.
Quinidine administration would probably help maintain sinus rhythm
which might be achieved by the DC discharge. Propranolol may be
useful in maintaining sinus rhythm following cardioversion in some
patients, but in this woman might conceivably suppress sinus node,
atrial,. and/or junctional automaticity (and possibly conduction velocities) to the point of causing post-cardioversion atrial standstill or
very slow sinus, atrial, or junctional rhythms. Atropine might, by
vagolysis, result in an increase in sinus and AV junctional automaticity and possibly even an improvement in sinoatrial conduction.
It appears to achieve these effects when administered within seconds
to minutes after DC discharge; however, it is unclear whether its
administration prior to DC discharge has beneficial or detrimental
effects.

Quinidine sulfate is administered orally in doses which achieve a
therapeutic serum level, digoxin 0.25 mg daily is continued, a temporary transvenous electrode catheter is positioned into the apex of
the right ventricle, and a 50 watt-second discharge is introduced at
the peak of the R wave. Sinus rhythm at a rate of about 60/minute
appears, with a PR interval of about 0.20 seconds. Three days
later the patient is discharged feeling well, and is advised to take
digoxin and quinidine sulfate. She has no arrhythmias until three
years after operation, when she has an episode of atrial flutter
which lasts several days and which is uneventfully converted electrically to sinus rhythm. When last seen five years postoperatively,
she is still taking digoxin and quinidine sulfate and is having no
arrhythmias.

BIBLIOGRAPHY

Daicoff GR, Brandenburg RO, Kirklin JW: Results of operation for
atrial septal defect in patients forty-five years of age and older.
Circulation 35: I-143, 1967.

Popper RW, Knott JMS, Selzer A, Gerbode F: Arrhythmias after
cardiac surgery. I. Uncomplicated atrial septal defect. Amer
Heart J 64:455, 1962.

Rabbino MD, Dreifus WL, Likoff W: Cardiac arrhythmias following
intracardiac surgery. Amer J Cardiol 7:681, 1961.

Rodstein M, Zeman FD, Gerber IE: Atrial septal defect in the aged.
Circulation 23:665, 1961.

Rose MR, Glassman E, Spencer FC: Arrhythmias following cardiac
surgery: relation to serum digoxin level. Amer Heart J 89:288,
1975.

CASE 5: Electrocardiographic abnormalities during treadmill
exercise testing in an asymptomatic man.

A 62-year-old man with neither symptoms nor signs of cardiovascular disease performs a graded treadmill exercise test as part of
a routine medical examination. His physical examination, chest
x-ray, and resting 12-Lead ECG are all within normal limits.

Figs. 5.1 and 5.2 show Leads V_1 and V_6 recorded in close temporal relationship at rest and at specified times during exercise.
During the third minute of exercise, when the patient feels entirely
well, wide bizarre QRS complexes begin to alternate with the normal-appearing QRS complexes (Fig. 5.1).

1. Which of the following describe the rhythm during the third
   minute of exercise (Fig. 5.1)?
   a) ventricular bigeminy, in which a ventricular premature beat
      follows each sinus-stimulated QRS complex
   b) fusion beats, in which the ventricles are activated in close
      temporal relationship by the sinus impulse and by an ectopic
      ventricular impulse.
   c) sinus impulses with intraventricular conduction that alter-
      nates between normal and left bundle branch block.

ANSWER: (c)   In the tracings recorded at rest, the rhythm is sinus
at a rate of about 86/minute, the PR interval is normal at about
0.17 seconds, and the QRS contour and duration are normal. In
the tracings recorded in the third minute of exercise, P waves occur
at regular intervals of about 0.48 seconds (corresponding rate about
125/minute), indicating sinus tachycardia. The wide, bizarre QRS
complexes alternating with normal-appearing QRS complexes have
left bundle branch block type contours, indicating that in these beats
ventricular activation is occurring via the right bundle branch. This
left bundle branch block pattern of ventricular activation could occur
because a ventricular ectopic beat originates in the area of the right
bundle branch, or because a sinus impulse is blocked in the left
bundle branch. However, since the QRS complexes with left bundle
branch block pattern follow P waves at intervals identical to the PR
intervals of the normal-appearing QRS complexes, they are not
occurring prematurely. The identical PR intervals preceding both
normal and left bundle branch block type QRS complexes make it
very unlikely that ventricular fusion beats are present. The alternation of QRS complexes with normal and left bundle branch block
intraventricular conduction patterns is, then, most likely due to
alternate sinus P waves being unable to traverse the left bundle
branch antegradely. The development of intraventricular conduction
abnormalities with changes in sinus rate may be explained by rate-
related conduction delays (or blocks). In this patient, the conduction
abnormality may be characterized as a tachycardia-dependent left
bundle branch block.

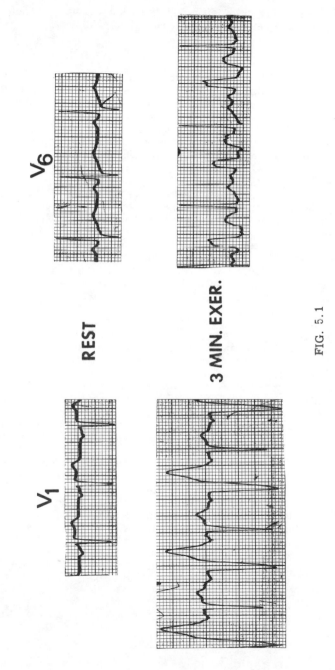

FIG. 5.1

2. Is the development of left bundle branch block during treadmill
   stress testing diagnostic of coronary artery disease?
   a) yes
   b) no

ANSWER: (b)   Rate-dependent intraventricular conduction abnormalities occur in three to five percent of all patients undergoing
treadmill exercise testing, and may involve either the right or left
bundle branch system.   The occurrence of exercise-related intraventricular conduction abnormalities does not per se correlate with
the presence of coronary artery disease, although it is possible for
exercise-induced acute ischemia of conduction tissue to cause the
phenomenon.

Since this patient is asymptomatic, the exercise test is continued.
During the sixth minute, when the sinus rate is about 150/minute,
the normal intraventricular conduction disappears and all QRS complexes now show left bundle branch block (Fig. 5.2). Although the
patient offers no complaints, exercise is terminated at this time.
Following exercise the sinus rate gradually slows and during the
fourth minute of the recovery period, when the heart rate is about
115/minute, ventricular activation continues to occur solely via
the right bundle branch (Fig. 5.2). At seven minutes of recovery,
when the sinus rate is about 110/minute, alternating normal and
left bundle branch block intraventricular conduction patterns recur.
The long Lead V_6 rhythm strip, recorded during the fourteenth
minute of recovery when the sinus rate is about 107/minute, begins
with 2:1 left bundle branch block conduction. (Fig. 5.3) Over a period of
several seconds intraventricular conduction changes to 3:1 left
bundle branch block conduction; and the last three QRS complexes
are of normal configuration indicating that the left bundle branch
is now capable of conducting at least three out of every four sinus
impulses. During the fifteenth minute of recovery, when the sinus
rate is about 105/minute, intraventricular conduction is normal.

The occurrence of normal and of left bundle branch block type intraventricular conduction at comparable heart rates illustrates
that although bundle branch conduction is rate-dependent, the exact
rate at which it changes may vary from moment to moment. This
lack of precision probably reflects the fact that conduction velocities and refractory periods of the intraventricular conduction
system tissue are dependent not only on heart rate but also on autonomic influences, the humoral environment, the presence or absence of ischemia, and mechanical factors such as tension in the
wall of the ventricle surrounding the conduction tissue.

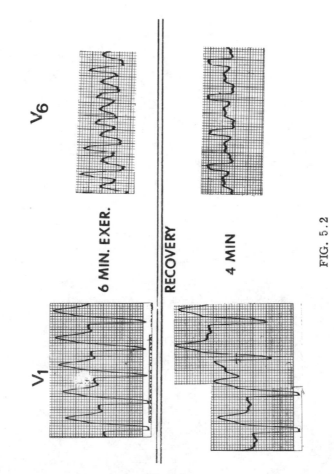

FIG. 5.2

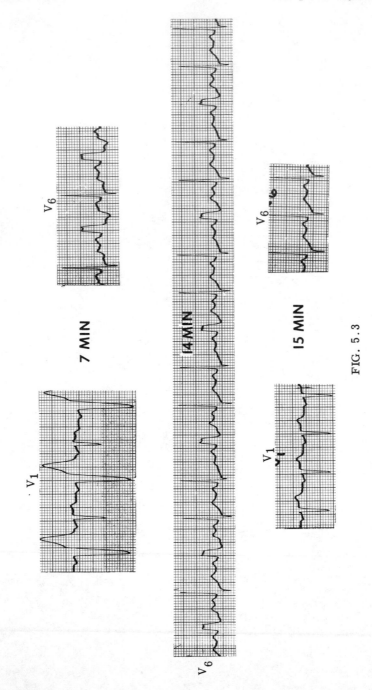

FIG. 5.3

BIBLIOGRAPHY

Bauer GE: Transient bundle-branch block. Circulation 29:730, 1964.

El-Sherif N: Tachycardia-dependent versus bradycardia-dependent intermittent bundle branch block. Brit Heart J 34:167, 1972.

Lewis CM, Dagenais GR, Friesinger GC: Coronary arteriographic appearance in patients with left bundle branch block. Circulation 41:299, 1970.

Neuss H, Thormann J, Schlepper M: Electrophysiological findings in frequency-dependent left bundle branch block. Brit Heart J 36:888, 1974.

Whinnery JE, Froelicher V Jr: Acquired bundle branch block and its response to exercise testing in asymptomatic aircrewmen: A review with case reports. Aviation, Space, and Environ Med 47: 1217, 1976.

Froelicher VF, Thomas MM, Pillow C, Lancaster MC: Epidemiologic study of asymptomatic men screened by maximal treadmill testing for latent coronary artery disease. Amer J Cardiol 34:770, 1974.

CASE 6:   Tachyarrhythmia in a patient with chronic obstructive
          pulmonary disease and respiratory failure.

A 64-year-old man with severe chronic obstructive pulmonary disease
is admitted to the Intensive Care Unit for treatment of respiratory
failure precipitated by acute respiratory infection. He is cyanotic
and in severe respiratory distress, with marked prolongation of the
expiratory phase of respiration. The pulse is irregularly irregular
at a rate of about 140 per minute, and the blood pressure is 120/90
in the sitting position. The cardiac output appears adequate. There
is mild jugular venous distension, mild hepatomegaly, and moderate
pretibial edema. Examination of the chest reveals movement of only
small amounts of air, and severe bronchospasm. Examination of the
heart shows right ventricular hypertrophy and loud gallop sounds
over the right ventricle. The chest x-ray shows hyperexpanded lung
fields, flat diaphragms, no pulmonary infiltrates, normal heart size,
and large proximal pulmonary arteries with a paucity of distal pulmonary vascular markings. An arterial blood gas with the patient
breathing room air reveals $pO2$ of 42 mm Hg, $pCO2$ of 64 mm Hg, and
pH of 7. 25. The serum potassium level is normal. The cardiac
rhythm is shown in the two continuous ML II rhythm strips of Fig. 6. 1.

1. Which terms describe the rhythm?
   a) atrial ectopic impulses   e) ventricular ectopic
   b) multifocal atrial tachycardia   impulses
   c) chaotic atrial tachycardia   f) atrial fibrillation
   d) aberrant intraventricular   g) wandering atrial pace-
      conduction   maker

ANSWER: (a, b, c, d) QRS complexes occur at irregular intervals
ranging from 0. 27 to 1. 04 seconds. Some QRS complexes are narrow
($\leq$ 0. 10 seconds), indicating that ventricular activation occurs relatively normally via the AV junction, while other QRS complexes
are wide, indicating that ventricular activation occurs abnormally.
Atrial activity is clearly identifiable throughout the tracing as irregularly and rapidly occurring P waves of varying contours indicating multiple sites of impulse formation. This atrial rhythm is referred to as "chaotic" or "multifocal" atrial tachycardia. The
presence of P waves excludes the diagnosis of atrial fibrillation.

P waves precede virtually all QRS complexes, and presumably stimulate them. Some P waves are blocked within the AV conduction system, but it is not clear exactly which of two P waves preceding a
QRS complex is the one actually conducted to the ventricles (e. g. , P
waves labeled "X" and "Y"). Since all QRS complexes are stimulated
by atrial impulses, wide complexes are more likely to be aberrantly
conducted atrial impulses rather than single or multiple ventricular
ectopic impulses.

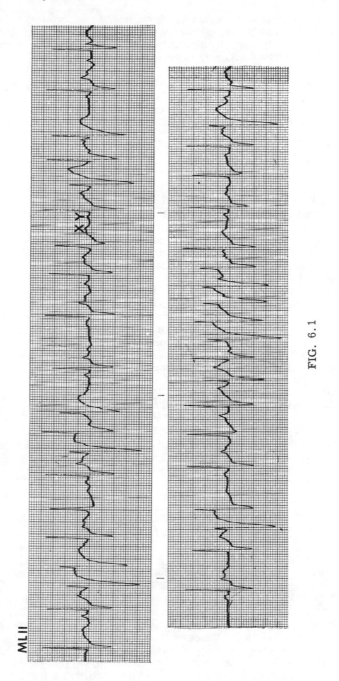

FIG. 6.1

"Wandering atrial pacemaker", a term used to describe the rhythm
in which P waves of varying contours occur in an irregular pattern
at slow rates contrasts with multifocal atrial tachycardia in which
the atrial impulses occur at rapid rate.

2. Reasonable management of this rhythm in this patient might
   include:
   a) achievement of adequate arterial blood gases
   b) digoxin administration
   c) quinidine administration
   d) lidocaine administration
   e) propranolol administration
   f) DC cardioversion

ANSWER: (a) Multifocal or chaotic atrial tachycardia occurs almost
exclusively in patients critically ill with respiratory failure or severe
end-stage congestive heart failure. Hypoxemia, elevated right heart
filling pressures, and electrolyte and acid-base disturbances are
felt to play a major role in its occurrence. Even though the rhythm
usually occurs in already extremely ill patients, it rarely causes
hemodynamic deterioration per se. Its recognition should prompt
aggressive therapy aimed at correcting the underlying disease process. In this patient with acute respiratory infection superimposed
upon severe chronic pulmonary disease, vigorous treatment of the
pulmonary process with supplemental inspired oxygen, expectorants,
intermittent positive pressure breathing, chest physiotherapy, and
antibiotics is in order; it may even become necessary to perform
endotracheal intubation in order to provide assisted mechanical ventilation. Achievement of adequate arterial blood gases will usually
be followed by the disappearance of the multifocal atrial tachycardia.
Administration of bronchodilator medications such as isoproterenol
and aminophylline may, by improving gas exchange, contribute to
disappearance of the arrhythmia. However, their administration in
the presence of abnormal arterial blood gases may result in an increase in the rate of the multifocal atrial tachycardia and/or the
appearance of ventricular arrhythmias.

The administration of antiarrhythmic medications is ill-advised in
patients with multifocal atrial tachycardia. Digoxin administration
to a hypoxemic patient who may have rapid and dramatic changes in
pH, pO2, and serum potassium level might precipitate more serious
arrhythmias. While quinidine administration has been reported to
contribute to the disappearance of multifocal atrial tachycardia, it
is not clear that the medication itself had this effect. Lidocaine
would not be expected to, nor has it been documented to, have any
effect on multifocal atrial tachycardia. Propranolol, a beta-blocking
agent which may itself result in bronchospasm, is contraindicated in
a patient critically ill from pulmonary disease with bronchospasm.
DC cardioversion has no place in the therapy of multifocal atrial
tachycardia, which is not due to sustained reentry or to a rapidly
firing ectopic focus. In cases where DC cardioversion of multifocal
atrial tachycardia has been attempted, the arrhythmia invariably
recurred within seconds.

The patient is treated with supplemental inspired oxygen, intermittent positive pressure breathing, expectorants, antibiotics, and
intravenous aminophylline. Over a period of four hours he appears
and feels more comfortable. His pO_2 is now 60 mm Hg, his pCO_2
48 mm Hg, and his pH 7.40. His cardiac rhythm is now sinus at a
rate of 105/minute with rare atrial premature beats. Over the ensuing two weeks the patient recovers from his pulmonary infection
and his pulmonary function returns to its baseline state. His
rhythm at the time of discharge from the hospital is sinus at a rate
of 80/minute, with no ectopic atrial activity.

BIBLIOGRAPHY

Chung EK: Appraisal of multifocal atrial tachycardia. Brit Heart
J 33:500, 1971.

Shine KI, Kastor JA, Yurchak PM: Multifocal atrial tachycardia.
Clinical and electrocardiographic features in 32 patients. New
Engl J Med 279:344, 1968.

CASE 7: Cardiac irregularity in a man acutely ill with diverticulitis.

A 75-year-old man is admitted to the hospital with fever and abdominal pain which are attributed to diverticulitis. Past medical history is noteworthy only in that the patient has had hypertension for many years, for which he now takes hydrochlorothiazide 100 mg each morning. He denies ever having had angina pectoris, symptoms of congestive heart failure, or awareness of cardiac action. Physical examination of the cardiovascular system reveals a pulse of about 85 per minute with occasional irregularity, and a blood pressure of 160/100 with minimal change on standing. The cardiac output appears adequate, the jugular venous pressure is normal and the chest is clear. There is evidence of left ventricular hypertrophy and a soft basal flow murmur. The abnormal laboratory findings are a moderately elevated white blood cell count with a shift to early forms, and a slightly low serum potassium level of 3.0 mEq/L. The chest x-ray shows moderate generalized cardiomegaly and dilatation of the ascending aorta. The ECG is shown in Fig. 7.1. Left ventricular hypertrophy is suggested by the large QRS voltage, the ST segment and T wave abnormalities, and evidence in Lead V1 of left atrial abnormality.

1. Which terms describe the rhythm?
    a) atrial premature beats with aberrant intraventricular conduction
    b) ventricular premature beats
    c) junctional premature beats with aberrant intraventricular conduction and retrograde atrial activation
    d) fascicular premature beats with retrograde atrial activation

ANSWER: (a) In Leads I, II, and III each QRS complex is preceded at an interval of about 0.14 seconds by a P wave of normal contour and axis, establishing the diagnosis of sinus rhythm. In all other Leads there is a premature QRS complex which has a duration, contour, and axis that differs from the sinus-stimulated QRS complexes. The increase in QRS duration from 0.09 to 0.11 seconds, and the change in contour in Lead V1 from rS to rSR' and in Lead V6 from qR to Rs suggest conduction delay in the right bundle branch; the shift in mean frontal plane QRS axis from about +40 degrees to about +105 degrees suggests conduction delay in the posterior fascicle of the left bundle branch. In these early beats, then, the ventricles are activated aberrantly, predominantly via the anterior fascicle of the left bundle branch.

A ventricular premature beat originating in Purkinje fibers would not be expected to be of such short duration.

The T waves of the QRS complexes preceding the premature QRS complexes have contours much sharper than those of the other sinus-stimulated QRS complexes, probably because there are superimposed P waves. As these premature P waves precede the premature QRS complexes by intervals somewhat longer than the PR intervals of

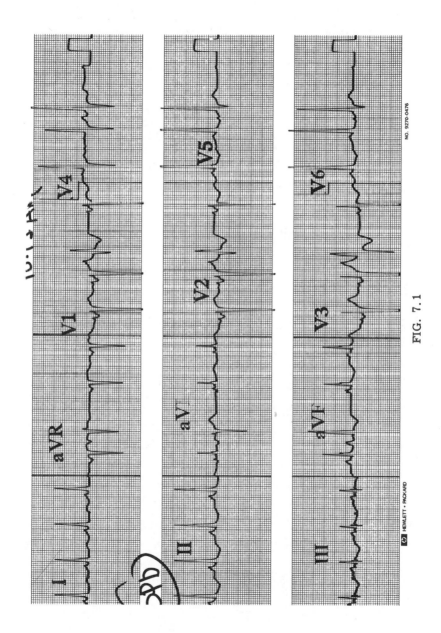

FIG. 7.1

sinus beats (0.19 vs. 0.15 seconds), they are likely to be atrial
premature beats. Junctional or fascicular premature beats with
retrograde atrial activation would be expected to have PR intervals
shorter than those of sinus beats, and to stimulate P waves which
are directed superiorly rather than inferiorly.

2. Are the atrial premature beats likely to be unifocal or multi-
    focal?

ANSWER: (Unifocal) The constant coupling intervals of premature
atrial beats to preceding sinus beats suggest that the premature
atrial beats originate in the same focus, a conclusion that would
be strengthened had several atrial premature beats of identical
contour and axis been recorded in a single Lead.

3. At this time, which part(s) of the AV conduction system have
    the longest refractory period(s)?
    a) AV node
    b) His bundle
    c) anterior fascicle of the left bundle branch
    d) posterior fascicle of the left bundle branch
    e) right bundle branch

ANSWER: (d, e) Since the refractory periods of the different portions
of the atrioventricular conduction system are usually unequal, an
atrial impulse introduced to the AV conduction system will antegradely traverse only those tissues which are no longer refractory.
In Fig. 7.1, the atrial impulses must have been conducted through
the AV node, His bundle, and a portion of the bundle branch system, for they stimulate QRS complexes. The fact that they are conducted with delays in the right bundle branch and in the posterior
fascicle of the left bundle branch suggests that the refractory periods
of these tissues are longer than those of the AV node, His bundle,
and anterior fascicle of the left bundle branch.

Although the AV node-His-Purkinje system is able to conduct the
atrial premature beats, the longer PR intervals of these beats than
sinus beats (0.19 vs. 0.15 seconds) indicate that AV conduction is
slower than in sinus beats. The AV conduction delay may be occurring in the AV node and/or His bundle and/or anterior fascicle
of the left bundle branch. The exact location(s) of conduction delay
cannot be determined from a surface electrocardiogram, but might
be more accurately defined by intracardiac recording of the His
bundle potential.

4. Does the fact that the atrial premature beats are conducted with
    delay in the right bundle branch and posterior fascicle of the left
    bundle branch indicate disease of these portions of the AV con-
    duction system?

ANSWER: (No) Studies aimed at measuring the refractory periods
of different portions of the AV conduction system at different heart

rates suggest that atrial premature beats may be conducted aberrantly into ventricular tissue in patients who have no demonstrable
cardiac disease.

5. How might this arrhythmia be managed in this patient?
   a) maintain normal serum potassium level
   b) administer a quinidine preparation
   c) maintain adequate fluid balance
   d) maintain the blood pressure at reasonable levels

ANSWER: (a, c, d) Atrial premature beats are commonly seen in
older patients, especially in the setting of acute febrile illness. As
they rarely produce symptoms or hemodynamic problems, they do
not require specific treatment. In this patient with diverticulitis
and mild hypokalemia, restoration of normal serum potassium
levels and maintenance of adequate fluid balance may well cause
disappearance of the atrial premature beats. While adequate control of blood pressure may also contribute to disappearance of the
atrial premature beats, presumably by lowering left atrial pressure,
administration of medications that may cause orthostatic hypotension
should be avoided. In an acutely ill elderly man, bedrest, salt restriction, and reassurance may be all that is needed to lower the
blood pressure to acceptable ranges.

If the atrial premature beats make the patient uncomfortable, or if
they precipitate atrial tachyarrhythmias, they might be suppressed
by administration of a quinidine preparation, with optimum therapeutic effect expected when the serum potassium level is within the
normal range.

The patient is treated with oral antibiotics and intravenous fluids
containing potassium chloride in doses which raise the serum potassium level to 4.3 mEq/L. Over a period of three days the
abdominal discomfort disappears, the temperature and white blood
cell count fall to normal, the blood pressure stabilizes at 150/90,
and the atrial premature beats now occur only rarely. After ten
days in the hospital the patient feels well and is discharged home
to take hydrochlorothiazide 100 mg each morning, and a potassium
chloride solution, 20 mEq three times daily. When seen for a
follow-up visit one month after discharge, he feels well and has
only rare atrial premature beats of which he is unaware.

BIBLIOGRAPHY

Damato AN, Lau SH, Helfant RH, Stein E, Berkowitz WD, Cohen
SI: Study of atrioventricular conduction in man using electrode
catheter recordings of His bundle activity. Circulation 39:287,
1969.

Damato AN, Lau SH, Patton RD, Steiner C, Berkowitz WD: A
study of atrioventricular conduction in man using premature atrial
stimulation and His bundle recordings. Circulation 40:61, 1969.

Dreifus LS, de Azevedo IM, Watanabe Y: Electrolyte and anti-arrhythmic drug interaction. Amer Heart J 88:95, 1974.

Goel BG, Han J: Atrial ectopic activity associated with sinus bradycardia. Circulation 42:853, 1970.

Goldreyer BN: Intracardiac electrocardiography in the analysis and understanding of cardiac arrhythmias. Ann Int Med 77: 117, 1972.

Kasser I, Kennedy JW: The relationship of increased left atrial volume and pressure to abnormal P waves on the electrocardiogram. Circulation 39:339, 1969.

Scott RC: The correlation between the electrocardiographic patterns of ventricular hypertrophy and the anatomic findings. Circulation 21:256, 1960.

Tarazi RC, Miller A, Frohlich ED, Dustan HP: Electrocardiographic changes reflecting left atrial abnormality in hypertension. Circulation 34:818, 1966.

Puech P, Grolleau R, Guimond C: Incidence of different types of A-V block and their localization by His bundle recordings. In: The Conduction System of the Heart, Eds. Wellens HJJ, Lie KI, and Janse MJ, Lea & Febiger, Philadelphia, pp. 467-484, 1976.

CASE 8: Palpitations, lightheadedness, and exertional shortness
of breath in a woman with mitral stenosis.

A 48-year-old woman who had had a closed mitral commissurotomy
for rheumatic mitral stenosis at twenty-seven years of age now complains of increasing shortness of breath on exertion, palpitations,
and occasional lightheadedness. Physical examination reveals a
regular pulse of about 115/minute which does not measurably increase on brisk walking, and signs of moderately severe mitral
stenosis. Her initial ECG is shown in Fig. 8.1.

1. What is the rhythm?
    a) atrial flutter with 2:1 AV conduction
    b) ectopic atrial tachycardia with 2:1 AV conduction
    c) sinus tachycardia with prolonged AV conduction
    d) ectopic atrial tachycardia with ventricular tachycardia and
       AV dissociation (double tachycardia)
    e) accelerated junctional rhythm with retrograde atrial
       activation

ANSWER: (a) QRS complexes occur at regular intervals at a rate
of about 115/minute. Atrial activity, most clearly seen in Lead
V1, appears to have a fixed temporal relationship to the QRS complexes, preceding them by about 0.23 seconds. In Lead V2, however, the RR interval transiently lengthens from about 0.56 to
about 0.67 seconds, allowing atrial activity, occurring at a rate of
230/minute, to be clearly seen between the last two QRS complexes.
Except in this Lead, therefore, every other atrial complex is
hidden within the QRS complexes. The presence of an undulating
baseline in Leads II, III, and aVF, and the absence of isoelectric
segments indicate that the atrial rhythm is slow atrial flutter. Slow
flutter rates in patients not receiving quinidine therapy may be
attributed to atrial fibrosis and possibly to rheumatic involvement
of the atria in mitral stenosis.

Whereas the atrial rate of 230/minute could be due to an ectopic
atrial tachycardia and the slower ventricular rate due to 2:1 AV
conduction with occasional periods of higher grades of AV block, such
rhythms occur almost exclusively in the setting of severe heart failure
and end-stage heart disease and may be a manifestation of digitalis
intoxication. The P waves in ectopic atrial tachycardia are usually of
peaked contour and short duration, and isoelectric segments are
usually seen in the TP or PR intervals in the inferior Leads.

Sinus tachycardia with prolonged AV conduction (first degree AV
block) is excluded by the very rapid rate and the presence of flutter
waves. In addition, the failure of the patient's heart rate to increase
with brisk walking would be most unusual in sinus rhythm. Accelerated junctional rhythm with retrograde atrial activation is excluded

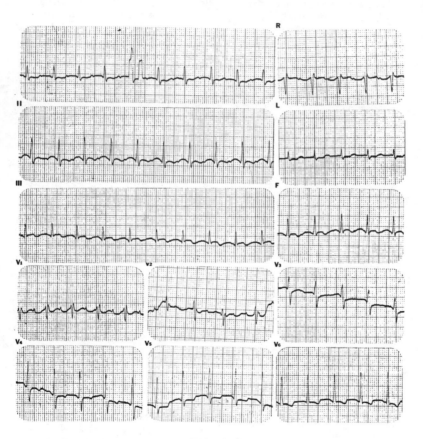

FIG. 8.1

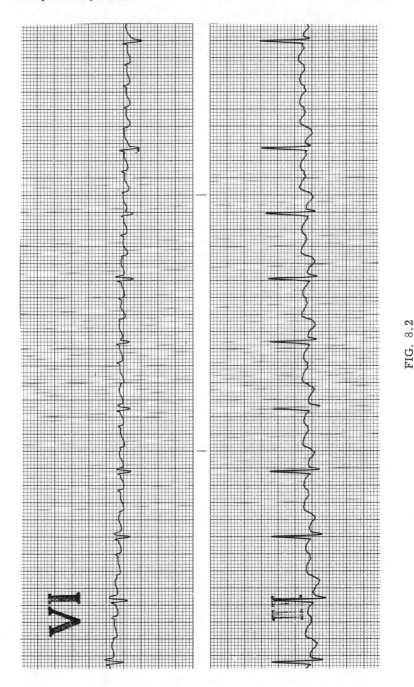

FIG. 8.2

by the atrial rate that exceeds the ventricular rate. Double tachycardia, or regular atrial (or sinus) tachycardia bearing no relationship to regular ventricular (or junctional) tachycardia is excluded
by the fixed temporal relationships between atrial and ventricular
activity.

2. How might this rhythm disturbance be managed in this patient?
    a) administer digoxin to slow the ventricular rate
    b) administer propranolol to slow the ventricular rate
    c) administer quinidine to slow the atrial rate
    d) administer quinidine to convert the rhythm to sinus
    e) perform DC cardioversion
    f) slow the ventricular rate with digitalis and/or propranolol,
       then perform DC cardioversion
    g) perform an operation to relieve her mitral stenosis that is
       probably a contributing factor to both onset and maintenance
       of the rhythm disturbance

ANSWER: (f) It is likely that the patient's symptoms are for the
most part due to the rapid heart rate in the presence of mitral
stenosis, although the mitral stenosis alone could conceivably account for them. It is therefore important to attempt to either slow
the ventricular response to the atrial flutter or to convert the flutter
to sinus rhythm before recommending mitral valve surgery. The
ventricular rate can be slowed with digitalis preparations alone,
with propranolol alone, or with a combination of the two; in the presence of significant left ventricular dysfunction, propranolol is to be
avoided and digitalis preparations preferred.

The patient is treated with oral digoxin and several days later the
rhythm strip shown in Fig. 8.2 is recorded. It more clearly shows
the atrial deflections in Lead II to be flutter waves. Digoxin has resulted in a slightly faster atrial rate of 240/minute and a change in
AV conduction ratio to 3:1 (increasing to 5:1 in the last beat). Both
phenomena are commonly seen when digoxin is used to treat atrial
flutter. Atrial flutter with 3:1 AV conduction, although rare, is
seen almost exclusively in patients with slow flutter rates in the
range of 200-240/minute.

DC cardioversion is planned within twenty-four hours. Digoxin is
discontinued and quinidine sulfate, 300 mg orally every six hours,
is ordered in an attempt to prevent post-cardioversion recurrence
of the atrial flutter. After two doses of the quinidine sulfate the
patient complains of transient lightheadedness upon arising from a
sitting position, and while walking. At this time the modified Lead
II rhythm strip shown in Fig. 8.3A is recorded by means of telemetry.

3. What is the rhythm?
    a) atrial fibrillation with rapid ventricular response
    b) atrial flutter with variable, but predominantly 1:1 AV
       conduction
    c) digitalis-induced accelerated junctional rhythm
    d) multifocal atrial tachycardia
    e) quinidine-induced ventricular tachycardia

ANSWER: (b) The QRS complexes are narrow (0.09 seconds in
duration) and the QRS rhythm is only slightly irregular at a rate of
about 190-200/minute. Atrial activity is not clearly identifiable.
The slightly irregular ventricular response could occur if the
atrial rhythm had changed from flutter to fibrillation; however,
a ventricular response this rapid is most unusual, especially in the
presence of digitalis. A more likely explanation is that the atrial
rhythm is still flutter, with the irregular ventricular response explained by penetration of the flutter impulses to variable depths
into the AV node, thereby affecting conduction through the AV node
of subsequent flutter impulses (concealed conduction); but almost
all flutter waves reach the ventricles.

Accelerated junctional rhythm would not have such a rapid ventricular rate and would be a perfectly regular tachycardia. Quinidine-
induced ventricular tachycardia is not likely in view of the normal
QRS duration and configuration. Multifocal atrial tachycardia is
not usually associated with valvular heart disease in the absence
of severe heart failure or a superimposed acute pulmonary process,
and clearly defined P waves of variable contour are usually readily
discernible.

4. What is the likely cause of the occurrence of this rhythm?
    a) acute pulmonary embolism
    b) slowing of the atrial rate by quinidine
    c) enhancement of AV conduction due to quinidine
    d) enhancement of AV conduction due to digitalis
    e) enhanced automaticity due to digitalis

ANSWER: (b) The cause of the rapid ventricular rate is most likely
a quinidine-induced slowing of the atrial rate (from 230/minute to
about 200/minute) to a level at which the AV node can transmit almost every flutter impulse. It is unlikely that the increased ventricular rate results from a vagolytic effect of quinidine at the dosages
used in this patient. Digoxin should neither enhance AV conduction
nor cause an automatic rhythm of this rate and with this degree of
irregularity.

5. How might the patient be managed now?
    a) add propranolol
    b) restart digoxin
    c) administer additional quinidine
    d) perform DC cardioversion
    e) none of the above

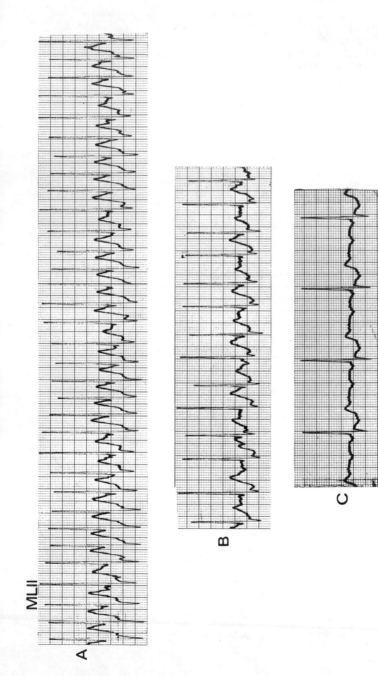

FIG. 8.3 A, B, C

ANSWER: (a, b, c, d) Since the patient's heart rate can be slowed by
increasing AV block at this time, either digoxin or propranolol can
be given. As DC cardioversion is planned, however, digoxin might
impose a slight risk to the patient with regard to the appearance of
postcardioversion arrhythmias; similar attendant risk has not been
associated with the use of propranolol. Additional quinidine sulfate
might convert this rhythm to sinus, but DC cardioversion is a safer
maneuver.

Ten milligrams of propranolol are administered orally, and one
hour later the tracing shown in Fig. 8.3B is recorded. This rhythm
strip shows atrial flutter with an atrial rate of about 200/minute,
3:2 AV Wenckebach periods, and an average ventricular rate of
about 140/minute. Two hours after the propranolol the rhythm strip
shown in Fig. 8.3C is recorded, showing 4:1 AV conduction and a
ventricular rate of about 50/minute. At this time the atrial flutter
is cardioverted to sinus rhythm with a 20 watt-second electrical
discharge.

The patient is discharged from the hospital in sinus rhythm with
occasional atrial premature beats. She continues to take digoxin
0.25 mg daily, and quinidine sulfate in doses which achieve therapeutic serum levels of 4.0 mg/L, but still has dyspnea on moderate
exertion. The development of severe diarrhea necessitates the discontinuation of the quinidine sulfate. Within a few days of stopping
this medication, slow atrial flutter with 2:1 AV conduction and ventricular rate of about 115/minute recurs. Propranolol, 5 mg twice
daily, is added to the digoxin and results in a slowing of the ventricular rate to 55/minute, but no change in the atrial rate or rhythm.

Because of the patient's continued symptoms reflecting pulmonary
venous congestion in the face of a normal ventricular rate, cardiac
catheterization is performed, revealing mitral stenosis of moderately
severe degree (mitral valve area of 1.1 cm^2), for which open mitral
commissurotomy is performed. In the four weeks following the
operation, her rhythm is atrial fibrillation, and the ventricular rate
is controlled at 70-80/minute with 0.25 mg of oral digoxin daily,
and oral propranolol 10 mg twice daily. Sinus rhythm appears spontaneously at this time and, with digoxin and propranolol being continued, lasts for three weeks. After this, the slow atrial flutter
with ventricular rate of about 55/minute recurs. Since the patient
is now relatively asymptomatic and has adequate effort tolerance,
no effort is made to convert the rhythm to sinus, since long-term
maintenance of sinus rhythm would almost certainly require administration of quinidine preparations, to which she is intolerant.

BIBLIOGRAPHY

Arani DT, Carleton RA: The deleterious role of tachycardia in
mitral stenosis. Circulation 36:511 , 1967.

Childers R: Concealed conduction. In: Symposium in cardiac rhythm disturbances I. The Med Clin No Am 60:149, 1976.

Harvey RM, Ferrer MI, Richards DW, Cournand A: Cardiocirculatory performance in atrial flutter. Circulation 12:507, 1955.

Langendorf R, Pick A: Concealed conduction. Further evaluation of a fundamental aspect of propagation of the cardiac impulse. Circulation 13:381, 1956.

Lindsay J, Hurst JW: The clinical features of atrial flutter and their therapeutic implications. Chest 66:114, 1974.

Lown B, Wyatt NF, Levine HD: Paroxysmal atrial tachycardia with block. Circulation 21:129, 1960.

Shine KI, Kastor JA, Yurchak PM: Multifocal atrial tachycardia. New Engl J Med 279:344, 1968.

CASE 9: Lightheadedness and palpitations in a woman with
         Prinzmetal's variant angina.

A 48-year-old previously healthy woman visits her physician for
evaluation of almost daily episodes of retrosternal burning discomfort of several weeks duration. The discomfort occurs only at
about 3 to 5 AM, awakens her from sleep with a gradually increasing and subsiding intensity lasting one to ten minutes. During the
episodes she frequently is aware of her heart "pounding" or "racing"
and at these times she often feels lightheaded even though she is
supine. The episodes have continued despite avoidance of alcoholic
beverages and foods which have previously caused dyspepsia. The
physical examination and chest x-ray are normal, and the 12-Lead
ECG shown in Fig. 9.1 is also normal.

Since the patient is having retrosternal discomfort almost every
morning, usually associated with an awareness of cardiac action,
Holter monitor recording is performed for a continuous 24-hour
period. Fig. 9.2A-E shows five MCL$_6$ rhythm strips recorded
over a 24-minute period beginning at 5 AM. Strip A is recorded
while the patient is asleep; and strips B through D are recorded
shortly thereafter when she has been awakened by retrosternal burning followed by a feeling of lightheadedness and awareness of her
heart "pounding"; strip E is recorded after disappearance of all
symptoms.

Strip A shows sinus rhythm at a rate of about 75/minute, with normal PQRST complexes and normal PR intervals. Strip B shows a
longer PR interval, a slightly faster heart rate, and depressed
downsloping ST segments suggesting acute myocardial ischemia.
Strip C shows 2:1 AV conduction with the PR interval of the conducted beats still longer than in Strip B. The reason for the unexpectedly longer PR interval despite the longer RR interval is presumably acute ischemic dysfunction of the AV node.

1. Which terms characterize Strip 9.2D?
    a) sinus tachycardia   e) AV dissociation
    b) first degree AV block   f) junctional escape beat
    c) second degree AV block   g) ventricular escape beat
    d) third degree AV block

ANSWER: (a,b,c,d,e,f) The QRS complexes, being narrow and
identical to those in Strips A, B, and C, indicate that they are conducted from the AV junction. The P waves, identical to P waves
in Strip A, B, and C, and occurring at short and somewhat variable
cycle length indicate that the atrial rhythm is sinus tachycardia.

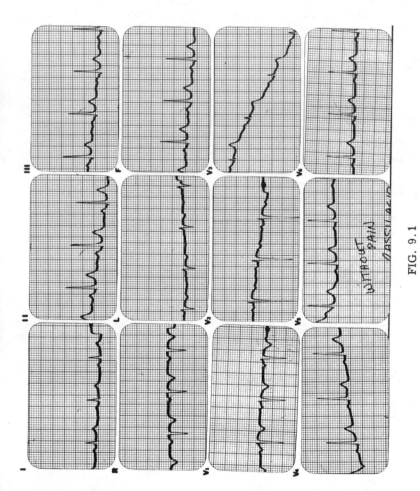

FIG. 9.1

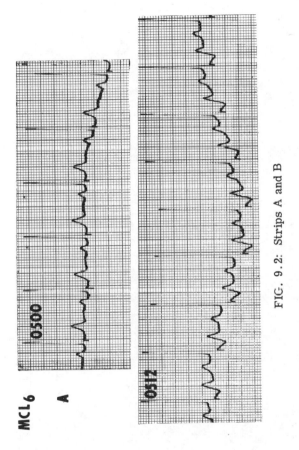

FIG. 9.2: Strips A and B

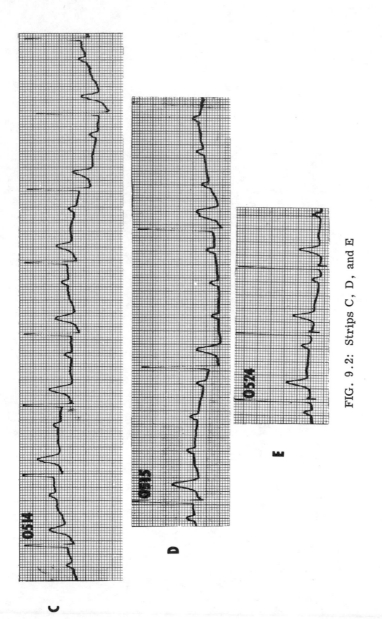

FIG. 9.2: Strips C, D, and E

The first two QRS complexes, preceded by P waves at intervals of about 0.24-0.25 seconds, are probably stimulated by these P waves, and are thus sinus beats conducted with first degree AV block. Since nonconducted P waves are occurring between the first and second QRS complexes, there is also second degree AV block at this time. The third QRS complex, terminating a pause in QRS rhythm of 2.07 seconds, while the preceding RR interval was slightly shorter (2.01 seconds) probably is a junctional escape beat. As nonconducted P waves precede and follow this last QRS complex, transient third degree (complete) AV block has resulted in AV dissociation. The fact that the third QRS complex is narrow excludes its being a ventricular escape beat. In Strip E sinus rate has slowed to about 60/minute, 1:1 AV conduction is now occurring with a PR interval that is still slightly prolonged, and the ST segments and T waves have returned almost to normal.

The patient is advised to come to the hospital, where she is monitored in the Coronary Care Unit. The normal physical examination, chest x-ray, and 12-Lead ECG are unchanged. At about 5 AM on her first hospital day she is awakened with a retrosternal burning sensation. Her limb lead ECG recorded at this time is shown in Fig. 9.3A. Sinus rhythm at a rate of about 76/minute is present. The QRS complexes are 0.12 seconds in duration, 0.04 seconds wider than those of her initial normal ECG in Fig. 9.1. There is marked ST segment elevation in the inferior Leads II, III, and aVF, and ST segment depression in Leads I and aVL, indicating acute inferior myocardial injury. The prolonged PR interval of about 0.25 seconds suggests acute ischemic dysfunction of the AV node.

The patient is given a nitroglycerin tablet, 1/150 gr sublingually, and over a period of about five minutes the burning discomfort disappears. The Lead II rhythm strip recorded at this time (Fig. 9.3B) shows that now the QRS duration is normal at 0.07-0.08 seconds, and the PR interval is normal at about 0.19 seconds. Only minimal ST segment elevation remains.

2. How might this patient be reasonably managed at this time?
    a) administer coronary vasodilator medications
    b) administer atropine
    c) administer phenoxybenzamine
    d) administer propranolol
    e) perform cardiac catheterization and coronary angiography

ANSWER: (a, e) This middle-aged woman with several weeks of burning chest discomfort occurring only at rest and only in the early morning, and associated with transient marked ST segment elevation localized to an area of myocardium supplied by a major coronary artery, fulfills the criteria for Prinzmetal's type of variant angina. Spasm of a coronary artery without significant anatomic obstruction may be occurring, considering that the patient is a middle-aged woman who has never had effort-related symptoms. Fixed high-grade stenosis in a coronary artery, with or without superimposed

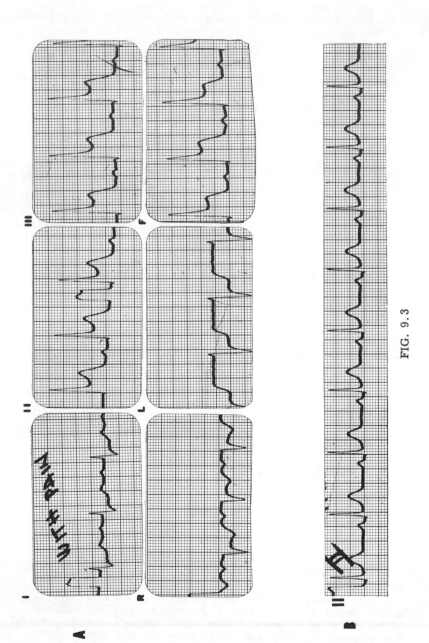

FIG. 9.3

spasm, could also be present. Since patients with "variant" angina
and fixed high-grade coronary artery stenoses tend to fare better
with coronary artery bypass graft surgery than without it, performance of cardiac catheterization and coronary angiography would
be reasonable at this time in order to define coronary artery anatomy.

Coronary artery vasodilator medications such as nitroglycerin and
isosorbide dinitrate, often extremely useful in the management of
patients with fixed anatomic obstruction, presumably by altering
myocardial oxygen demands, may also be effective in preventing
and treating coronary artery spasm. While knowledge of the neuro-
humoral control of coronary artery dynamics is limited, the available data suggest that in some patients cholinergic and alpha-adrenergic stimulation increase vascular tone, thus tending to cause
coronary artery vasoconstriction; while cholinergic blockade (as
with, for example, atropine), alpha-adrenergic blockade (as with,
for example, phenoxybenzamine), and beta-sympathetic stimulation
may cause coronary artery dilatation which may prevent spasm;
propranolol might possibly facilitate the occurrence of spasm as it
is a beta-sympathetic blocking agent. However, since individual
clinical responses to these medications differ from patient to patient and are not always reproducible in the same patient, the effects
of the administration of such medications should be clearly documented.

The patient is treated with isosorbide dinitrate 5 mg sublingually
every three hours while awake, and over the next 72 hours the early
morning episodes of retrosternal burning, ST segment elevation,
and periods of high-grade AV block disappear. Cardiac catheterization, left ventricular cineangiography, and selective coronary
arteriography reveal normal intracardiac and intravascular pressures and normal left ventricular performance; the only abnormality
seen on coronary angiography is mild focal irregularity in the mid-
descending portion of the right coronary artery.

After she has had no further retrosternal burning episodes for seven
days, she is discharged home and advised to take isosorbide dinitrate in the previously effective doses. She continues to be free of
symptoms for about six weeks, during which time she gradually stops
taking the isosorbide dinitrate. Two weeks later the early morning
episodes recur, so she reinstitutes the isosorbide dinitrate.

One morning when the patient is at her job on a particularly stress-
ful day, she has the sudden onset of retrosternal burning followed by
awareness of rapid heart action, syncope, and grand mal seizure.
Cardiopulmonary resuscitation is successfully performed, and the
patient admitted to the hospital for observation. On the first hospital
day she has several of her typical non-effort related retrosternal
burning episodes. During one of these she becomes lightheaded at
a time when the rhythm strips shown in Fig. 9.4A-D are recorded.
Strip A is recorded just prior to the onset of the retrosternal burning
and lightheadedness, and Strips B, C, and D are recorded serially
a few seconds apart during the episode.

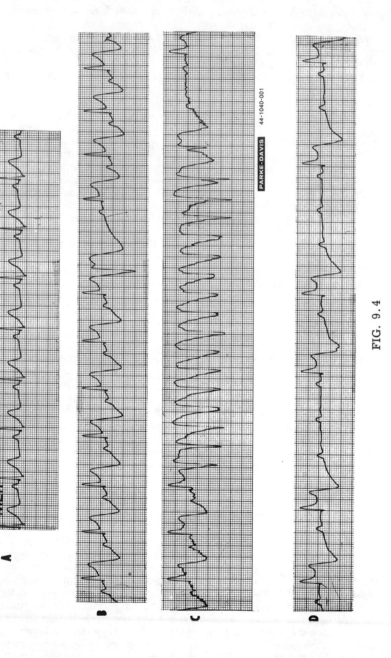

FIG. 9. 4

3. What are the rhythms in Fig. 9.4C?
   a) ventricular tachycardia
   b) junctional tachycardia with aberrant intraventricular
      conduction
   c) sinus rhythm with first degree AV block

ANSWER: (a, c) In Fig. 9.4C three QRS complexes occurring at intervals that are essentially equal to those in Fig. 9.4B are preceded by P waves at intervals of about 0.26 seconds, establishing
the diagnosis of sinus rhythm with first degree AV block. A wide,
bizarre QS complex, falling at the peak of the T wave of the third
QRST complex initiates a six-second burst of similar wide QS complexes at a rate of about 167/minute. The rate, width, and contour
of these QS complexes, and their initiation by a QRS complex falling
on the peak of a T wave suggest that the rhythm is ventricular tachycardia.

In junctional tachycardia with aberrant intraventricular conduction
the QRS complexes would not be expected to be so wide and bizarre,
to occur at this rapid a rate, or to occur in such a brief burst.

4. How might this patient's arrhythmias reasonably be managed?
   a) perform coronary artery bypass graft surgery
   b) administer increasing doses of coronary artery vasodilator
      medications
   c) administer antiarrhythmic medications specifically aimed at
      preventing the ventricular tachycardia

ANSWER: (b, c) Since the ventricular tachycardia is related to myocardial ischemia presumably induced by coronary artery spasm,
prevention of arterial spasm with increasing doses of coronary vasodilator medications is the most reasonable treatment. If such measures do not prevent the episodes of ventricular tachycardia, antiarrhythmic medication such as a quinidine preparation or procainamide might be tried. Although patients with variant angina and
normal coronary arteries do not seem to develop myocardial infarction,
they do have syncope and sudden unexpected death, due presumably to
ventricular tachycardia or ventricular fibrillation.

The results of coronary artery bypass graft surgery in patients who
have variant angina without fixed high-grade anatomic obstruction
have been unsatisfactory, presumably because such surgery has no
effect on coronary artery spasm; episodes of myocardial ischemia,
arrhythmias, syncope, and sudden death are thus not prevented.

The patient is treated with increasing doses of isosorbide dinitrate
until she is taking 20 mg sublingually every three hours while awake,
and a 40 mg sustained-release tablet at bedtime. Quinidine sulfate,
300 mg four times daily, is also administered. Over a ten-day
period, her episodes of burning chest discomfort, AV conduction disturbances, and ventricular tachycardia gradually disappear. The

patient returns to her normal life at home and at work uneventfully.
Over the next six months she takes smaller and variable amounts of
the isosorbide dinitrate and the quinidine sulfate, and is troubled
only occasionally by her typical episodes.

BIBLIOGRAPHY

Berman ND, et al.: Prinzmetal's angina with coronary artery
spasm. Angiographic, pharmacologic, metabolic, and radionuclide
perfusion studies. Amer J Med 60:727, 1976.

Endo M, et al.: Prinzmetal's variant angina. Coronary arteriogram
and left ventriculogram during angina attack induced by methacholine.
New Engl J Med 294:252, 1976.

Higgins CB, et al.: Clinical and arteriographic features of Prinzmetal's variant angina: documentation of etiologic factors. Amer
J Cardiol 37:831, 1976.

Levene DL, Freeman MR: Alpha-adrenoreceptor-mediated coronary
artery spasm. JAMA 236:1018, 1976.

MacAlpin RN, et al.: Angina pectoris at rest with preservation of
exercise capacity. Circulation 47:946, 1973.

Maseri A, et al.: Coronary artery spasm as a cause of acute myocardial ischemia in man. Chest 68:625, 1975.

Gensini GG: Coronary artery spasm and angina pectoris. Chest
68:709, 1975.

Gaasch WH, et al.: Surgical management of Prinzmetal's variant
angina. Chest 66:614, 1974.

Oliva PB, et al.: Coronary arterial spasm in Prinzmetal's angina.
Documentation by coronary arteriography. New Engl J Med 288:
745, 1973.

Prinzmetal M, et al.: Angina pectoris I. A variant form of angina
pectoris. Amer J Med 27:375, 1959.

Selzer A, et al.: Clinical syndrome of variant angina with normal
coronary arteriogram. New Engl J Med 295:1343, 1976.

Silverman ME, Flamm MD: Variant angina pectoris. Anatomic
findings and prognostic implications. Ann Int Med 75:339, 1971.

Yasue H, et al.: Role of autonomic nervous system in the pathogenesis of Prinzmetal's variant form of angina. Circulation 50:
534, 1974.

CASE 10:   Thirty-two year-old jogger with a "thumping" sensation
in his chest.

A 32-year-old healthy jogger visits his physician complaining of a
fleeting "thumping" sensation in his chest, and wishes to know if he
can continue jogging.   He does not smoke cigarettes, and drinks
only one cup of coffee daily.   Physical examination, chest x-ray,
screening laboratory data, and a 12-Lead electrocardiogram are
all within normal limits.   Fig. 10.1 shows two continuous rhythm
strips in which Leads V_1 and II are simultaneously recorded.

1.   Which of the following describe(s) the rhythm?
    a) sinoatrial exit block
    b) atrial premature beat
    c) sinus arrhythmia
    d) ventricular premature beat
    e) retrograde atrial activation

ANSWER: (c,d,c) Except for the wide, bizarre (fourth) QRS complex in the bottom two strips, all QRS complexes are narrow, of
normal contour, and preceded by normal-appearing P waves at normal intervals, indicating that they are sinus beats. The marked
variability of the intersinus interval, with cyclical lengthening and
shortening, indicates sinus arrhythmia.

The wide, bizarre QRS complex most likely originates in the ventricles, and, occurring at shorter cycle length than any other QRS
complex, is premature.   The notching in the ST segment of this
ventricular premature beat, which causes a negative deflection in
Lead II (●), is most likely a retrograde P wave stimulated by ventriculoatrial conduction of the ventricular impulse. However, in
the presence of such dramatic sinus arrhythmia, the possibility that
this is a sinus P wave cannot be absolutely excluded.

While it is difficult to define atrial prematurity in the presence of
marked sinus arrhythmia, the observation that all P waves are of
identical contour and precede QRS complexes by identical intervals
suggests that atrial premature beats are not present.

A diagnosis of sinoatrial exit block can be established only when (1)
during reasonably constant PP intervals there is a sudden disappearance of atrial activity which then reappears at an interval that is a
multiple of the preceding sinus cycle length (Type II sinoatrial exit
block); or (2) there is group beating in which P waves occurring at
progressively shorter cycle length are separated by intervals less
than twice the shortest PP interval (Wenckebach Type sinoatrial
exit block).   In this tracing, neither criterion is met.

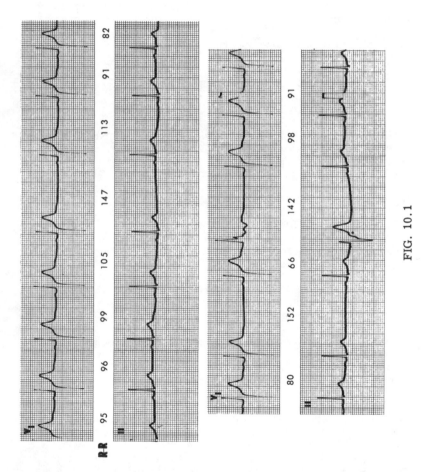

FIG. 10.1

2. How might this patient be reasonably managed at this time?
   a) perform a treadmill exercise test
   b) perform ambulatory cardiac rhythm monitoring
   c) advise him to stop jogging
   d) prescribe antiarrhythmic medication
   e) reassure him that his rhythm disturbance is of no consequence

ANSWER: (a, b) Dramatic sinus arrhythmia occurs in healthy, well-conditioned individuals of this age, and requires no specific treatment. Whether or not ventricular premature beats should be treated depends on the clinical setting in which they occur. In this patient, the ventricular premature beat occurs only after a sinus beat that terminates a long pause (presumably because the long pause predisposed to reentry within the distal Purkinje system); simply preventing long pauses may suppress them. Although the probability that this young man has significant arrhythmias is very small, since he wishes to continue jogging it is reasonable to perform ambulatory cardiac rhythm monitoring and maximal treadmill exercise testing in order to more clearly assess the seriousness of the rhythm disturbance. It does not seem reasonable to advise him to stop jogging, to place him on antiarrhythmic medication, or to simply reassure him that his rhythm disturbance is inconsequential before more detailed arrhythmia evaluation has been undertaken.

The patient performs maximal treadmill exercise, achieving a heart rate of 190 beats per minute and an appropriate blood pressure response, without ventricular premature beats or ST segment abnormalities appearing. He is reassured that a serious cardiac problem is not present. He continues jogging and when last seen six weeks after the exercise test, feels well but still experiences occasional "thumping" sensations in his chest.

BIBLIOGRAPHY

Friedberg CK: Disturbances in impulse formation: Premature beats. In: Diseases of the Heart, W. B. Saunders Company, Philadelphia, pp. 496-514, 1966.

Han J, Millet D, Chizzonitti B, et al.: Temporal dispersion of recovery of excitability in atrium and ventricle as a function of heart rate. Amer Heart J 71:481, 1966.

Han J, DeTraglia J, Millet D, et al.: Incidence of ectopic beats as a function of basic rate in the ventricle. Amer Heart J 72:632, 1966.

Han J: The concepts of reentrant activity responsible for ectopic rhythms. Amer J Cardiol 28:253, 1971.

Schamroth L, Rosenzweig D: Reciprocal ventricular extrasystoles. Brit Heart J 24:805, 1962.

Scherf D: The mechanism and treatment of extrasystoles.   Prog
Cardiovasc Dis 2:370, 1960.

Surawicz B, MacDonald MG: Ventricular ectopic beats with fixed
and variable coupling. Incidence, clinical significance and factors
influencing the coupling interval. Amer J Cardiol 13:198, 1964.

Myburgh DP, Lewis BS: Ventricular parasystole in healthy hearts.
Amer Heart J 82:307, 1971.

Romero CA: Holter monitoring in the diagnosis and management of
cardiac rhythm disturbances. Med Clin No Amer 60:299, 1976.

McHenry PL, Fisch C, Jordan JW, Corya BR: Cardiac arrhythmias observed during maximal treadmill exercise testing in clinically
normal men. Amer J Cardiol 29:331, 1972.

Blackburn H, Taylor HL, Hamrell B, Buskirk E, Nicholas WC, Thor-
sen RD: Premature ventricular complexes induced by stress testing.
Their frequency and response to physical conditioning. Amer J
Cardiol 31:441, 1973.

Hinkle LE, Carver ST, Stevens M: The frequency of asymptomatic
disturbances of cardiac rhythm and conduction in middle-aged men.
Amer J Cardiol 24:629, 1969.

CASE 11: Lightheadedness and syncope in a woman with a normal
cardiac examination.

A 54-year-old woman with a twelve-year history of frequent episodes
of lightheadedness has four syncopal spells within a three-month
period. There is no history of congestive heart failure or coronary
artery disease, and no evidence of valvular dysfunction. Except for
the rhythm (Fig. 11.1) the 12-Lead ECG is normal.

1. Which of the following terms describe the rhythm in Fig. 11.1?
    a) sinus pauses   d) sinus arrest
    b) group beating   e) second degree AV block
    c) sinoatrial exit block

ANSWER: (a, b, c) The QRS complexes are of normal duration and
contour, indicating that ventricular activation is occurring normally via the AV junction-His-Purkinje system. They are preceded
at intervals of 0.14-0.15 seconds by normal-appearing P waves that
stimulate them. Since all P waves are followed by QRS complexes,
second degree AV block is not present. There is group beating, in
which three P waves are followed by pauses in sinus rhythm ("sinus
pauses"). Since these pauses are almost exactly twice the interval
between consecutive P waves within a group, the sinus node presumably discharged on time during the pause but did not cause atrial
depolarization. The failure of an on-time sinus impulse to depolarize non-refractory atrial tissue is due to conduction delay or block
of the impulse in the area surrounding the sinus node, a phenomenon
called "sinoatrial exit block". "Sinus arrest" is said to occur when
the sinus node unexpectedly and randomly fails to discharge, and the
pauses occasioned by the sinus arrest are usually terminated by a
slow and irregular sinus, atrial, or junctional rhythm. In Fig. 11.1,
the regular group beating of the sinus rhythm suggests that sinus
arrest is not occurring.

2. Which of the following might help to establish whether sinus node
    function is or is not normal in this patient?
    a) measurement of the sinus node recovery time
    b) analysis of the behavior of the sinus rhythm in the 10-15
       second period following cessation of rapid atrial pacing
    c) the response of sinus rate to intravenous atropine administration
    d) the response of sinus rate to intravenous isoproterenol ad-
       ministration
    e) the response of sinus rate to exercise

ANSWER: (a, b) Both measurement of sinus node recovery time and
analysis of the behavior of the sinus rhythm in the ten to fifteen
second period following cessation of rapid atrial pacing are useful
in evaluating sinus node function. Measurement of sinus node recovery time involves pacing the right atrium at rates of 100-140 bpm

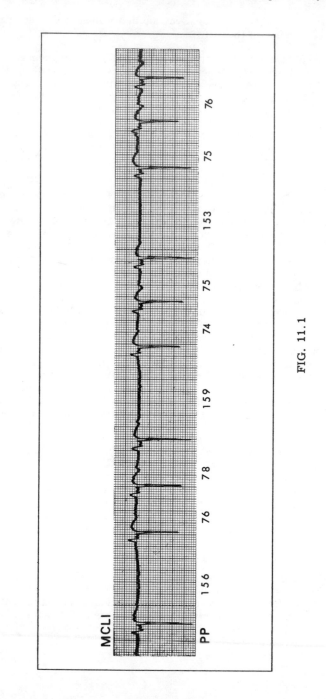

FIG. 11.1

for at least two minutes. Pacing is then abruptly terminated, and
the sinus node recovery time is measured as the interval from the
last paced P wave to the first spontaneously occurring sinus P wave.
Normal sinus node recovery time is less than 1.50 seconds. About
50% of patients with sinus node dysfunction electrocardiographically
documented by profound sinus bradycardia, sinoatrial exit block,
and/or sinus arrest will have abnormally prolonged sinus node recovery times. The rhythm which returns following cessation of
atrial pacing is normally characterized by sinus P waves occurring
at more or less progressively shorter cycle length such that a gradual increase in sinus rate occurs. In about 90% of patients with
electrocardiographically documented sinus node dysfunction, however, the initial progressive shortening of sinus cycle length is interrupted by one or more unexpected pauses in sinus rhythm. These
later pauses have been termed "secondary pauses" to distinguish
them from the initial pause which is the sinus node recovery time.

In many patients with sinus node dysfunction the response of the
sinus rate to intravenous administration of atropine and/or isoproterenol, and to exercise, is blunted due to abnormalities in sinus
node automaticity and/or sinoatrial conduction. However, experience with these maneuvers suggests that they do not adequately
separate normal from abnormal sinus node function, and may not
be reproducible in individual patients.

Fig. 11.2, which displays simultaneously recorded Lead II, Lead
V_1, and a His bundle electrogram (HBE) shows the events surrounding cessation of two minutes of right atrial pacing at a rate of about
100/minute.

3. Which of the following statements can be made on the basis of
    these events?
    a) sinus node recovery time is prolonged
    b) there are secondary pauses in sinus rhythm
    c) sinus node function is normal
    d) sinus node function is abnormal
    e) sinoatrial exit block is present following pacing

ANSWER: (a, b, d, e) The first three atrial beats are stimulated by
pacing artifacts (s). Following cessation of pacing there is a 2.9
second pause in atrial rhythm which is terminated by a sinus P wave.
Thus, the sinus node recovery time is abnormally long. As the interval between the last two sinus P waves is much longer than either
of the two immediately preceding sinus cycle lengths, there is a
secondary pause in sinus rhythm. Since the secondary pause is
exactly twice the preceding sinus cycle length, it is probably due
to 2:1 sinoatrial exit block. The prolonged sinus node recovery
time, the presence of secondary pauses in sinus rhythm, and the
2:1 sinoatrial exit block indicate abnormal sinus node function.

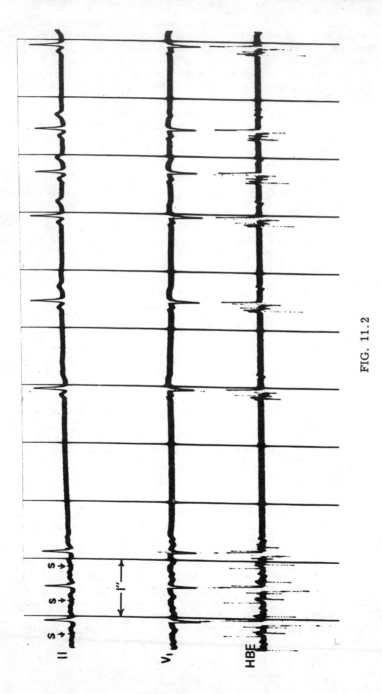

FIG. 11.2

4. How might the patient be reasonably managed at this time?
   a) evaluation of possible non-cardiac causes of syncope
   b) chronic oral administration of a parasympatholytic agent
   c) chronic sublingual administration of isoproterenol
   d) watchful waiting
   e) implantation of a permanent demand ventricular pacemaker

ANSWER: (a, e) Although syncope in this patient with abnormal
sinus node function might well be due to bradycardia-related inadequate cerebral perfusion, the possibility that the syncope is due
to other mechanisms such as orthostatic hypotension, seizure dis-
order, and cerebrovascular disease should be investigated.   If
other causes are not found, then prevention of bradycardia is reasonable, although it must be recognized that bradycardia profound
enough to cause syncope has not been documented in this patient.
While intravenously administered parasympatholytic agents have
been documented to acutely enhance sinus node automaticity and
improve sinoatrial conduction, their chronic oral administration
generally causes unpleasant side effects much more often than the
desired improvement in sinus node function.   Sublingual administration of isoproterenol may result in an increase in sinus rate and
enhancement of sinoatrial conduction, but is not reliably absorbed
and the effectiveness of each dose lasts only two to three hours.
Permanent ventricular demand pacing is currently the only practical,
reliable, and effective means of preventing symptomatic bradycardia.
The risks of watchful waiting in a patient with documented sinus node
dysfunction and syncopal episodes may exceed the morbidity of permanent pacemaker implantation.

A permanent transvenous right ventricular pacemaker is implanted
and the patient discharged on no cardiac medications. Over the next
five months she has no syncopal episodes but continues to experience
occasional episodes of lightheadedness.

BIBLIOGRAPHY

Abbott JA, Hirschfeld DS, Kunkel FW, Scheinman MM, Modin G:
Graded exercise testing in patients with sinus node dysfunction.
Amer J Med 62:330,1977.

Benditt DG, Strauss HC, Scheinman MM, Behar VS, Wallace AG:
Analysis of secondary pauses following termination of rapid atrial
pacing in man. Circulation 54:436, 1976.

Dhingra RC, Amat-y-Leon F, Wyndham C, Deedwania PC, Wu D,
Denes P, Rosen KM: Clinical significance of prolonged sinoatrial
conduction time. Circulation 55:8, 1977.

Dhingra RC, Amat-y-Leon F, Wyndham C, Denes P, Wu D, Miller
RH, Rosen KM: Electrophysiologic effects of atropine on sinus node
and atrium in patients with sinus nodal dysfunction. Amer J Cardiol
38:848, 1976.

Dighton DH: Sinus bradycardia. Autonomic influences and clinical assessment. Brit Heart J 36:791, 1974.

Easley RM Jr, Goldstein S: Sino-atrial syncope. Amer J Med 50:166, 1971.

Mandel WJ, Hayakawa H, Allen HN, Danzig R, Kermaier AI: Assessment of sinus node function in patients with the sick sinus syndrome. Circulation 46:761, 1972.

Narula OS, Samet P, Javier RP: Significance of the sinus-node recovery time. Circulation 45:140, 1972.

Rubenstein JJ, Schulman CL, Yurchak PM, DeSanctis RW: Clinical spectrum of the sick sinus syndrome. Circulation 46:5, 1972.

Sigurd B, Jensen G, Meibom J, Sandoe E: Adams-Stokes syndrome caused by sinoatrial block. Brit Heart J 35:1002, 1973.

Wan SH, Lee GS, Toh CCS: The sick sinus syndrome. A study of 15 cases. Brit Heart J 34:942, 1972.

CASE 12: Pulse of 140 per minute in an asymptomatic man.

An asymptomatic elderly man sees his physician for an annual routine examination at which time his pulse is found to be regular at a rate of about 140/minute. The chest x-ray shows normal lung fields and a normal cardiac silhouette. The only abnormality in the 12-Lead ECG is the presence of atrial flutter with 2:1 AV conduction, the ventricular rate being about 140/minute. The patient is admitted to the hospital. On the first hospital day he is treated with digoxin 0.5 mg orally, and on each of the next two days he receives digoxin 0.25 mg orally, and quinidine sulfate 300 mg orally four times daily. As a result, the atrial rate slows from about 280/minute to about 240/minute, but there is no change in AV conduction. The decision is then made to attempt electrical conversion of the atrial flutter to sinus rhythm. The two continuous Lead II rhythm strips in Fig. 12.1 are recorded during this procedure. In the initial portion of the top strip the rhythm is atrial flutter with 2:1 AV conduction and the ventricular rate is about 120/minute. At the arrow, a 10 watt-second discharge, synchronized to the R wave, is delivered. After a 1.05 second period during which the ECG machine is not recording, cardiac electrical activity reappears.

1. What rhythm emerges following the 10 watt-second discharge?
    a) sinus tachycardia with atrial premature beats
    b) atrial flutter with variable AV conduction
    c) atrial fibrillation
    d) junctional rhythm
    e) multifocal atrial tachycardia

ANSWER: (c)   The coarse irregular baseline without P waves or flutter waves excludes the diagnoses of sinus rhythm, multifocal atrial tachycardia, and atrial flutter. The irregularly irregular ventricular rhythm at a rate of about 120/minute in the presence of this coarse irregular baseline suggests the diagnosis of atrial fibrillation. Junctional rhythm emerging after DC cardioversion would be expected to begin at a much slower rate and gradually accelerate over several seconds to a regular rhythm at a rate of about 50-70 minute.

The electrical conversion of atrial flutter to atrial fibrillation usually occurs only if the discharge energy applied is below 50 watt-seconds. However, initial use of low energy discharges (10-50 watt-seconds) is justified by the accumulated experience that in most instances atrial flutter can be successfully converted to sinus rhythm at these low energy levels, and the suggestion that low energy discharges apparently result in less cardiac damage and in fewer postcardioversion arrhythmias than do high energy discharges.

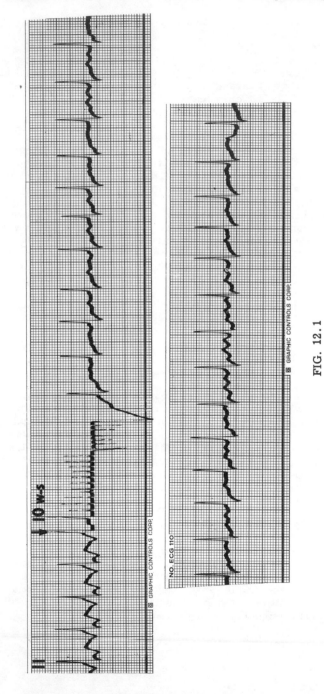

FIG. 12.1

2. How might the atrial fibrillation reasonably be managed at this
   time?
   a) repeat the DC discharge using higher energy
   b) administer digoxin and/or propranolol to control the
      ventricular rate
   c) wait a few minutes to see if spontaneous conversion to sinus
      rhythm will occur

ANSWER: (a, c) Since it is not uncommon for atrial fibrillation that
occurs following attempts at DC cardioversion of atrial flutter to
convert spontaneously to sinus rhythm within minutes, it is reasonable to wait a few minutes to see if sinus rhythm will appear. As
the original aim of DC cardioversion was to restore sinus rhythm,
it is reasonable to attempt to electrically convert the atrial fibrillation to sinus rhythm. This maneuver usually requires higher
energy levels than does conversion of atrial flutter to sinus rhythm,
probably because the termination of fibrillation requires depolarization of a large amount of atrial tissue, while the termination of
atrial flutter only requires interruption of impulses traversing a reentrant circuit within the atria.

There are a few patients with atrial flutter in whom sinus rhythm
cannot be maintained and who are symptomatic because the ventricular response to the flutter impulses cannot be adequately slowed
with digoxin and/or propranolol. Since the ventricular response to
atrial fibrillation is generally easier to control than is the ventricular response to atrial flutter, the conversion of atrial flutter to
atrial fibrillation in such patients may be desirable. This conversion may be achievable by low energy DC discharge or by rapid
right atrial stimulation using an electrode catheter. Since in this
case the patient is asymptomatic in atrial flutter despite the rapid
ventricular rate, there is no justification for allowing him to remain
in atrial fibrillation which exposes him to the very low but unnecessary risk of systemic embolization.

The two continuous Lead II rhythm strips shown in Fig. 12.2 are continuous with the strips of Fig. 12.1. The decision has been made to
deliver a 100 watt-second DC discharge at this time rather than watch
the rhythm for four to five minutes, for the patient would probably
require additional anesthesia if repeat DC cardioversion were then
necessary.

3. Which terms characterize the rhythm following the 100 watt-
   second electrical discharge?
   a) sinus rhythm   e) AV dissociation
   b) junctional rhythm   f) sinus arrest
   c) warmup phenomenon   g) AV block
   d) escape rhythm   h) escape beat

ANSWER: (a, b, c, d, e, f, h) Following the 100 watt-second discharge
there is a period of 1.2-1.8 seconds during which the ECG machine

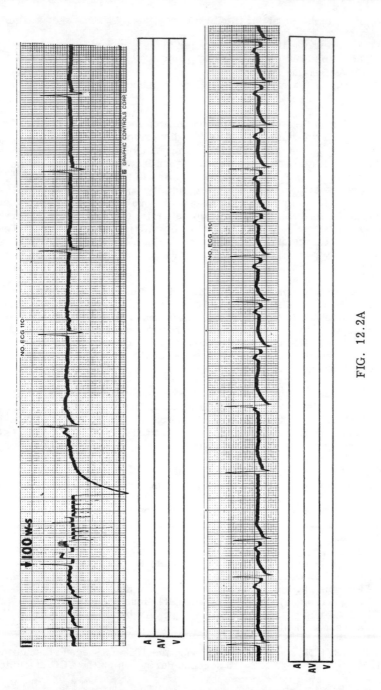

FIG. 12.2A

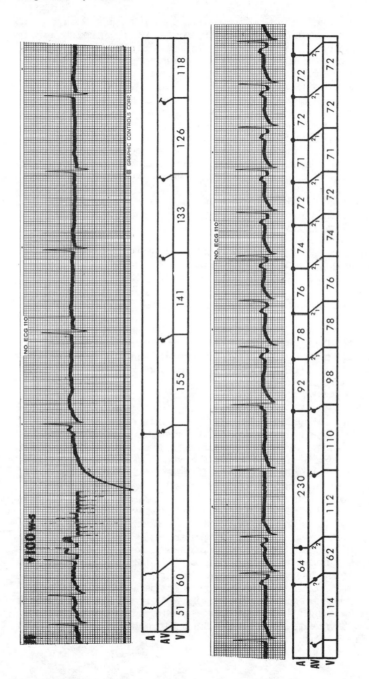

FIG. 12.2B

is not recording. The first recognizable complex is a P wave which
is followed by a narrow, normal-appearing QRS complex about 0.14
seconds later. The next five complexes are probably junctional in
origin as they are of normal contour and duration and occur in the
absence of P waves. Since QRS complexes rather than P waves terminate the pauses, the junctional rhythm qualifies as an "escape"
rhythm. The gradually shortening cycle lengths demonstrate a
rhythm of development, or "warmup" phenomenon, in which an
emerging pacemaker occurs at gradually shortening cycle lengths.
The second QRS complex in the bottom strip, occurring at about the
time the next junctional complex is expected, could be a junctional
complex, but since it is preceded by a normal-appearing P wave at
an interval of about 0.20 seconds, it could also be a sinus-stimulated complex. The subsequent P wave, having a contour slightly
different from the preceding P wave, and occurring at the shortest
PP interval in these tracings, is probably an ectopic, and premature, atrial beat which stimulates a normal QRS complex. A
junctional escape beat and then a sinus P wave which is superimposed on a normal QRS complex follow. The dissociation of this P
wave from this QRS complex is caused by lack of opportunity of the
sinus impulse to capture the AV junction before it discharged. The
subsequent QRS complexes are sinus-stimulated, with the sinus
rhythm also showing a warmup phenomenon.

The absence of atrial activity for about 2.32 seconds following the
ectopic atrial impulse could be due either to spontaneous sinus
arrest or to premature depolarization of the sinus node by the ectopic atrial impulse. Since there is no instance in which an appropriately timed P wave is not conducted to the ventricles, there is
no evidence of AV block.

The patient is discharged from the hospital two days later. He is
advised to take digoxin 0.25 mg daily, and quinidine sulfate 300 mg
four times daily. He has no cardiovascular symptoms but begins to
suffer frequent diarrheal episodes for which he seeks medical assistance. His rhythm is again atrial flutter with 2:1 AV conduction
despite a serum quinidine level which is in the therapeutic range.
The quinidine sulfate is discontinued, and the gastrointestinal symptoms subside; so the patient refuses to take any quinidine preparation.
Inasmuch as his atrial flutter doubtless reflects sinus node and/or
atrial disease which will probably progress, it is unlikely that sinus
rhythm will be maintained for any prolonged period of time in the
absence of quinidine administration. Digoxin 0.25 mg daily and propranolol 10 mg three times daily are administered for control of the ventricular rate. Over the next 10 months the patient continues to feel
well; his rhythm continues to be atrial flutter, and AV conduction is
now predominantly 4:1, with periods of alternating 4:1 and 2:1 conduction. The ventricular rate is about 70/minute at rest and about
95/minute with exertion.

BIBLIOGRAPHY

Castellanos A Jr, Lemberg L, Gosselin A, Fonseca EJ: Evaluation of countershock treatment of atrial flutter. With special reference to arrhythmias related to this procedure. Arch Int Med 115:426, 1965.

Guiney TE, Lown B: Electrical conversion of atrial flutter to atrial fibrillation. Flutter mechanism in man. Brit Heart J 34:1215, 1972.

Lemberg L, Castellanos A Jr., Swenson J, Gosselin A: Arrhythmias related to cardioversion. Circulation 30:163, 1964.

Lown B: Electrical reversion of cardiac arrhythmias. Brit Heart J 29:469, 1967.

Cheng TO: Rapid atrial pacing in conversion of atrial flutter. Amer J Cardiol 31:287, 1973.

Haft J, Kosowsky BD, Lau SH, Stein E: Termination of atrial flutter by rapid electrical pacing of the atrium. Amer J Cardiol 20:239, 1967.

Pittman ED, Makar JS, Kooros KS, Joyner CR: Rapid atrial stimulation. Successful method of conversion of atrial flutter and atrial tachycardia. Amer J Cardiol 32:700, 1973.

Preston TA: Atrial pacing to convert atrial flutter. Amer J Cardiol 32:737, 1973.

Mower MM, Mirowski M: Phenomenon of delayed reversion following atrial cardioversion. Circulation 49-50 (Suppl III): III-194, 1974.

CASE 13: Cardiac irregularity in a healthy merchant seaman.

A 45-year-old merchant seaman is referred for cardiac evaluation
before being allowed to return to work aboard ship. He is aware of
frequent cardiac irregularity, but leads an active life and has never
had syncope, presyncope, angina pectoris, or symptoms of congestive heart failure. The cardiac irregularity was detected at age 40
by a physician who was seeing the patient for treatment of an upper
respiratory infection. Since that time he has carried the diagnosis
of "myocarditis" despite the fact that, except for the cardiac irregularity, the electrocardiograms have always been within normal
limits. Over the past five years the patient has been treated with
digoxin, quinidine sulfate, procainamide, diphenylhydantoin, and
potassium chloride, alone and in combination, without any noticeable effect on the cardiac irregularity, despite the achievement of
therapeutic blood levels. The physical examination, chest x-ray,
and 12-Lead ECG are within normal limits. Three non-continuous
rhythm strips, recorded over a period of about 30 seconds, are
shown in Fig. 13.1.

1. Which terms characterize the wider QRS complexes in the
    middle strip of Fig. 13.1?
    a) atrial premature beats with aberrant intraventricular con-
       duction
    b) junctional premature beats with aberrant intraventricular
       conduction
    c) ventricular premature beats

ANSWER: (c) In the top strip the rhythm is sinus with normal P-
QRST complexes. In the middle strip there is group beating, characterized by two sinus-stimulated QRS complexes followed by a
wide (0.16 seconds) QRS complex. The wide QRS complex, occurring at a coupling interval shorter than the intersinus interval, is
premature. While the premature complexes have the same general
rS contour as sinus-stimulated complexes, the magnitudes of the
initial and terminal forces are quite different, the contour suggesting a LBBB pattern. According to guidelines developed from clinical
observations and confirmed by His bundle recordings, a wide premature QRS complex is likely to be supraventricular in origin (that
is, conducted into the ventricles from the AV junction) only if in
Lead V_1 or MCL_1 it has a RBBB pattern and/or its initial forces
are identical to the initial forces of sinus-stimulated QRS complexes.
Since neither of these criteria are met here, the wide bizarre complexes are more likely to be ventricular premature beats than aberrantly conducted atrial or junctional premature beats. The absence
of P waves preceding the premature QRS complexes excludes the
presence of atrial premature beats.

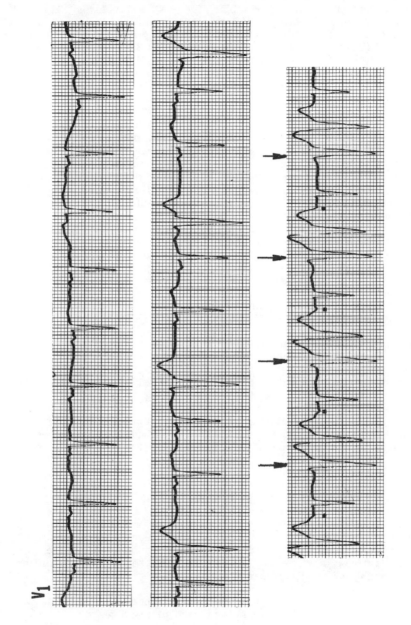

V_1

FIG. 13.1

The bottom strip in Fig. 13.1 also shows group beating, but here
one sinus beat is followed by a pair of wide QRS complexes. The
second complex of each pair has a contour similar to the first, but
occurs at shorter cycle length than the coupling interval of the first
wide QRS complex to the preceding sinus beat (0.35 vs. 0.38 seconds).

2. What term best describes the second of the two wide QRS complexes in the bottom strip of Fig. 13.1?
   a) ventricular ectopic beat
   b) aberrantly conducted sinus impulse

ANSWER: (a) The similarity of the contours of both wide QRS complexes indicates that ventricular activation is occurring via similar
pathways, and suggests that the second QRS complex is a ventricular ectopic beat arising in the area of origin of the preceding beat.
Conceivably, a sinus impulse that enters the His-Purkinje system
shortly after a ventricular premature beat might also initiate ventricular activation in the area of origin of the preceding ventricular
beat, because it should be the earliest area of ventricular tissue to
be repolarized. In the bottom strip of Fig. 13.1, however, the intersinus interval of about 0.60 seconds, estimated as one-half the
time between clearly seen consecutive P waves (●) indicates that
the sinus P wave that might stimulate the second wide QRS complex
would occur in the early portion of the first wide QRS complex
(arrow), when the His-Purkinje system would be expected to be refractory and therefore unable to conduct the impulse.

In order to evaluate whether or not underlying coronary artery disease might be responsible for the arrhythmia, a multistage treadmill exercise test is performed (Fig. 13.2). At rest (strip A) the
rhythm is sinus at a rate of about 83/minute and no ventricular premature impulses are present.

During exercise the patient achieves maximum predicted heart rate
and has a normal blood pressure response and no symptoms of myocardial ischemia. The electrocardiogram reveals no arrhythmias,
no conduction abnormalities, and no ST segment depression. The
test is terminated at the end of Stage IV, when the heart rate is
180/minute (strip B). At about thirty seconds into the recovery
period a ventricular premature beat initiates sustained ventricular
tachycardia at a rate of about 230/minute (strip C). The patient
feels faint and almost loses consciousness during the ventricular
tachycardia, which continues for about forty seconds (strip D) until
spontaneous termination occurs (strip E). The remainder of the recovery period is uneventful. At no time do ST segment abnormalities
suggesting myocardial ischemia occur.

3. Is the occurrence of ventricular tachycardia during treadmill
   exercise testing indicative of coronary artery disease?
   a) yes
   b) no
   c) uncertain

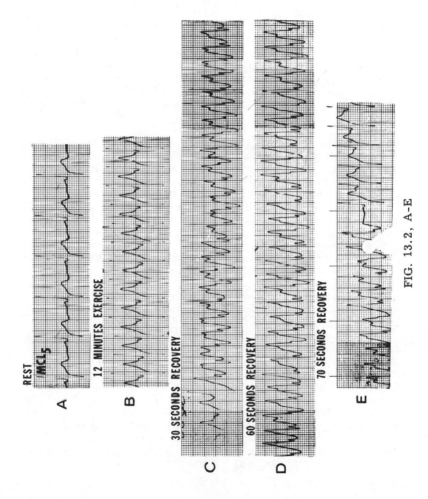

FIG. 13.2, A-E

ANSWER: (c) Currently available information suggests that exercise-induced ventricular ectopic activity, especially bursts of ventricular tachycardia, occurs most commonly in patients whose subsequent coronary, arteriograms reveal significant two- and three-vessel coronary disease. Such patients are likely to have <u>symptomatic</u> coronary disease, to have the ventricular ectopy occur at heart rates well below the predicted maximum heart rate, and to have electrocardiographic evidence of myocardial ischemia during exercise testing. Although about one-third of normal subjects have exercise-induced ventricular ectopy, it tends to appear only at or near maximum predicted heart rate. Furthermore, the occurrence of ventricular tachycardia is most unusual, and exercise-induced symptoms and electrocardiographic evidence of myocardial ischemia are virtually always lacking in such individuals. In this asymptomatic patient who has no symptoms or electrocardiographic evidence of myocardial ischemia during maximal effort, the chance of coronary artery disease being present is small.

Inasmuch as the patient's status for sea duty is in question, cardiac catheterization with left ventricular and selective coronary cine-angiography is performed, revealing normal resting and supine exercise hemodynamic data, normal left ventricular function, and normal coronary arteriogram. During the study the patient has frequent spontaneous premature beats and a His bundle electrogram is therefore recorded. Fig. 13.3 displays the X, Y, and Z orthogonal Leads of the Frank system and the His bundle electrogram during bigeminal rhythm in which each sinus beat is followed by a wide bizarre QRS complex. As Lead Z is similar to Lead V_1 except that the complexes are inverted, the complexes are identical to those in Fig. 13.1. The His bundle electrogram, demonstrating that a His deflection does not precede the wider QRS complexes, excludes supraventricular origin of these beats, and confirms the diagnosis of ventricular ectopic beats.

The antiarrhythmic agent disopyramide phosphate (Norpace®), administered in gradually increasing doses to the point of causing unpleasant side effects including blurred vision, dry mouth, difficulty urinating, and rapid regular heart action during modest exertion, has no effect on the arrhythmia. The patient, who now has not been working for four months, requests that he be allowed to return to sea; the request is granted, and the patient returns to duty taking no medications. When last seen several years later he continues to have the ventricular ectopic beats, but has had no syncope or presyncopal symptoms, and is feeling entirely well.

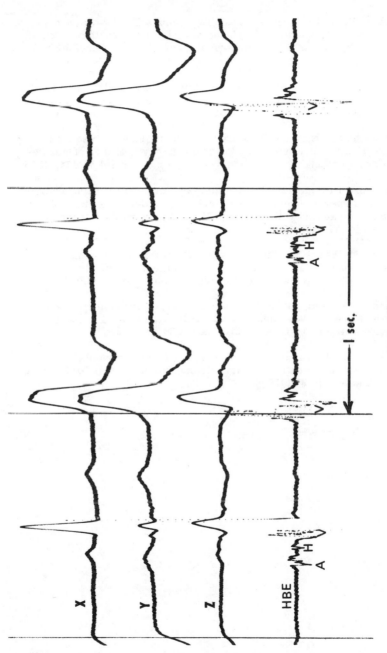

FIG. 13.3

BIBLIOGRAPHY

Faris JV, McHenry PL, Jordan JW, Morris SN: Prevalence and reproductibility of exercise-induced ventricular arrhythmias during maximal exercise testing in normal men. Amer J Cardiol 37:617, 1976.

Froelicher VF Jr, Thompson AJ, Wolthuis R, et al. : Angiographic findings in asymptomatic aircrewmen with electrocardiographic abnormalities. Amer J Cardiol 39:32, 1977.

Goldschlager N, Cake D, Cohn K: Exercise induced ventricular arrhythmias in patients with coronary artery disease. Their relationship to angiographic findings. Amer J Cardiol 31:434, 1973.

McHenry PL, Morris SN, Kavalier M, Jordan JW: Comparative study of exercise-induced ventricular arrhythmias in normal subjects and patients with documented coronary artery disease. Amer J Cardiol 37:609, 1976.

Lesch M, Lewis E, Humphries JO, Ross RS: Paroxysmal ventricular tachycardia in the absence of organic heart disease. Report of a case and review of the literature. Ann Int Med 66:950, 1967.

Sandler IA, Marriott HJL: The differential morphology of anomalous ventricular complexes of RBBB-type in lead V_1: ventricular ectopy versus aberration. Circulation 31:551, 1965.

Kistin AD: Problems in the differentiation of ventricular arrhythmia from supraventricular arrhythmia with abnormal QRS. Prog Cardiovasc Dis 9:1, 1966.

CASE 14:   Physician with acute myocardial infarction and unruly
behavior.

A 45-year-old physician with a history of inferior wall myocardial
infarction at age 42 and mild stable angina pectoris for the past year
comes to the hospital because of severe chest discomfort which he
feels is due to an acute myocardial infarction.   His cardiac output
appears adequate and there is no evidence of congestive heart failure.   His 12-Lead ECG, recorded about one hour after the onset of
symptoms, is shown in Fig. 14.1A.   There are small q waves and
slight ST segment elevation in Leads II, III, and aVF, ST segment
depression in Leads V2-V3, and ST segment straightening and T
wave flattening in Leads V5-V6, all of which are compatible with
acute inferior wall ischemic injury and old inferolateral wall myocardial infarction.   The patient is given morphine sulfate with minimal change in his chest discomfort, but two hours later his discomfort becomes more severe, at which time the 12-Lead ECG shown
in Fig. 14.1B is recorded.   Compared to the ECG recorded two
hours earlier, the PR interval has lengthened from about 0.14 to
0.21 seconds, and the ST segment depression is more pronounced
and more extensive.

1.   The increase in PR interval most likely reflects slower conduction in which part(s) of the AV conduction system?
a) AV node
b) His-Purkinje system

ANSWER: (a)   The increase in PR interval reflects prolonged conduction time from onset of atrial activation to onset of ventricular
activation. In the setting of acute inferior wall myocardial ischemia
and infarction, this slowing of AV conduction occurs almost invariably within the AV node, which generally receives blood flow from
the same vessels which supply the inferior wall of the heart.

2.   Reasonable management of the patient at this time might include:
a) administration of atropine
b) administration of isoproterenol
c) watchful waiting
d) insertion of a temporary transvenous pacing catheter into the
right ventricle

ANSWER: (c)   Since a change in PR interval from 0.14 to 0.21
seconds is unlikely to cause hemodynamic deterioration, specific
therapy aimed at shortening it is not indicated.   However, since
higher grades of AV block occurring in the setting of acute inferior
wall myocardial infarction are virtually always preceded by PR interval prolongation, close observation is warranted.

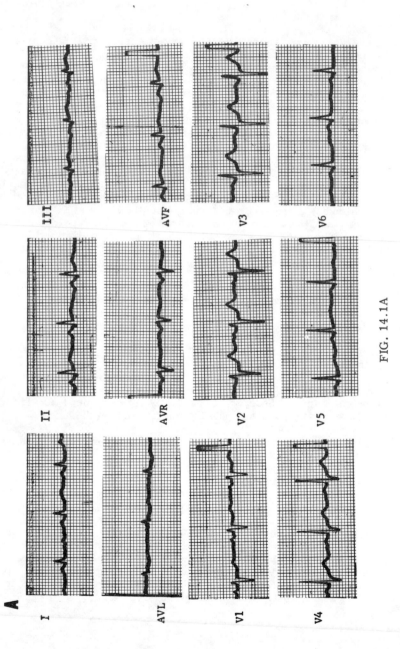

FIG. 14.1A

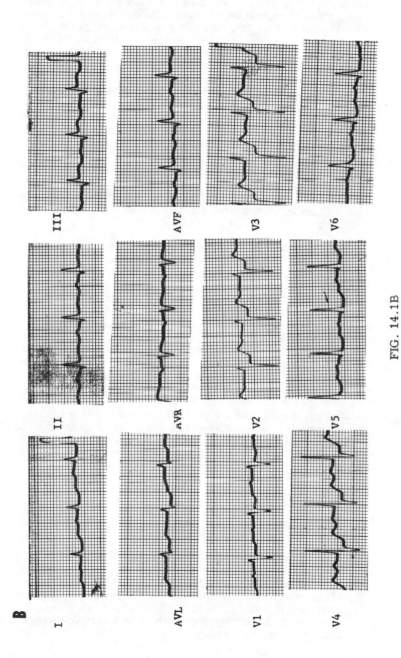

FIG. 14.1B

The parasympatholytic agent atropine will shorten AV conduction time when there is significant parasympathetic input into the AV node; the patient's sinus rate of about 100/minute suggests, however, that vagal influence at this time may be minimal. Isoproterenol might shorten the PR interval and even prevent the occurrence of higher grades of AV block, but it would also be expected to increase the heart rate and the contractile state of the ventricle, both of which would tend to increase myocardial oxygen demand thereby possibly increasing the extent of ischemic injury. Temporary transvenous right ventricular pacing would ensure adequate ventricular rate should second and third degree AV block occur. However, since many patients who develop first degree AV block never progress to higher grades of AV block, insertion of a pacing catheter at this time is premature. In those patients who do develop high grade AV block, intravenous isoproterenol can usually be relied upon to either improve AV conduction or increase the rate of the emerging escape pacemaker such that an adequate hemodynamic state can be maintained until right ventricular pacing is achieved.

The patient is anxious and hostile, demands more medication for relief of his chest discomfort, and states that under no circumstances will he consent to pacemaker insertion. He is given additional morphine sulfate following which he becomes diaphoretic and nauseated and begins to vomit, so 1.0 mg of atropine is administered intravenously. About 30 minutes later 2:1 AV block with ventricular rate of about 60/minute occurs and the patient's blood pressure falls from 110/80 to 90/70. Atropine, 1.0 mg, is again administered intravenously, and the Lead II rhythm strip shown in Fig. 14.2A is recorded. The sinus rate has increased to about 120/minute, the PR interval of the conducted beats has lengthened to about 0.24 seconds, and ventricular ectopic beats have appeared. The patient is now disoriented and combative, probably due to the combination of morphine sulfate, atropine, hypotension, and emotional stress. Isoproterenol, administered intravenously in doses up to 4 μg/min in an attempt to improve the hemodynamic state results in an increase in the sinus rate to about 130/minute but does not prevent the occurrence of complete AV block (Fig. 14.2B).

3. Which term(s) describe the QRS rhythm in Fig. 14.2B?
    a) junctional escape rhythm
    b) ventricular escape rhythm
    c) accelerated junctional rhythm

ANSWER: (a) The QRS complexes have no fixed temporal relationship to the P waves, indicating complete AV block. As they are narrow and have identical contours to those stimulated by P waves in Fig. 14.2A, their origin must be in the AV junction. The somewhat long QRS cycle length of 1.73-1.76 seconds (rate about 34-35/minute) for a junctional escape rhythm may be due to depression of automaticity caused by ischemia.

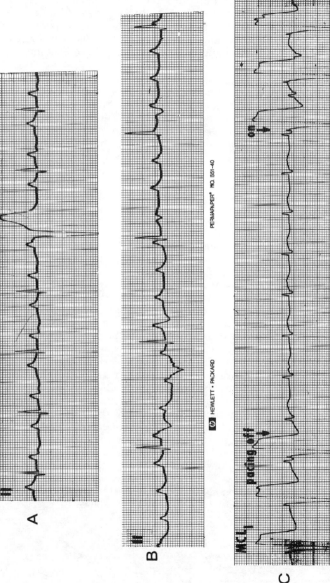
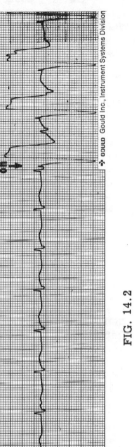

FIG. 14.2

As the patient is doing very poorly and apparently realizes it, he agrees to allow pacemaker insertion. A temporary transvenous electrode catheter is advanced into the right ventricular apex where stable pacing is achieved and employed at a rate of 80/minute; the isoproterenol is then discontinued. The blood pressure increases to acceptable levels, the ventricular ectopic beats disappear, and the patient's general appearance improves. Over the next 12 hours the hemodynamic state remains stable and the patient becomes alert and cooperative.

Every twelve hours the pacemaker is turned off in order to assess the state of AV conduction, as shown in Fig. 14.2C, which is recorded 48 hours after pacemaker insertion. Following cessation of ventricular pacing P waves are seen to be occurring at intervals of about 0.68 seconds (rate about 86/minute), but since no QRS complexes occur over a period of about 5.2 seconds, ventricular pacing is resumed.

4. Is AV block likely to be permanent in this patient?
    a) yes
    b) no

ANSWER: (b) AV nodal dysfunction causing AV block in the setting of acute inferior wall myocardial infarction is almost invariably a transient phenomenon, as the underlying pathologic process appears to be reversible ischemic injury rather than irreversible fibrosis. Improvement in AV nodal function usually occurs gradually over a period of several days to one-two weeks, and is typically characterized by a regression from complete AV block to 2:1 AV conduction, then to 1:1 AV conduction with prolonged PR interval, and finally, the PR interval shortens to normal. Occasionally, and most typically when the PR interval is still prolonged, AV Wenckebach periods may occur. In the small number of patients with inferior wall myocardial infarction and transient complete AV block whose AV nodal conduction time has been measured following return of 1:1 AV conduction with normal PR interval, AH times have usually been within normal limits. Permanent ventricular pacemaker implantation is required only very rarely, as it is extremely rare for a patient who develops complete AV block during acute inferior wall myocardial infarction to have persistent high grade AV block.

When the ventricular pacemaker is temporarily turned off on the fourth hospital day, the Lead V1 rhythm strip shown in Fig. 14.3A is recorded.

5. What terms describe the rhythm?
    a) sinus tachycardia
    b) first degree AV block
    c) Type I second degree AV block
    d) Type II second degree AV block
    e) 2:1 AV block of uncertain type
    f) complete AV block
    g) ventriculophasic sinus arrhythmia

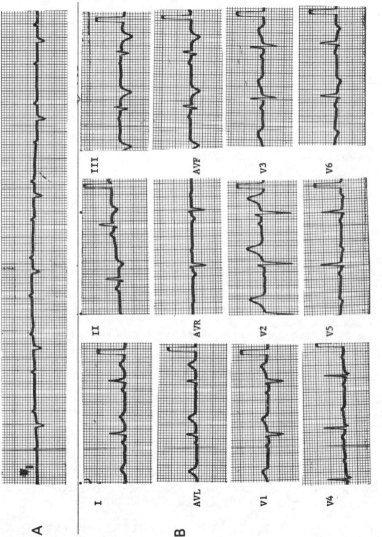

FIG. 14.3

ANSWER: (a, b, e, g) Narrow, normal-appearing QRS complexes occur at regular intervals of about 1.15-1.16 seconds (rate about 52/minute) and P waves occur at intervals about half this (0.57-0.59 seconds). Atrial activity has a fixed temporal relationship to the QRS complexes, a P wave preceding each of them by an abnormally long interval of 0.35 seconds. The rhythm is thus sinus tachycardia with 2:1 AV conduction, with the conducted P wave showing first degree AV block. The differential diagnosis of Type I from Type II second degree AV block cannot be established with certainty in an isolated rhythm strip showing 2:1 AV block. The response of AV conduction to changes in atrial rate may allow accurate diagnosis.

Intervals between consecutive P waves which include a QRS complex are about 0.02 seconds shorter than intervals between consecutive P waves which do not (0.57 vs. 0.59 seconds), a commonly observed but incompletely understood phenomenon known as "ventriculophasic sinus arrhythmia".

Sinus rhythm with 2:1 AV conduction persists until the eleventh hospital day when 1:1 AV conduction with normal PR interval appears, and one day later the electrode catheter is removed. The remainder of the hospitalization is unremarkable. The patient is discharged on the 21st hospital day at which time the 12-Lead ECG (Fig. 14.3B) shows a normal PR interval of about 0.15 seconds. In comparison with tracings shown in Fig. 14.1A and B, the q waves are larger, the ST segment elevation less marked, and the T waves inverted in Leads II, III, and aVF, indicating evolution of inferior wall myocardial infarction. The patient was last heard from 18 months after his myocardial infarction, at which time he was doing well and had no angina, no symptoms of congestive heart failure, and no arrhythmias.

BIBLIOGRAPHY

Das G, Talmers FM, Weissler AM: New observations on the effects of atropine on the sinoatrial and atrioventricular nodes in man. Amer J Cardiol 36:281, 1975.

Dreifus LS, Watanabe Y, Haiat R, Kimbiris D: Atrioventricular block. Amer J Cardiol 28:371, 1971.

Hope RR, Scherlag BJ, El-Sherif N, Lazzara R: Hierarchy of ventricular pacemakers. Circulation Res 39:883, 1976.

Narula OS, Scherlag BJ, Samet P, Javier RP: Atrioventricular block. Localization and classification by His bundle recordings. Amer J Med 50:146, 1971.

Langendorf R, Cohen H, Gozo EG Jr: Observations on second degree atrioventricular block including new criteria for the differential diagnosis between type I and type II block. Amer J Cardiol 41:111, 1970.

Rosen KM, Loeb HS, Chuquimia R, Sinno MZ, et al.: Site of heart block in acute myocardial infarction. Circulation 42:925, 1970.

Sutton R, Davies M: The conduction system in acute myocardial infarction complicated by heart block. Circulation 38:987, 1968.

Norris RM: Heart block in posterior and anterior myocardial infarction. Brit Heart J 31:352, 1968.

Courter SR, Moffat J, Fowler NO: Advanced atrioventricular block in acute myocardial infarction. Circulation 27:1034, 1963.

CASE 15:   Prolonged intraventricular conduction time in an
           asymptomatic forty-three-year-old woman.

A 43-year-old asymptomatic woman has a thorough routine medical
examination.   Her physical examination and chest x-ray are within
normal limits, and the 12-Lead ECG is shown in Fig. 15.1.   The
rhythm is sinus at a rate of about 72/minute.   The P wave axis is
just within the normal range at about 0 degrees, and the PR interval is normal at about 0.17 seconds.   The QRS complexes have an
abnormally prolonged duration of 0.12-0.13 seconds, and the mean
frontal plane QRS axis is about +95 degrees.   The ST segments are
downsloping in Leads III and aVF, and straightened in Leads II and
V_6, and the T waves are somewhat flattened in these four Leads.

1. Which of the following is (are) likely to account for the right
    axis deviation in this tracing?
    a) right ventricular hypertrophy
    b) normal variant
    c) left posterior fascicle block
    d) right bundle branch block
    e) left bundle branch block
    f) ventricular preexcitation

ANSWER: (c) Right axis deviation in adults may rarely be seen as
an isolated finding.   It is much more commonly the result of right
ventricular hypertrophy, unusual chest cage configuration, or left
posterior fascicle conduction delay (or block).   Right ventricular
hypertrophy and unusual chest cage configuration are excluded by
the patient's normal physical examination, and in view of the prolonged QRS duration indicating intraventricular conduction delay,
the right axis deviation here is most likely attributable to conduction
delay within the posterior fascicle of the left bundle branch.   Since
this degree of QRS prolongation is much greater than expected
solely on the basis of left posterior fascicle block (the development
of which might increase QRS duration by up to 0.02 seconds), unusually slow conduction through the peripheral Purkinje system is
also probably present.

Although rightward axis may occur in the presence of isolated right
bundle branch block, the absence of right bundle branch block pattern
in the precordial Leads indicates that right bundle branch conduction
delay is not present.   The QRS contours in this tracing do not support
the diagnosis of conduction delay in the main left bundle branch, and
left bundle branch block itself is not a cause of right axis deviation.
While ventricular preexcitation via an accessory AV conduction pathway might conceivably cause both right axis deviation and intraventricular conduction delay, the absence of delta waves makes this
diagnosis very unlikely.

The patient continues to feel well, and electrocardiograms recorded at ages 45, 47, 48, and 50 years are unchanged from that shown in Fig. 15.1. However, at age 53 the patient sees her physician with complaints of a two-year history of awareness of rapid irregular heart action lasting seconds to minutes, and one recent episode of "near fainting" which occurred while she was sitting down. Physical examination at this time is again within normal limits, and the 12-Lead ECG is shown in Fig. 15.2.

2. Which of the following has (have) developed in the ten-year period since the ECG in Fig. 15.1 was recorded?
   a) left anterior fascicle block
   b) right bundle branch block
   c) left ventricular hypertrophy
   d) right ventricular hypertrophy

ANSWER: (b) The abnormally rightward QRS axis that was attributed to left posterior fascicle block has progressed from about +95 degrees to about +120 degrees, the QRS duration has lengthened from about 0.12-0.13 seconds to about 0.18 seconds, and the QRS contours in the precordial Leads now indicate right bundle branch conduction delay, all of which suggest progressive dysfunction of the intraventricular conduction system. There is no evidence, however, of interim development of left anterior fascicle block which, occurring in the presence of left posterior fascicle block, would be expected to have resulted in the QRS pattern of left bundle branch block; and, as the PR interval has not changed there is no evidence that the disease process involves the AV node. While it is conceivable that the progressive right axis deviation and the development of the large R wave in Lead V_1 could be due to the interval development of right ventricular hypertrophy, widening of the QRS complex to this degree would be a most unusual manifestation of right ventricular hypertrophy which, again, is excluded by the patient's normal physical examination. Neither QRS voltage nor ST and T wave abnormalities suggesting left ventricular hypertrophy are present in this tracing.

3. How might this patient be reasonably managed at this time?
   a) perform His bundle recording to measure the His-Purkinje system conduction (HV) time
   b) perform a Holter monitor recording
   c) implant a permanent demand ventricular pacemaker
   d) reassure her that the episode of "near fainting" is not likely to have been cardiac in origin

ANSWER: (a, b, c) Within the framework of the trifascicular intraventricular conduction system, when block is present in the right bundle branch and in the posterior fascicle of the left bundle branch, AV conduction can occur only via the anterior fascicle of the left bundle branch, whose function can be assessed by recording the His bundle potential and measuring the HV (His-Purkinje system conduction) time. Failure of conduction in the left anterior fascicle

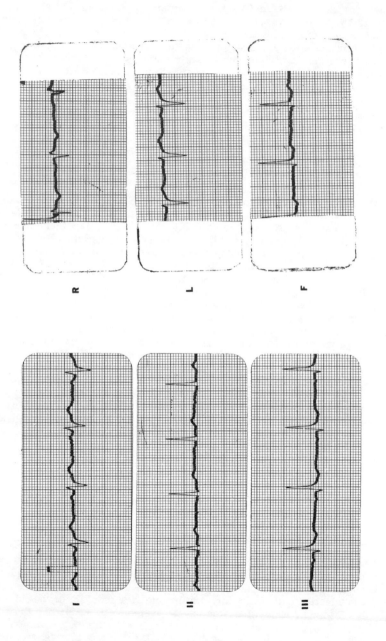

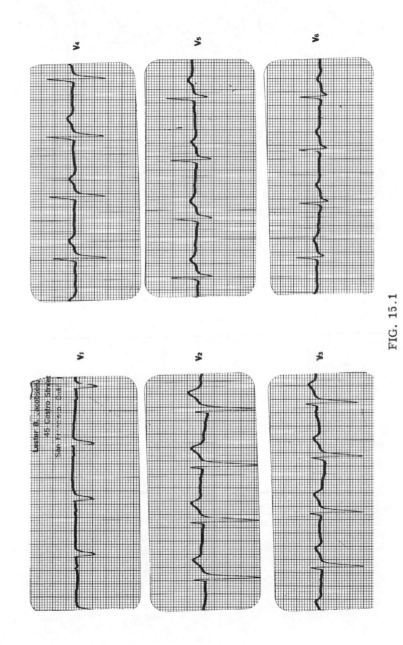

FIG. 15.1

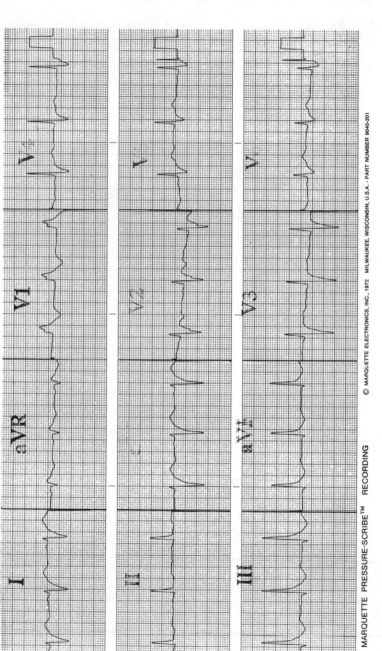

MARQUETTE PRESSURE-SCRIBE™   RECORDING   © MARQUETTE ELECTRONICS, INC., 1972   MILWAUKEE, WISCONSIN, U.S.A. - PART NUMBER 8040-201

FIG. 15.2

would lead to complete AV block which might result in near-syncope
or syncope (Stokes-Adams-Morgagni attacks). The QRS duration of
about 0.18 seconds is longer than can be attributed simply to the left
posterior fascicle block and right bundle branch block, indicating that
conduction is abnormally slow in Purkinje fibers in the ventricles
as well. The electrocardiographic evidence of extensive intraventricular conduction system disease makes it unreasonable to reassure the patient that the episode of "near fainting" is not likely to
have been cardiac in origin.

Currently, the most effective and only reliable therapy for intermittent or established complete AV block is permanent ventricular
pacing. However, in this patient who has not had syncope it seems
reasonable to defer permanent ventricular pacemaker implantation
until Holter monitoring recording can be performed to see if periods
of complete AV block or Type II second degree AV block are indeed
occurring, and to observe the rhythm occurring at the time of the
awareness of rapid heart action.

A 24-hour Holter monitor recording is obtained, during which time
the patient has several three- to four-minute episodes of rapid heart
action, but no presyncopal symptoms and no syncope. Fig. 15.3,
strip A, recorded at a time when the patient is asymptomatic, shows
sinus rhythm at a rate of about 72/minute, while strip B is recorded
during a time when the patient was aware of rapid heart action.

4. The sensation of rapid heart action is likely to have been due to
    which of the following?
    a) atrial fibrillation
    b) atrial flutter
    c) ventricular tachycardia
    d) sinus tachycardia

ANSWER: (a) In Fig. 15.3B wide, bizarre QRS complexes are occurring in an irregularly irregular pattern at an average rate of
about 120/minute. These QRS complexes have contours identical
to the sinus-stimulated QRS complexes in Fig. 15.3A, indicating
that ventricular activation proceeds via the AV junction. Although
atrial activity is not clearly identifiable, atrial fibrillation accounts
best for the irregularity of the ventricular rhythm. While atrial
flutter waves might not be easily discerned in a modified Lead I,
the ventricular rhythm in atrial flutter would be expected to be much
less irregular. The irregularity of the QRS rhythm also excludes
the diagnosis of sinus tachycardia.

5. How might the paroxysmal atrial fibrillation be reasonably
    managed in this patient at this time?
    a) prescribe no medication and simply reassure the patient that
       the rhythm is not serious
    b) administer digoxin
    c) administer a quinidine preparation

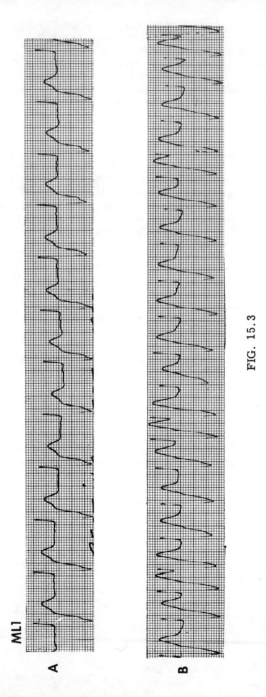

FIG. 15.3

d) administer propranolol
e) perform His bundle recording before starting any medication
f) implant a permanent ventricular demand pacemaker

ANSWER: (b, c, d, e, f) Since the patient is made uncomfortable by
the episodes of rapid heart action which have been documented to be
due to paroxysms of atrial fibrillation, prevention of the atrial fibrillation and/or control of the ventricular rate during atrial fibrillation is reasonable. As atrial fibrillation is usually initiated
by atrial premature beats, preventing atrial ectopic activity is
reasonable, and quinidine preparations and propranolol are often
effective in this regard. While there has been some concern that
both these medications may depress intraventricular conduction
and thus predispose this patient to periods of high grade and/or
complete AV block, studies of their effect on His-Purkinje system
conduction time in man have demonstrated a depressant effect on
AV nodal but not on His-Purkinje system conduction. His bundle
recording before and after intravenous administration of one or
both of these medications to this patient might help predict whether
or not they are likely to significantly worsen atrioventricular conduction, but implantation of a permanent ventricular demand pacemaker would allow their use without concern that untoward depressant effects on AV conduction would cause symptomatic bradycardia.
Propranolol, by slowing AV nodal conduction, would be expected to
slow the ventricular rate in atrial fibrillation, and digoxin, which
slows AV nodal conduction but does not alter intraventricular conduction velocity, may safely be used for this purpose, but is not
likely to prevent the onset of atrial fibrillation.

The patient is treated with digoxin 0.25 mg every morning, and
quinidine sulfate in doses which achieve a low therapeutic serum
level. Over the next two months she has no further episodes of
rapid or irregular heart action, but she has four presyncopal episodes. A His bundle electrographic study is therefore performed.
Fig. 15.4, displaying simultaneously recorded surface Leads II
and V1, the His bundle electrogram (HBE) and the high right atrial
electrogram (HRAE), shows normal AV nodal conduction time of
about 90 msec (normal 70-120 msec) and markedly prolonged His-
Purkinje system conduction (HV) time of about 100 msec (normal
35-55 msec). Since the patient is having the presyncopal spells
and has evidence of dysfunction in all portions of the intraventricular conduction system, a permanent ventricular demand pacemaker
is implanted the following day. Postoperatively, the digoxin and
quinidine sulfate are continued. The patient is asymptomatic for
the next twelve months, until frequent brief episodes of rapid heart
action occur. During repeat Holter monitor recording, the patient
has rapid heart action most of the time, and the tracings reveal a
normally sensing and normally pacing demand ventricular pacemaker, and atrial fibrillation with an average ventricular rate of
about 100/minute. The digoxin 0.25 mg daily is continued, and the

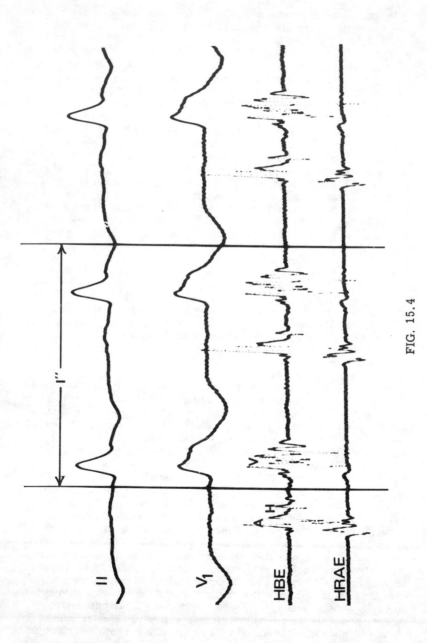

FIG. 15.4

Simple Arrhythmias   Case 15/ 127

dosage of quinidine sulfate is increased to achieve a higher therapeutic serum level. When last seen two months after the second
Holter monitor recording, the patient has had only two very brief
episodes of irregular heart action, and no presyncope or syncope.

BIBLIOGRAPHY

Berkowitz WD, Wit AL, Lau SH, Steiner C, Damato AN: The effects
of propranolol on cardiac conduction. Circulation 40:855, 1969.

Denes P, Dhingra RC, Wu D, Chuquimia R, Amat-y-Leon F, Wyndham C, Rosen KM: H-V interval in patients with bifascicular block.
Amer J Cardiol 35:23, 1975.

Dhingra RC, Denes P, Wu D, Chuquimia R, Amat-y-Leon F, Rosen
KM: Syncope in patients with chronic bifascicular block. Significance,
causative mechanisms, and clinical implications. Ann Int Med
81:302, 1974.

Dhingra RC, Denes P, Wu D, Chuquimia R, Amat-y-Leon F, Wyndham C, Rosen KM: Chronic right bundle branch block and left posterior hemiblock. Amer J Cardiol 36:867, 1975.

Hirschfeld DS, Ueda CT, Rowland M, Scheinman MM: Clinical and
electrophysiological effects of intravenous quinidine in man. Brit
Heart J 39:309, 1977.

Ranganathan N, Dhurandhar R, Phillips JH, Wigle ED: His bundle
electrogram in bundle-branch block. Circulation 45:282, 1972.

Josephson ME, Seides SF, Batsford WP, et al.: The electrophysiological effects of intramuscular quinidine on the atrioventricular
conducting system in man. Amer Heart J 87:55, 1974.

Sokolow M, Perloff DB: The clinical pharmacology and use of
quinidine in heart disease. Prog Cardiovasc Dis 3:316, 1961.

Spurrell RAJ, et al.: Study of right bundle-branch block in association with either left anterior hemiblock or left posterior hemiblock using His bundle electrograms. Brit Heart J 34:800, 1972.

Wu D, et al.: Bundle branch block. Demonstration of the incomplete nature of some "complete" bundle branch and fascicular
blocks by the extrastimulus technique. Amer J Cardiol 33:583, 1974.

Pamintuan JC, Dreifus LS, Watanabe Y: Comparative mechanisms
of antiarrhythmic agents. Amer J Cardiol 26:512, 1970.

Narula OS: His Bundle Electrocardiography and Clinical Electrophysiology. F.A. Davis Company, Philadelphia, pp. 112-115, 1975.

Narula OS, Samet P: Right bundle branch block with normal, left
or right axis deviation. Amer J Med 51:432, 1971.

CASE 16: Young woman with paroxysmal rapid heart action of
          ten years' duration.

A 35-year-old woman with a 10-year history of paroxysmal rapid
heart action is referred for evaluation and treatment of these
episodes. Rapid heart action occurs only when she is up and about,
has an abrupt onset, lasts minutes to hours, and terminates abruptly.
During these episodes she feels weak and lightheaded, but has no
symptoms of congestive heart failure or myocardial ischemia. She
had recently been experiencing three to four such episodes daily,
but the administration of 0.25 mg digoxin daily and 10 mg propranolol three times daily has decreased their frequency to once or
twice daily. Her cardiovascular examination and chest x-ray are
normal. Her 12-Lead ECG is shown in Fig. 16.1.

The abnormalities in this tracing include a short PR interval of
about 0.11 seconds, non-diagnostic T flattening in the inferior and
mid and lateral precordial leads, and prominent U waves.

On the first hospital day while washing she experiences the sudden
onset of rapid heart action shortly after which the two continuous
Lead II rhythm strips in Fig. 16.2 are recorded.

1. What is the rhythm?
    a) atrial flutter with 2:1 AV conduction
    b) supraventricular tachycardia (SVT)
    c) atrial fibrillation
    d) ventricular tachycardia

ANSWER: (b) Narrow QRS complexes occurring at regular intervals at a rate of 187-193 beats per minute (RR intervals about
0.31-0.32 seconds) suggest that the rhythm is supraventricular
tachycardia (SVT). P waves are not clearly identifiable. The
regularity of the QRS rhythm indicates that it is not related to
atrial fibrillation. Atrial flutter is excluded by the isoelectric segments in Lead II; in addition, the QRS rate would be unusually fast
for atrial flutter with 2:1 AV conduction, and unusually slow for atrial
flutter with 1:1 AV conduction, as the atrial rate in flutter is usually
250-350/minute. While ventricular tachycardia may have narrow
QRS complexes if the rhythm originates in the proximal area of a
fascicle of the intraventricular conduction system, in the few reported
cases the ventricular rates have been slower than in this case (around
100/minute), and the patients have had underlying heart disease such
as myocardial infarction or congestive heart failure.

2. What therapeutic interventions might appropriately be used to
    terminate the tachycardia in this hemodynamically stable patient?
    a) carotid sinus massage
    b) Vasoxyl ® administration

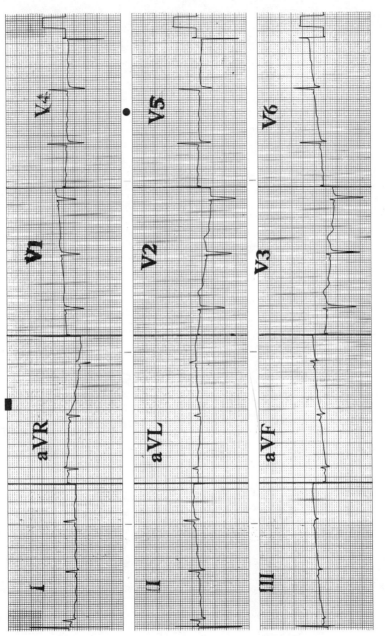

FIG. 16. 1

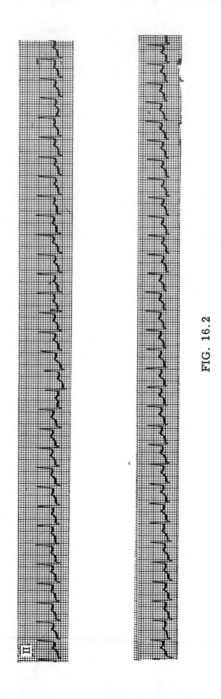

FIG. 16.2

c) lidocaine administration
d) Tensilon ® (edrophonium) administration
e) additional propranolol administration
f) additional digoxin administration

ANSWER: (a, b, d, e, f) The exact mechanism of supraventricular tachycardia in patients with short PR interval and normal QRS duration is unclear. It may involve (1) antegrade conduction via an accessory AV conduction pathway or via an AV node which is anatomically shorter than normal and/or physiologically able to conduct impulses faster than normal AV nodal tissue; and (2) retrograde impulse conduction via the AV node and/or an accessory ventriculoatrial conduction pathway. If the tachycardia impulses traverse the AV nodal tissue (as is the case in the majority of patients with SVT) then any therapeutic modality which slows AV nodal conduction time or alters AV nodal refractory period might terminate the supraventricular tachycardia. Thus, carotid sinus massage, edrophonium, Vasoxyl®, and additional propranolol might help terminate the tachycardia. Lidocaine, which has little effect on the AV node, would likely be ineffective. Additional digoxin administration might convert the SVT, and if given in small doses is unlikely to cause serious arrhythmias in a patient without organic heart disease.

Carotid sinus massage was performed without effect, so Tensilon®, 2 mg, was injected rapidly intravenously and the tracing shown in Fig. 16.3 recorded. The strip begins with the narrow QRS complexes occurring at intervals of about 0.34 seconds (rate about 176/minute). The last three QRS complexes of the tachycardia occur at somewhat longer RR intervals of 0.36, 0.39, and 0.38 seconds, following which the tachycardia terminates. Following a pause of about 1.0 second sinus rhythm resumes, and gradually accelerates ("warmup" phenomenon). It is not possible to say whether the last complex of the tachycardia is a QRS or P wave since P waves are not clearly identifiable during the tachycardia. The lengthening RR intervals preceding termination of the tachycardia suggest that the Tensilon® in some manner altered conduction and probably also refractory periods in the tachycardia circuit such that the mechanism could not be sustained.

Many patients with short PR interval, normal QRS duration, and paroxysmal supraventricular tachycardia have been studied using atrial and ventricular pacing and His bundle recordings. In most patients, the AV nodal conduction (AH) time is at or below the lower limits of normal, and the His-Purkinje system conduction (HV) time is usually at the lower limits of normal. The short AH time could be due to (1) an anatomically short AV node, (2) atrial fibers which bypass the AV node and insert near the His bundle, and/or (3) fibers within the AV node that conduct impulses more rapidly than normal. Atrial pacing studies indicate that the majority of patients behave as if AV conduction occurs via an anatomically small AV node, or one which conducts impulses more rapidly

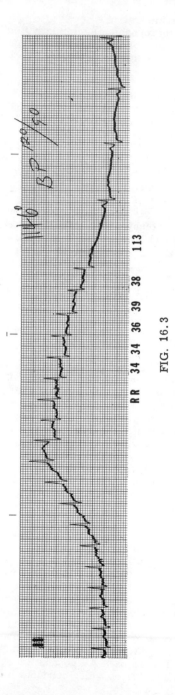

FIG. 16.3

than normal. Only in rare instances can an AV nodal bypass tract with antegrade conduction be demonstrated. The reason for the low normal HV time in these patients is unclear.

Another finding in these patients (as well as in patients with normal PR intervals and paroxysmal supraventricular tachycardias) is that the majority of them, when paced from the right ventricular apex, have 1:1 ventriculoatrial conduction at very rapid ventricular rates, and VA conduction time that is independent of pacing rate. Pacemaker-induced premature ventricular depolarizations may also be conducted retrograde to the atria with constant VA time at all coupling intervals. These findings indicate that a retrograde pathway having properties different from the normal AV node is present. It therefore appears likely that in the majority of patients with short PR interval, normal QRS duration, and paroxysmal SVT, antegrade conduction during the tachycardia occurs via the AV node, while retrograde conduction occurs via an accessory pathway which can conduct impulses only from ventricle to atrium.

In this patient, electrophysiologic studies demonstrated a low-normal AH time, AV conduction occurring via a pathway behaving like AV nodal tissue, no antegrade accessory AV pathway, low-normal HV time, and a retrograde accessory pathway. Although the onset of SVT was never recorded in this patient, 72 hours of telemetry monitoring of cardiac rhythm revealed only premature ventricular beats. It is attractive to hypothesize that in this patient supraventricular tachycardia is initiated by a premature ventricular impulse which conducts to the atrium via the accessory VA pathway (blocking retrogradely in the AV node), and then activates the ventricles antegradely via the AV node-His-Purkinje system.

The patient is treated with propranolol, 40 mg orally four times daily and digoxin 0.25 mg daily. When last examined six weeks later, she has had no episodes of rapid heart action.

BIBLIOGRAPHY

Bissett JK, Thompson AJ, de Soyza N, Murphy ML: Atrioventricular conduction in patients with short P-R interval and normal QRS complex. Brit Heart J 35:123, 1973.

Caracta AR, Damato AN, Gallagher JJ, Josephson ME, et al.: Electrophysiological studies in the syndrome of short P-R interval, normal QRS complex. Amer J Cardiol 31:245, 1973.

Castellanos A, Castillo CA, Agha AS, Tessler M: His bundle electrograms in patients with short P-R intervals, narrow QRS complex and paroxysmal tachycardia. Circulation 43:667, 1971.

Clerc A, Levy R, Cristesco C: A propos du raccourcissement permanent de l'espace P-R de l'electrocardiogramme sans deformation du complexe ventriculare. Arch Mal Coeur 31:569, 1938.

Cohen HC, Gozo EG Jr, Pick A: Ventricular tachycardia with narrow QRS complexes (left posterior, fascicular tachycardia). Circulation 45:1035, 1972.

Durrer D, Schuilenburg RM, Wellens HJJ: Pre-excitation revisited. Amer J Cardiol 25:690, 1970.

Lown B, Ganong WF, Levine SA: The syndrome of short P-R interval, normal QRS complex, and paroxysmal rapid heart action. Circulation 5:693, 1952.

Narula OS: Electrophysiologic evaluation of accessory conduction pathways. In: His Bundle Electrocardiography and Clinical Electrophysiology. Narula OS, Ed.,F.A. Davis Co., Philadelphia, pp. 314-322, 1975.

Roelandt J, Willems J, DeGeest H: Ventricular tachycardia with normal QRS duration diagnosed by reciprocal beats. Dis Chest 56:166, 1969.

Seigel L, Breithardt L, Both A: Atrioventricular (AV) and ventriculoatrial (VA) conduction pattern in patients with short P-R interval and normal QRS complex. In: Cardiac Pacing. Diagnostic and Therapeutic Tools. Luderitz B, Ed., Springer-Verlag, Berlin-Heidelberg, pp. 151-163, 1976.

CASE 17: Acute myocardial infarction in a sixty-three year-old
          woman.

A 63-year-old woman is admitted to the Coronary Care Unit because
of symptoms suggesting acute myocardial infarction. Her 12-Lead
ECG indicates extensive anterior and lateral wall myocardial infarction. She appears to have barely adequate cardiac output with
scattered rales, mild jugular venous distension, and blood pressure
of 90/70. She is treated with supplemental inspired oxygen and
morphine sulfate, and her cardiac rhythm is monitored. Suddenly
she complains of feeling lightheaded, at which time the Lead II
rhythm strip shown in Fig. 17.1 is recorded.

1. Which terms describe the rhythm?
    a) sinus tachycardia
    b) ventricular tachycardia
    c) concealed conduction
    d) group beating
    e) accelerated ventricular rhythm

ANSWER: (a, b, c) Positively-directed normal-appearing QRS complexes are separated by runs of negatively-directed wide, bizarre
QRS complexes. P waves precede the first, second, fourth, fifth,
and last normal QRS complexes by about 0.13 seconds, indicating
sinus tachycardia. The wide bizarre complexes, occurring at
short, slightly irregular cycle length (about 0.36 seconds, rate
about 167/minute) constitute bursts of ventricular tachycardia that
are initiated by premature ventricular beats and terminate spontaneously.

The next to last QRS complex (X) is preceded by a P wave (P) at an
interval longer than PR intervals of other sinus beats (about 0.18
vs. 0.13 seconds), probably because of delay in antegrade AV nodal
conduction occasioned by retrograde penetration of the preceding
ventricular ectopic beat into the AV node, an event which would be
electrocardiographically silent. This electrocardiographically
silent event, manifest only by its aftereffects (in this case by prolongation of the PR interval of the subsequent sinus beat) is called
"concealed conduction".

The phrase "group beating", used to describe rhythms in which there
is a regular grouping of beats, does not apply to this tracing in which
salvos of varying numbers of ventricular ectopic beats irregularly
interrupt the sinus rhythm.

Accelerated ventricular rhythm occurs commonly within the first
24-36 hours of the onset of symptoms of myocardial infarction. It
consists of regularly occurring wide QRS complexes, the first of
which occurs at a coupling interval longer than the preceding sinus

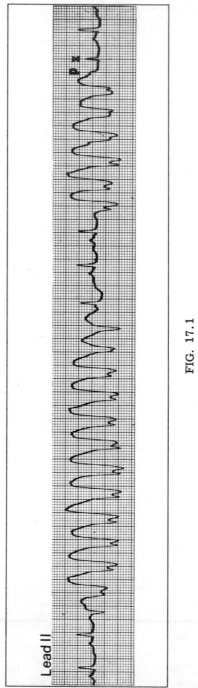

FIG. 17.1

cycle length, and is thus in essence an acelerated escape rhythm. Its rate of about 60 to 100 beats per minute is usually within a few beats per minute of the sinus rate. Accelerated ventricular rhythm has not been documented to initiate ventricular tachycardia, and is of little or no hemodynamic consequence. None of the features of accelerated ventricular rhythm are present in this tracing.

2. Reasonable management of this patient at this time might include:
a) watchful waiting
b) intravenous lidocaine administration
c) intravenous procainamide administration
d) oral quinidine sulfate administration
e) intravenous atropine administration

ANSWER: (b, c) In this critically ill woman with acute myocardial infarction, therapy aimed at preventing premature ventricular beats is crucial to avoid the occurrence of catastrophic ventricular tachycardia and ventricular fibrillation. Lidocaine, a most effective and minimally toxic agent in this setting, might be extremely useful and should be administered intravenously in a 50-100 mg bolus, followed by a continuous infusion of up to 2-4 mg/min. If the rhythm disturbance is refractory to lidocaine, it would be reasonable to administer procainamide intravenously at a rate of 50-100 mg/minute to a dose of about one gram, followed by a continuous intravenous infusion of 1-2 mg/min. While oral quinidine sulfate has been shown to diminish the frequency of ventricular arrhythmias in acute myocardial infarction, medication administered orally to a critically ill patient is unlikely to be rapidly effective because of slow gastrointestinal absorption. Atropine, useful in suppressing ventricular ectopic beats occurring during slow sinus rhythm, presumably by increasing the sinus rate, is unlikely to be useful here, where the sinus rate is about 115-120/minute. There is no place for watchful waiting while a patient critically ill with acute myocardial infarction has ventricular tachycardia.

Lidocaine, administered in the manner described above, has no effect on the premature ventricular beats or on the ventricular tachycardia. On several occasions over a 20-minute period, the ventricular tachycardia degenerates into ventricular fibrillation which is easily converted to sinus rhythm with 400 watt-second electrical discharges. Procainamide is therefore administered intravenously in a dose of one gram over a 30-minute period, again without effect on the episodes of ventricular tachycardia and ventricular fibrillation, which are now occurring every ten minutes. Diphenylhydantoin is therefore administered intravenously at a rate of 50 mg/min to a dose of one gram, and results in substantial reduction of ventricular premature beats and disappearance of the episodes of ventricular tachycardia and ventricular fibrillation. About three hours later the salvos of ventricular tachycardia and episodes of ventricular fibrillation recur, and despite administration of additional lidocaine,

procainamide, and diphenylhydantoin, frequent electrical defibril-
lations, closed-chest cardiac massage and adequate respiratory
support, the patient has an episode of ventricular fibrillation from
which she cannot be converted, and she expires.

BIBLIOGRAPHY

Bigger JT, Dresdale RJ, Heissenbuttel RH, Weld FM, Wit AL:
Ventricular arrhythmias in ischemic heart disease: Mechanism,
prevalence, significance, and management. Prog Cardiovasc Dis
19:255, 1977.

Bigger JT: Pharmacologic and clinical control of antiarrhythmic
drugs. Amer J Med 58:479, 1975.

Giardina EV, Bigger JT: Procaine amide against re-entrant ventricular arrhythmias. Circulation 48:959, 1973.

Giardina EV, Heissenbuttel RH, Bigger JT: Intermittent intravenous procaine amide to treat ventricular arrhythmias. Ann Int
Med 78:183, 1973.

Han J: Mechanisms of ventricular arrhythmias associated with
myocardial infarction. Amer J Cardiol 24:800, 1969.

Miller RR, Hilliard G, Lies JE, Massumi RA, Zelis R, et al.:
Hemodynamic effects of procainamide in patients with acute
myocardial infarction and comparison with lidocaine. Amer J
Med 55:161, 1973.

Norris RM, Mercer CJ: Significance of idioventricular rhythms in
acute myocardial infarction. Prog Cardiovasc Dis 16:455, 1974.

Pfeifer HJ, Greenblatt DJ, Koch-Weser J: Clinical use and toxicity of intravenous lidocaine. Amer Heart J 92:168, 1976.

Schumacher RR, Lieberson AD, Childress RH, Williams JF Jr:
Hemodynamic effects of lidocaine in patients with heart disease.
Circulation 37:965, 1968.

Schwartz ML, Webb NC, Covino BG, Finck EM, Haider B: Comparative antiarrhythmic effects of intravenously administered lidocaine and procainamide and orally administered quinidine. Amer
J Cardiol 26:520, 1970.

CASE 18:   Palpitations occurring in a man with heavy alcohol
           beverage consumption.

A 46-year-old man who admits to heavy alcoholic beverage con-
sumption for years comes to the Emergency Room mildly intoxicated, complaining of "palpitations" which he has had intermittently
for several months. There is no history to suggest angina pectoris
or congestive heart failure, and his cardiovascular examination is
normal except for an irregular pulse which is alternately rapid and
slow. The chest x-ray and serum potassium level are normal. The
12-Lead ECG shows mild diffuse nondiagnostic T wave abnormalities. Three continuous Lead II rhythm strips are shown in Fig.
18.1.

1. Which of the following are present in these strips?
    a) sinus rhythm
    b) rhythm of development ("warmup" phenomenon)
    c) atrial premature beats
    d) ventricular premature beats
    e) atrial fibrillation
    f) atrial flutter
    g) multifocal atrial tachycardia
    h) aberrant intraventricular conduction

ANSWER: (a, b, c, e, h) QRS complexes of differing contours and
duration occur at markedly variable cycle length. QRS complexes
occurring at cycle length greater than about 0.50 seconds have normal contour and duration, while those occurring at shorter cycle
length often have abnormal contour and duration. Discrete, normal-appearing P waves probably originating in the sinus node, are
seen in each strip. These P waves which precede by about 0.15
seconds the first, third, and last QRS complexes in the top strip,
the first, second, third, fourth, sixth, and eighth QRS complexes
in the middle strip, and the thirteenth, fourteenth, and fifteenth
QRS complexes in the bottom strip presumably stimulate these QRS
complexes, establishing the presence of sinus rhythm. The second
and fourth QRS complexes in the top strip, the fifth, seventh, and
ninth QRS complexes in the middle strip, and the last QRS complex
in the bottom strip have contours similar to each other but different
from the sinus beats, indicating that the sequence of ventricular
activation is abnormal at these times. These abnormal QRS complexes follow sinus-stimulated QRS complexes whose T waves are
more peaked than the T waves of other sinus beats because they
contain P waves. These P waves, occurring prematurely, encounter delays in AV node-His-Purkinje system conduction such that the
PR interval is longer than in sinus beats (0.22-0.25 seconds vs.
0.15 seconds) and intraventricular conduction is aberrant.

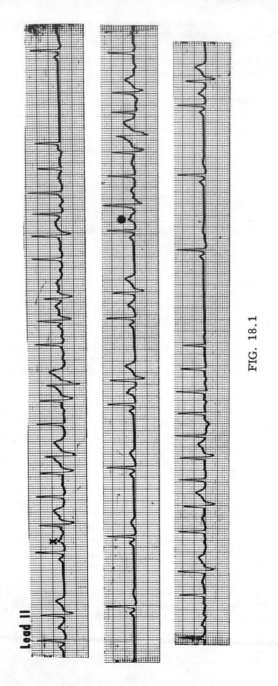

lead II

FIG. 18.1

Following the second atrial premature beat in the top strip (X) the
QRS rhythm becomes rapid and irregularly irregular, and the baseline becomes coarsely irregular for a period of about seven seconds
until, near the end of the top strip, atrial and ventricular activity
cease until a sinus impulse terminates the pause about 1.4 seconds
later. This same course of events follows the third atrial premature beat in the middle strip (●). The irregularly irregular
QRS rhythm and irregular baseline suggest the diagnosis of atrial
fibrillation, which in these strips is transient and self-terminating.
The sinus rhythm which emerges following cessation of these two
brief paroxysms of atrial fibrillation shows gradually shortening
cycle length, or, a rhythm of development ("warmup" phenomenon).

Multifocal atrial tachycardia can often be confused with atrial fibrillation when a rapid ventricular rate precludes accurate analysis of
atrial activity. However, it occurs almost exclusively in patients
critically ill with respiratory failure or heart failure and is associated with rapid rather than slow sinus rates. The absence of
flutter waves in this Lead II rhythm strip excludes the diagnosis
of atrial flutter.

The differential diagnosis of the wider, somewhat bizarre QRS complexes appearing during the paroxysms of atrial fibrillation includes
ventricular ectopic beats and aberrantly conducted fibrillatory impulses. The fact that these wider complexes resemble the aberrantly
conducted atrial premature beats, and invariably occur at cycle
length shorter than the preceding cycle length favor the diagnosis
of aberrantly conducted fibrillatory impulses.

2. How might this patient reasonably be managed at this time?
    a) advise him to stop his alcohol intake
    b) perform DC cardioversion
    c) administration of a quinidine preparation
    d) administration of digoxin
    e) administration of propranolol
    f) administration of atropine

ANSWER: (a) Removal of toxic substances is essential in the management of all cardiac rhythm disturbances, and cessation of alcohol in
gestion might be followed by disappearance of the arrhythmia. Since
in this case the atrial fibrillation spontaneously converts to sinus
rhythm after a period of several seconds, DC cardioversion is not
necessary; rather, prevention of the events which precipitate the
atrial fibrillation is in order. As atrial fibrillation is initiated by
an atrial premature impulse which occurs at very short cycle length
(presumably falling in the atrial vulnerable period) its prevention
requires suppression of atrial premature beats. In this patient, the
atrial premature beats may be the result of the slow sinus rate, thus
reflecting primary sinus node dysfunction rather than primary atrial
irritability. While quinidine preparations are often effective in
suppressing atrial premature beats occurring in the presence of

normal sinus node function, our impression is that they are much
less effective in the setting of abnormal sinus node function.

Atrial premature beats occurring in the setting of sinus bradycardia
can usually be abolished by increasing the sinus rate, and atropine,
administered intravenously, has been documented to do this. However, orally administered parasympatholytic agents usually cause
unpleasant side effects more often than the desired increase in sinus
rate. Administration of digoxin might slow the ventricular rate during atrial fibrillation but would not per se be likely to prevent its
onset. Propranolol, often effective in suppressing atrial premature
beats, might have the opposite effect in this patient if it results in
further slowing of sinus rate.

In patients with normal cardiac function, atrial fibrillation usually
causes no problem so long as the ventricular rate is controlled.
Some patients with paroxysmal atrial fibrillation feel uncomfortable
because of the changes in rhythm rather than the cardiac irregularity occurring during the periods of atrial fibrillation. If sinus rhythm
cannot be maintained in such patients, withdrawing the medication
aimed at sustaining sinus rhythm, allowing atrial fibrillation to
occur, and controlling the ventricular rate with digoxin and/or propranolol might alleviate the symptoms.

The patient is admitted to the hospital where, despite no alcoholic
beverage intake, the paroxysms of atrial fibrillation continue.
Digoxin and quinidine sulfate, administered in doses which achieve
therapeutic serum levels, result in slow sinus rhythm and occasional
atrial premature beats, but not the cessation of the bursts of atrial
fibrillation. When the patient is discharged he is advised to take
digoxin and quinidine, but he discontinues them a few days later.
He is seen on several occasions over the next twenty months, usually
for problems related to alcohol ingestion. Initially, sinus rhythm
with paroxysms of atrial fibrillation identical to that in Fig. 18.1 is
present, but eventually atrial fibrillation with a resting ventricular
rate of about 120/minute becomes established. The patient is advised to take digoxin 0.25 mg daily, but shortly thereafter is lost
to follow-up.

BIBLIOGRAPHY

Goel BG, Han J: Atrial ectopic activity associated with sinus bradycardia. Circulation 42:853, 1970.

Haft JI, Lau SH, Stein E, Kosowsky BD, Damato AN: Atrial fibrillation produced by atrial stimulation. Circulation 37:70, 1968.

Killip T, Gault JH: Mode of onset of atrial fibrillation in man.
Amer Heart J 70:172, 1965.

Marriott HJL, Sandler IA: Criteria, old and new, for differentiating between ectopic ventricular beats and aberrant ventricular conduction in the presence of atrial fibrillation. Prog Cardiovasc Dis 9:18, 1966.

Lamb LE, Pollard LW: Atrial fibrillation in flying personnel. Report of 60 cases. Circulation 29:694, 1964.

Lau SH, Damato AN, Berkowitz MD, Patton RD: A study of atrioventricular conduction in atrial fibrillation and flutter in man using His bundle recordings. Circulation 40:71, 1969.

Bennett MA, Pentecost BL: The pattern of onset and spontaneous cessation of atrial fibrillation in man. Circulation 41:981, 1970.

CASE 19: Elderly woman with recent onset of paroxysmal rapid
         heart action.

A 73-year-old woman comes to her physician for evaluation of episodes of rapid regular heart action that have occurred about once
monthly for the past six months, but have caused the unpleasant
symptom of lightheadedness only within the past week. The episodes,
which occur only when the patient bends forward, begin abruptly and
are associated with a feeling of weakness and discomfort. She then
lies down and waits for the abrupt termination of the rapid heart
action which occurs after about one or two hours, leaving her feeling
fatigued. She has never had ischemic heart pain, syncope, or symptoms of congestive heart failure. The physical examination and
chest x-ray are within normal limits. A 12-Lead electrocardiogram, shown in Fig. 19.1, reveals mostly a bigeminal rhythm in
which sinus beats are followed by atrial premature beats.

1. Reasonable management of this patient at this time might include:
   a) administration of digoxin
   b) administration of quinidine sulfate
   c) administration of propranolol
   d) ambulatory cardiac rhythm monitoring
   e) instruction of the patient in the performance of Valsalva
      maneuver
   f) admission to the hospital for continuous cardiac rhythm
      monitoring

ANSWER: (d, e) While the awareness of rapid regular heart action
that begins and ends abruptly almost certainly represents paroxysmal
supraventricular tachycardia (SVT) in a patient with atrial premature
beats, reasonable management includes documentation and accurate
interpretation of an arrhythmia before potentially dangerous medications such as digoxin, quinidine, and propranolol are administered.
In a patient whose arrhythmia is not associated with serious symptoms such as presyncope, syncope, chest discomfort, or congestive
heart failure, ambulatory cardiac rhythm monitoring using a device
such as the Holter monitor would be recommended, and the patient
would be encouraged to perform those activities during the recording
period which are known to precipitate the episodes of rapid heart
action. She might also be taught how to perform the Valsalva maneuver, and perhaps other vagal maneuvers, so as to observe their
effects on the episode.

A 12-hour Holter monitor recording is performed, during which time
the patient has an episode of rapid heart action which begins when she
bends forward. The episode is unaffected by performance of what
the patient feels are several maximum Valsalva maneuvers. After
about two hours, spontaneous termination of the episode occurs.
Fig. 19.2 displays Lead MCL$_5$ recorded during the episode of tachycardia.

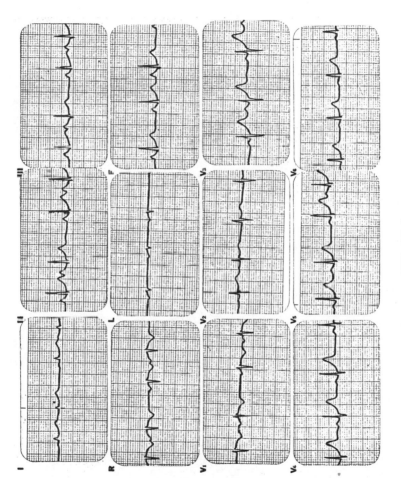

FIG. 19.1

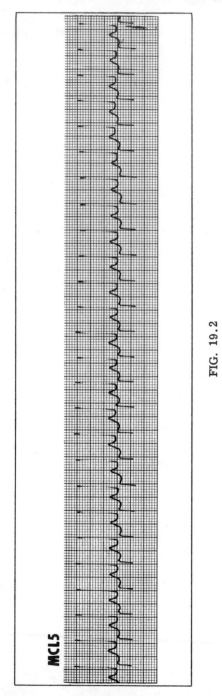

FIG. 19.2

2. What is the rhythm?
   a) atrial fibrillation
   b) atrial flutter with 2:1 AV conduction
   c) ectopic atrial tachycardia
   d) supraventricular tachycardia
   e) ventricular tachycardia

ANSWER: (d) Narrow QRS complexes occur at regular intervals of
about 0.38 seconds (rate about 158/minute). The normal duration
(0.07 seconds) of the QRS complexes essentially excludes the diagnosis of ventricular tachycardia, and the regularity of the rhythm
excludes the diagnosis of atrial fibrillation. While atrial activity
is not unequivocally demonstrable, the small, sharp, upright deflections at the J point (junction of the QRS complex with the ST segment) of almost all QRS complexes suggests that atrial activity has
a fixed temporal relationship to the QRS complexes. The rhythm
could conceivably be atrial flutter with 2:1 AV conduction, with the
alternate flutter waves occurring in the T waves, and the isoelectric T-P segment could be attributed to the MCL$_5$ Lead, in which
the baseline often is isoelectric even in atrial flutter. In view of
the regular narrow QRS complexes occurring at this rate, however,
the most likely rhythm is supraventricular tachycardia (SVT).
Supraventricular tachycardia, which usually occurs in paroxysms,
has until recently been called paroxysmal atrial tachycardia. Electrophysiologic studies in animals and in man indicate that SVT can
be initiated by premature impulses arising in the atrium, the AV
junction, or even in the ventricles; but regardless of the origin of
the initiating beat, ventricular activation during tachycardia occurs
in an antegrade manner via the His-Purkinje system, such that the
QRS rhythm is, in effect, "supraventricular". The mechanism
sustaining SVT in most patients who do not have an accessory AV
conduction pathway is reentry within the AV node, in contrast to
the mechanism of ectopic atrial tachycardia, in which there is rapid
repetitive firing of an ectopic atrial focus.

Fig. 19.3 shows the spontaneous onset (top strip) and termination
(bottom strip) of the two hour paroxysm of SVT. The top strip begins with bigeminal group beating, in which a sinus beat with PR interval of about 0.13 seconds is followed by an atrial premature beat
with PR interval of about 0.17 seconds. The bigeminal rhythm is
interrupted by the eighth P wave (P$_8$), which occurs prematurely and
is conducted to the ventricles with a PR interval of about 0.16 seconds,
and by the ninth P wave (P$_9$), which occurs with even greater prematurity, and is superimposed on the T wave of the preceding QRS
complex. The PR interval following the ninth P wave cannot be
accurately measured, but is certainly greater than 0.16 seconds and
is probably greater than 0.22 seconds. The next P wave (arrow) is
seen in the early portion of the ST segment of the preceding QRS
complex, and is followed by the regular tachycardia at cycle length
of about 0.41 seconds (rate about 146/minute) in which P waves may
be seen to occur at the J point. The increasing PR intervals of the

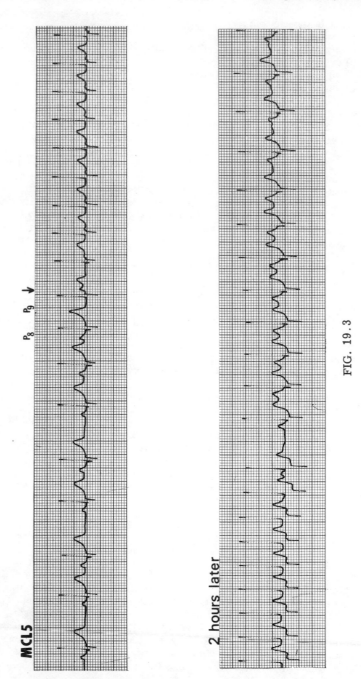

FIG. 19.3

beats preceding the onset of SVT reflect lengthening of AV nodal conduction time in response to shortening of the cycle length of the atrial
rhythm. Although it is not possible from this rhythm strip to be certain which event initiates the SVT, it is clear that an atrial premature
beat must be the inciting factor.

During the tachycardia, the cycle length gradually shortens from
about 0.41 seconds (rate about 146/minute) to about 0.37 seconds
(rate about 162/minute), probably because of the effects of catecholamine stimulation and/or vagolysis occurring in response to adverse
hemodynamic effects of the SVT. Spontaneous termination of the episode of SVT is seen in the lower strip of Fig. 19.3.

3. Termination of the episode of SVT involves interruption of the
    reentry circuit by which of the following?
    a) atrial impulse
    b) premature junctional complex
    c) ectopic ventricular complex
    d) changes in autonomic nervous system traffic

ANSWER: (a) The last QRS complex of the SVT is on time, but is
preceded by a P wave (the origin of which is unclear) at an interval
of about 0.09 seconds, suggesting that the atrial impulse somehow
interrupts the reentry circuit. The very short interval between this
P wave and the final on-time tachycardia QRS complex indicates that
the P wave does not stimulate this QRS complex. It is likely that
this P wave is conducted into the reentry circuit, depolarizing a part
of it such that a returning impulse finds the pathway refractory and
the tachycardia therefore stops. Conduction of the atrial impulse
into the AV node is electrocardiographically silent, and is hypothesized to occur on the basis of subsequent events (the termination of
SVT); it is thus an example of concealed conduction of an impulse
into the AV node.

Following termination of SVT, progressively slowing sinus rhythm
results - but at a rate much more rapid than prior to the SVT, probably because of changes in catecholamine levels and autonomic nervous system traffic induced by the relatively adverse hemodynamic
state during SVT.

Since neither a premature junctional complex nor an ectopic ventricular complex is present in this strip, they are not playing a role
in termination of SVT. And while changes in autonomic nervous
system traffic per se can cause termination of SVT, it would be most
fortuitous for this to have been the mechanism of termination here,
just at the time when an atrial premature beat occurred.

4. Administration of which of the following medications might be
    useful in the management of this patient at this time?
    a) digoxin   d) diphenylhydantoin
    b) quinidine preparation   e) procainamide
    c) propranolol

150/ Case 19   Simple Arrhythmias

ANSWER: (a, b, c, e) Since SVT in this patient is initiated by atrial
premature beats, their suppression should prevent its onset. Quinidine preparations are most likely to achieve suppression of atrial
premature beats, but procainamide and propranolol have also been
reported to be useful in this regard. Should these medications not
completely suppress atrial ectopic activity, they may nevertheless
prevent the development of AV nodal reentry by altering conduction
velocities and refractory periods of AV nodal tissue. Digoxin may
also prevent onset of SVT by altering conduction velocities and refractory periods within the AV node even though it is not likely to
suppress atrial premature beats. Although these medications might
not prevent the onset of SVT, they might facilitate its termination
in response to performance of vagal maneuvers. While diphenylhydantoin has been reported to terminate "atrial tachycardias", careful review of these reports indicates that the effectively treated
rhythms were atrial tachycardias associated with the use of digitalis,
and were not SVT. To our knowledge, the effectiveness of diphenylhydantoin in preventing and terminating SVT is not documented.

The patient is treated with digoxin 0.25 mg every morning, which results in her having fewer episodes of rapid heart action, which now
lasts only seconds to minutes, and can be easily terminated by performing the Valsalva maneuver.

BIBLIOGRAPHY

Bigger JT Jr, Goldreyer BN: The mechanism of supraventricular
tachycardia. Circulation 42:673, 1970.

Denes P, Wu D, Dhingra RC, Chuquimia R, Rosen KM: Demonstration of dual A-V nodal pathways in patients with paroxysmal supraventricular tachycardia. Circulation 48:549, 1973.

Goldreyer BN, Bigger JT Jr: Site of reentry in paroxysmal supraventricular tachycardia in man. Circulation 43:15, 1971.

Goldreyer BN, Bigger JT Jr: Spontaneous and induced reentrant
tachycardia. Ann Int Med 70:87, 1969.

Kastor JA, Goldreyer BN, Moore EN, Spear JF: Reentry - an important mechanism of cardiac arrhythmias. Cardiovasc Clinics
6:111, 1974.

Wu D, Wyndham C, Amat-y-Leon F, Denes P, Dhingra RC, Rosen
KM: The effects of ouabain on induction of atrioventricular nodal
reentrant paroxysmal supraventricular tachycardia. Circulation
52:201, 1975.

Conn RD: Diphenylhydantoin sodium in cardiac arrhythmias. New
Engl J Med 272:277, 1965.

CASE 20: Acute abdominal pain followed by syncope in an elderly
man.

A 72-year-old man with mild chronic stable angina pectoris but no
other cardiovascular symptoms has a routine medical examination,
at which time the physical examination and chest x-ray are normal.
The 12-Lead ECG is shown in Fig. 20.1.

1. Which of the following characterize this tracing?
    a) sinus rhythm
    b) first degree AV block
    c) junctional rhythm
    d) retrograde atrial activation
    e) left anterior fascicle block
    f) atrial fibrillation
    g) atrial flutter with 2:1 AV conduction

ANSWER: (a, b, e) All QRS complexes are narrow and of normal
contour, indicating that ventricular activation occurs via the AV
junction, but the abnormally leftward mean frontal plane QRS axis
of about -60 degrees suggests that intraventricular conduction occurs
with delay (or block) in the anterior fascicle of the left bundle branch.
The QRS rhythm is reasonably regular at intervals of about 0.62 -
0.64 seconds (corresponding rate 94-97/minute). Atrial activity,
identifiable in the ST segments and T waves of all QRS complexes,
occurs in 1:1 temporal relationship to them. The presence of discrete P waves at this rate excludes the diagnoses of atrial fibrillation and atrial flutter. Although accurate assessment of P wave
contour and axis is precluded by the superimposition of P waves on
ST segments and T waves, the atrial deflections appear to be upright
in all Limb Leads except Lead aVR, suggesting that the P wave axis
is normal. In junctional rhythm the P wave axis is almost invariably superior because atrial activation occurs in a retrograde manner. The rhythm is therefore likely to be sinus. The markedly
long PR interval of about 0.51 seconds indicates first degree AV
block.

2. How might this patient be reasonably managed at this time?
    a) reassure him that the conduction disturbance is not likely to
       result in sudden death without premonitoring symptoms
    b) prescribe an oral parasympatholytic agent
    c) warn him about bradycardia-related symptoms, and advise
       him to seek medical assistance if and when they occur
    d) discuss with him the availability of permanent demand ventri-
       cular pacemaker implantation as a way to prevent and to
       treat bradycardia-related symptoms

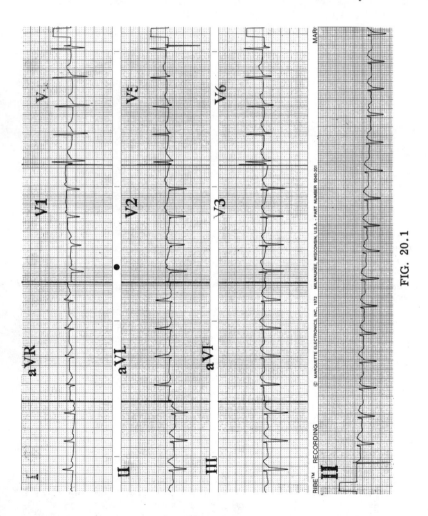

FIG. 20.1

ANSWER: (a, c, d) Although first degree AV block may result from
conduction delay in the atria, AV node, and/or His-Purkinje system, PR interval prolongation to the extent seen here is almost invariably due to abnormally slow conduction within the AV node. It
is usually due to AV nodal dysfunction caused by primary degenerative
disease or to an ischemic process. Since progression of these processes may result in Type I (Wenckebach) second degree or complete
AV block which might produce symptomatic bradycardia, the patient
should be advised to seek medical assistance if and when fatigue,
weakness, presyncope, syncope, symptoms of congestive heart failure, or awareness of cardiac action appear. However, since the
ventricular rate during both Type I (Wenckebach) second degree AV
block and complete AV block due to block in the AV node is usually
not so slow as to result in syncope, it is reasonable to reassure the
patient that his conduction abnormality is not likely to result in unheralded sudden death. He might also be informed that bradycardia-
related symptoms may effectively be prevented by a permanent demand ventricular pacemaker, which can be implanted with negligible
morbidity. Since oral parasympatholytic agents induce unpleasant
side effects much more often than the desired improvement in AV
conduction, it does not seem reasonable to prescribe such medication to an asymptomatic man of this age.

The patient is informed of his conduction disturbance and of the potential problems which might result from it. Permanent ventricular demand pacemaker implantation is offered but the patient declines.
He continues to have no bradycardia-related symptoms and when he
returns for a followup visit two months later the 12-Lead ECG shown
in Fig. 20.2 is recorded.

3. Which of the following rhythms are present in this tracing?
    a) sinus bradycardia with first degree AV block
    b) complete AV block
    c) sinus rhythm with second degree AV block
    d) AV dissociation

ANSWER: (a) The QRS complexes are supraventricular in origin,
and the RR intervals are reasonably constant at 1.20-1.22 seconds
(corresponding rate 49-50/minute). Each QRS complex is preceded
at an interval of about 0.47-0.48 seconds by a normal-appearing P
wave which is probably sinus in origin. The constant 1:1 relationship between atrial and ventricular activity excludes the diagnoses
of AV dissociation and complete AV block, in both of which atrial
and ventricular rhythms occur independently. The absence of non-
conducted P waves excludes the diagnosis of second degree AV
block. The rhythm is therefore sinus bradycardia with first degree AV block, and, except for the slower rate, is unchanged from
the tracing recorded two months earlier.

The patient does well for about ten months until he is awakened one
night with severe abdominal pain followed by diarrhea, a feeling of

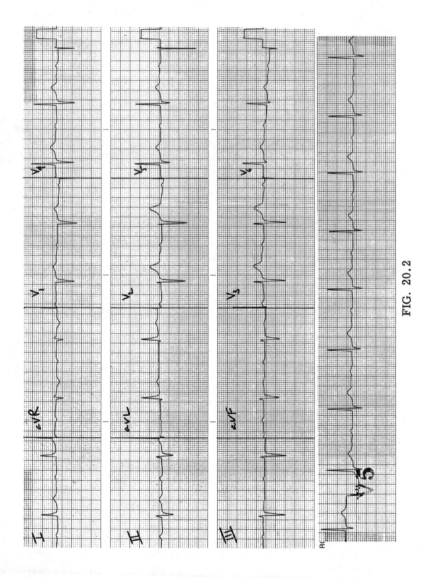

FIG. 20.2

profound weakness, and finally an episode of syncope. When he regains consciousness he feels generally weak and comes to the hospital by ambulance. The patient is somewhat pale, but the physical
examination is otherwise unremarkable. The ECG shown in Fig.
20.3 is then recorded, and during Leads V4 and V5 the patient complains of feeling weak.

4. Which of the following describe the rhythm(s) in Fig. 20.3?
   a) sinus rhythm with first degree AV block
   b) complete AV block
   c) sinus rhythm with second degree (2:1) AV block
   d) AV dissociation

ANSWER: (a, c) The rhythm in the Limb Leads and in Leads V_1-V_3
is sinus at a rate of about 60/minute, with first degree AV block
(PR interval about 0.54 seconds). In Leads V_4 and V_5 normal QRS
complexes occur with reasonable regularity at intervals of about
2.0 seconds (corresponding rate about 30/minute). Each QRS complex is preceded at an interval of about 0.58 seconds by a sinus P
wave which probably stimulates it. The dependence of the ventricular rhythm on the sinus impulse indicates that AV dissociation is
not present, and, since some P waves do stimulate QRS complexes,
complete AV block is not present. Following each T wave, and occurring at half the interval between P waves which stimulates QRS
complexes, are identical P waves which are not conducted to the
ventricles, establishing the diagnosis of 2:1 second degree AV block.

5. The development of 2:1 AV conduction in this patient is likely to
   be due to block in which of the following portions of the AV conduction system?
   a) AV node
   b) His bundle and bundle branches

ANSWER: (a) Second degree AV block may be due to conduction
block within the AV node and/or His bundle and bundle branches,
but in this patient, whose markedly prolonged PR intervals have
suggested severe AV nodal dysfunction during 1:1 AV conduction,
the development of 2:1 AV conduction almost certainly is due to block
within the AV node. The conducted P waves have longer PR intervals during 2:1 AV conduction than during 1:1 AV conduction, further
demonstrating an acute depression of AV nodal conduction.

The Lead II rhythm strips shown in Fig. 20.4 are recorded serially
but not continuously just after Lead V5 of Fig. 20.3, at which time
the patient becomes pale and sweaty, and loses consciousness.

6. Which of the following are present in strips A, B, and C of
   Fig. 20.4?
   a) sinus pauses   d) ventricular premature beat
   b) junctional escape beat   e) junctional premature beat
   c) ventricular escape beat   f) AV dissociation

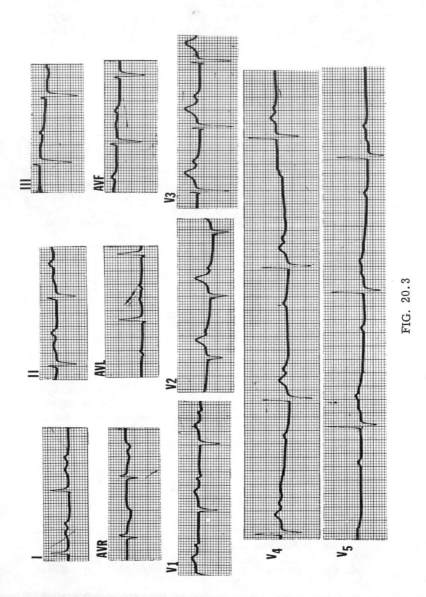

FIG. 20.3

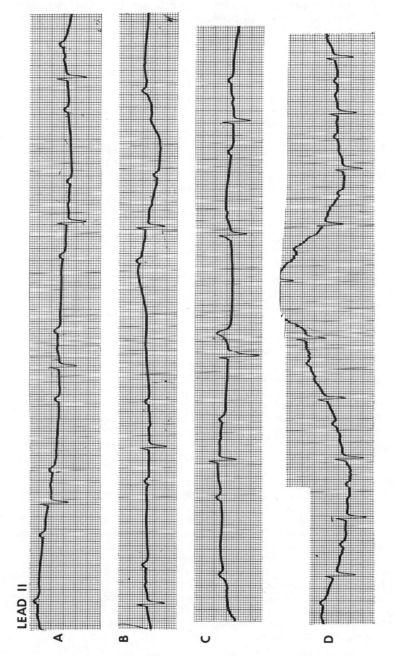

LEAD II

A

B

C

D

FIG. 20. 4

ANSWER: (a, b, c, f) In strip A, all QRS complexes are stimulated
by the P waves which precede them. There is mild irregularity of
the PP intervals, and 2:1 AV conduction is present.

In strip B, the PP intervals are longer than in strip A, and the extremely long PP interval of about 2.4 seconds which occurs in the
middle of the strip qualifies as a sinus pause. Whether a sinus pause
is due to sinoatrial exit block and/or depressed sinus node automaticity cannot be established with certainty in man, and in this
patient the irregularity of the sinus rhythm precludes accurate assessment of the mechanism.

In strip C the second QRS complex is of similar contour but of much
longer duration than the preceding sinus-stimulated QRS complex
(0.14 vs. 0.10 seconds). This wide QRS complex probably originates in the fascicles or the ventricles and, occurring about 1.71
seconds after the preceding QRS complex, is an escape beat. The
initial portion of the third QRS complex is deformed by a superimposed P wave which precedes it by an interval too brief to have
stimulated it; this third QRS complex, otherwise identical to sinus-
stimulated QRS complexes, probably originates in the AV junction
and, terminating a pause in ventricular rhythm of about 2.0 seconds,
is a junctional escape beat. Since at the time of this junctional escape beat the atrial and ventricular rhythms are unrelated, transient
AV dissociation is present. There are no premature beats present
in these strips, in which neither ventricular nor junctional complexes occur earlier than expected.

7. How might this patient be reasonably managed at the time of this
   episode of profound symptomatic bradycardia?
   a) intravenous administration of atropine
   b) subcutaneous administration of adrenalin
   c) intravenous administration of isoproterenol
   d) closed chest cardiac massage

ANSWER: (a, d) This patient's bradycardia is related primarily to
AV nodal block, although the slow sinus rhythm may be a contributing factor. Treatment aimed at improving AV nodal conduction is
therefore in order, and intravenous administration of a parasympatholytic agent such as atropine is likely to be the most rapid,
effective, and safest means of achieving this goal. In the presence
of slow sinus rhythm which suggests vagotonia, atropine will probably also result in an increase in sinus rate. Until the atropine can
be administered, closed chest cardiac massage might ensure adequate cardiac output, and may be performed so long as the patient
remains unconscious. Although the intravenous administration of
isoproterenol and the subcutaneous administration of adrenalin will
enhance AV nodal conduction by their beta-stimulating effects, they
are more difficult to use than atropine because appropriate dosage
cannot be accurately predicted and excessive dosage may cause
serious tachyarrhythmias.

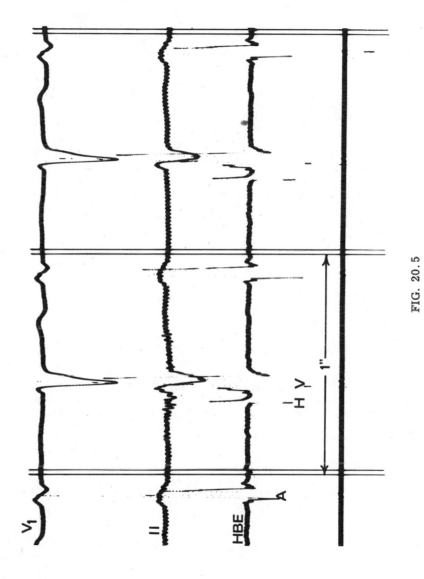

FIG. 20.5

The patient is given atropine, 2 mg intravenously, and within one minute the rhythm shown in Fig. 20.4 D is recorded. It shows sinus arrhythmia at an average rate of about 65/minute, and variably prolonged PR intervals of about 0.40-0.45 seconds. Temporary transvenous pacemaker insertion is recommended to the patient, who accepts the offer. Fig. 20.5 shows surface Leads MCL1 and II, and a His bundle electrogram (HBE) recorded simultaneously during passage of a bipolar electrode pacing catheter into the right ventricle, at a time when the sinus rate is about 58/minute and the PR interval about 0.51 seconds. It indicates markedly prolonged AV nodal conduction (AH) time of 450 msec (normal 70-120 msec) and normal His-Purkinje system conduction (HV) time of 50 msec (normal 35-55 msec). The pacing catheter is then positioned into the right ventricular apex and demand ventricular pacing is instituted. Following several days of pacing, during which time the patient feels well, the underlying ECG remains unchanged, and no enzymatic evidence of acute myocardial necrosis is documented. A permanent ventricular demand pacemaker is then implanted, and over the next ten months the patient feels well and has no symptoms of bradycardia. His ECG on several occasions shows ventricular pacing almost all of the time, but when sinus impulses do stimulate QRS complexes, the PR interval is still markedly prolonged.

BIBLIOGRAPHY

Damato AN, Lau AH, Helfant R, Stein E, Patton RD, Scherlag BJ, Berkowitz WD: A study of heart block in man using His bundle recordings. Circulation 39:297, 1969.

Dreifus LS, Watanabe Y, Haiat R, Kimbiris D: Atrioventricular block. AmerJ Cardiol 28:371, 1971.

Lister JW, Stein E, Kosowsky BD, Lau SH, Damato AN: Atrioventricular conduction in man. Effect of rate, exercise, isoproterenol and atropine on the P-R interval. Amer J Cardiol 16:516, 1965.

Narula OS, Scherlag BJ, Samet P, Javier RP: Atrioventricular block: localization and classification by His bundle recordings. Amer J Med 50:146, 1971.

Narula OS: Current concepts of atrioventricular block. In: His Bundle Electrocardiography and Clinical Electrophysiology. F.A. Davis Company, Philadelphia, 1975.

II. ARRHYTHMIAS OF INTERMEDIATE COMPLEXITY

CASE 21:   Sixty-two-year-old woman with acute inferior wall myocardial infarction.

A 62-year-old woman with past history of hypertension, but no previous symptoms of cardiovascular disease, comes to an Emergency Room with complaints suggesting acute myocardial infarction. She appears seriously ill but the physical examination suggests an adequate hemodynamic state. The 12-Lead ECG recorded shortly after the examination (Fig. 21.1) shows sinus arrhythmia at an average rate of 60/minute, and normal P waves and PR interval. The marked ST segment elevations and tall T waves in Leads II, III, and aVF, and the ST segment depression in Leads I, aVL, V_2 and V_3 indicate acute inferior wall epicardial injury. The patient is admitted to a Coronary Care Unit where she is treated with morphine sulfate and supplemental inspired oxygen. In the initial twenty-four hours of hospitalization the chest discomfort disappears, and the pulse, blood pressure, and physical examination remain normal. Serum enzyme determinations and repeat 12-Lead ECG establish the diagnosis of acute inferior wall myocardial infarction. Thirty hours after admission pauses in QRS rhythm are noted on the monitor, and the Lead II rhythm strip shown in Fig. 21.2 is recorded. The three strips are continuous.

1.   Which of the following describe the rhythm in Fig. 21.2?
   a) sinus arrest
   b) non-conducted atrial premature beat
   c) non-conducted sinus impulse
   d) first degree AV block
   e) Type I (Wenckebach) second degree AV block
   f) Type II second degree AV block
   g) group beating

ANSWER: (c, d, e, g) All QRS complexes are of normal duration, indicating that ventricular activation occurs normally via the AV junction-His-Purkinje system. The 0.04-second and deep Q wave and the T wave inversion reflect the evolving inferior wall myocardial infarction. In the top two strips there is group beating in which QRS complexes occurring at intervals of about 0.81-0.90 seconds are periodically separated by pauses in QRS rhythm of about 1.56-1.60 seconds. All QRS complexes are preceded at intervals of about 0.19-0.29 seconds by P waves which presumably stimulate them. The normal P wave contour indicates that the atrial rhythm is sinus, and the mild irregularity of PP intervals (0.80-0.86 seconds, corresponding rate 70-75/minute) indicates sinus arrhythmia. Since there are neither pauses in sinus rhythm nor premature P waves, neither sinus arrest nor atrial premature beats are present. All QRS complexes are stimulated by P waves, but not

161

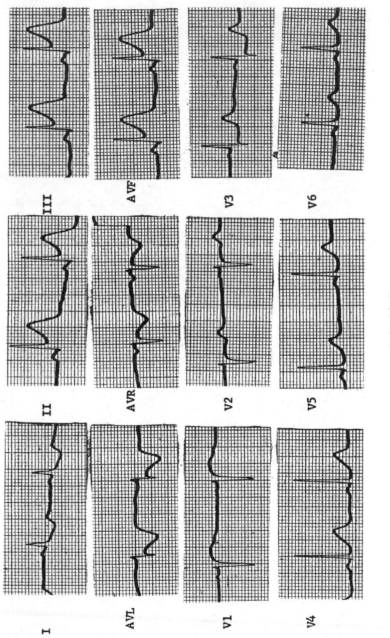

FIG. 21.1

all P waves stimulate QRS complexes, establishing the diagnosis of second degree AV block. The type of second degree AV block can be determined by analyzing the events in the middle strip of Fig. 21.2, as shown in the ladder diagram on page 165.

The strip begins with a sinus P wave that stimulates a QRS complex with prolonged AV conduction time (0.29 seconds), but the next P wave is blocked within the AV conduction system. Since the third, fourth, and fifth P waves are conducted to the ventricles but the sixth P wave is not, there is a period of 4:3 AV conduction. The progressively longer PR intervals (0.19, 0.23, and 0.25 seconds) preceding the non-conducted sinus impulse establish the diagnosis of Type I (Wenckebach) second degree AV block, and exclude the diagnosis of Type II second degree AV block, in which non-conducted sinus impulses occur without preceding prolongation of PR intervals. The successive PR intervals of 0.19, 0.23, and 0.25 seconds, reflecting increments in PR interval of 0.04 and 0.02 seconds, respectively, illustrate a phenomenon that is characteristic of AV Wenckebach periods, namely that the greatest increment in PR interval occurs between the first and second beats of a sequence, with the succeeding increments generally being less. This 4:3 AV Wenckebach period also illustrates the characteristic progressive shortening of RR intervals (from 0.86 to 0.85 seconds). The RR interval of 0.86 seconds is equal to the sum of the intersinus interval of 0.82 seconds and the 0.04 second increment in PR interval; and the subsequent RR interval of 0.85 seconds is equal to the sum of the intersinus interval of 0.83 seconds and the 0.02 second increment in PR interval. Thus, the progressive shortening of RR intervals that characteristically occurs during an AV Wenckebach sequence is due to the progressively smaller increments in PR interval.

The increments in PR interval are also responsible for another characteristic phenomenon of AV Wenckebach periods, namely that the length of the RR interval enclosing the non-conducted P wave is less than the sum of the two sinus cycle lengths enclosing the non-conducted P wave. In this 4:3 AV Wenckebach sequence, the duration of the pause (1.58 seconds) can be calculated as the sum of the two sinus cycle lengths enclosing the non-conducted P wave (1.64 seconds) minus the sum of the increments in PR intervals (0.04 + 0.02 seconds = 0.06 seconds) in the preceding conducted beats of the AV Wenckebach sequence.

Continuing in the middle strip, the seventh through eleventh P waves are conducted to the ventricles with progressively longer PR intervals, but the twelfth P wave is blocked, establishing a period of 6:5 AV conduction. In this 6:5 sequence the successive PR intervals of 0.19, 0.22, 0.24, 0.24, and 0.25 seconds represent progressive increments of 0.03, 0.02, 0.00, and 0.01 seconds in PR interval, and establish an AV Wenckebach period. The increase in PR interval

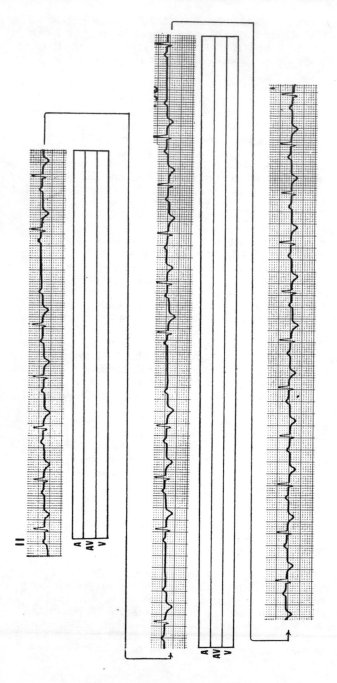

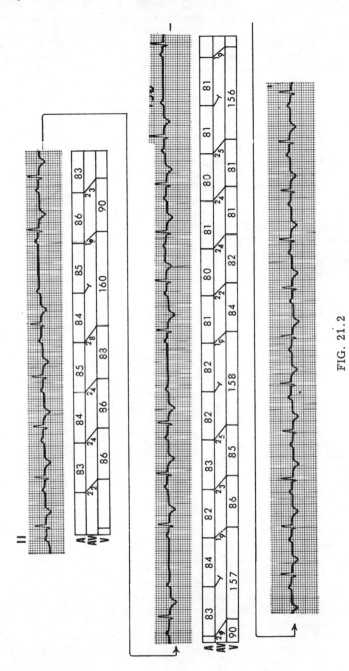

FIG. 21.2

increment in the beat preceding the non-conducted sinus impulse, and the occurrence of identical PR intervals in two successive beats of the AV Wenckebach sequence are phenomena commonly observed when the AV conduction ratio is 5:4 or greater. Nevertheless, in this 6:5 AV Wenckebach sequence as in the 4:3 sequence, the RR intervals can be calculated as the sum of the intersinus interval and the increment in PR interval; and the pause of 1.56 seconds terminating this sequence is about equal to the sum of the sinus cycle lengths during the pause (0.81 + 0.81 = 1.62 seconds) minus the sum of the increments in PR interval in the preceding conducted beats of the AV Wenckebach sequence (0.03 + 0.02 + 0.00 + 0.01 = 0.06 seconds). In the bottom strip AV conduction is consistently 1:1 with prolonged PR intervals of 0.23-0.24 seconds, establishing the presence of first degree AV block.

2. In this patient, the AV Wenckebach periods are most likely due to abnormal conduction within which of the following portion(s) of the AV conduction system?
   a) His bundle
   b) bundle branches
   c) AV node

ANSWER: (c) While AV Wenckebach periods have been reported to occur within the His bundle, and within the bundle branches of the intraventricular conduction system, in the vast majority of patients they occur within the AV node. Thus, AV Wenckebach periodicity may be considered to be an AV nodal phenomenon.

3. With which of the following might this hemodynamically stable patient be reasonably managed at this time?
   a) intravenous isoproterenol administration
   b) intravenous atropine administration
   c) placement of a temporary transvenous right ventricular pacemaker
   d) watchful waiting

ANSWER: (c, d) AV conduction disturbances occur commonly in the setting of acute inferior wall myocardial infarction, and are almost invariably due to ischemia within the AV node, presumably because the artery to the AV node arises from the same coronary arteries which supply the inferior wall of the heart. In some patients the disturbance in AV conduction will be limited to prolongation of the PR interval, but in others Type I second degree AV block or complete AV block may occur. Almost invariably, second degree AV block is preceded by the development of first degree AV block, and complete AV block by periods of second degree AV block. While occasionally the progression from normal AV conduction to complete AV block occurs over a period of just a few minutes, more commonly it evolves over a period of many minutes to hours. So, it is reasonable to simply observe this patient carefully at this time. So long as the sinus rate remains adequate and AV conduction remains 3:2 or greater (e.g., 4:3, 5:4, etc.) it is unlikely that hemodynamic

deterioration will be caused by the rhythm disturbance itself. However, if AV conduction changes to a 2:1 ratio or to complete AV
block, the resulting ventricular rate may be too slow to maintain
an adequate hemodynamic state. If either of these occur, atropine
and/or isoproterenol may be administered intravenously in an
attempt to increase ventricular rate by enhancing AV conduction
and/or by increasing the rate of an escape pacemaker, which would
probably arise in the AV junction (His bundle). However, the potential side effects of parasympatholysis (dry mouth, blurred vision,
urinary retention) and beta-adrenergic stimulation (ventricular
arrhythmias, anxiety) probably do not warrant use of these agents
at this time when the hemodynamic state of the patient is adequate.
Temporary transvenous right ventricular pacing is the most reliable means of preventing bradycardia in this setting, but considera-
tions for its placement at this time include patient acceptability,
the facility with which it can be done on an elective basis, the ease
with which it can be performed in an emergency setting, and the
potential of a transvenous pacemaker to mechanically induce ventricular arrhythmias.

No specific treatment is given, and the patient continues to have AV
Wenckebach periods intermittently for a period of about forty-eight
hours, until consistent 1:1 AV conduction with mildly prolonged PR
interval of about 0.21 seconds occurs. When she is transferred
from the Coronary Care Unit six days after the onset of symptoms
of the inferior wall myocardial infarction, her rhythm is sinus with
1:1 AV conduction and normal PR interval. After tolerating progressive increases in activity without difficulty, the patient is discharged from the hospital on the twentieth post-infarction day. When
last seen three months after the infarction she is feeling well, and
her rhythm and PR intervals are normal.

BIBLIOGRAPHY

Dreifus LS, Watanabe Y, Haiat R, Kimbiris D: Atrioventricular
block. Amer J Cardiol 28:371, 1971.

Narula OS, Samet P: Wenckebach and Mobitz Type II A-V blocks
due to lesions within the His bundle and bundle branches.   Circulation 42:925, 1070.

Langendorf R, Cohen H, Gozo EG: Observations on second degree
atrioventricular block, including new criteria for the differential
diagnosis between type I and type II block. Amer J Cardiol 29:111,
1972.

Narula OS: Wenckebach type I and type II atrioventricular block (revisited). Cardiovasc Clinics 6:137, 1974.

Biddle TL, Ehrich DA, Yu PN, Hodges M: Relation of heart block
and left ventricular dysfunction in acute myocardial infarction.
Amer J Cardiol 39:961, 1977.

Mullins CB, Atkins JM: Prognosis and management of ventricular conduction blocks in acute myocardial infarction. Mod Concepts Cardiovasc Dis 45:129, 1976.

Rosen KM, Loeb HS, Chuquimia R, Sinno MZ, Rahimtoola SH, Gunnar RM: Site of heart block in acute myocardial infarction. Circulation 42:925, 1970.

Katz LN, Pick A: Electrocardiography. Part I. The Arrhythmias. Lea and Febiger, Philadelphia, pp. 526-654, 1956.

CASE 22: Bradycardia in a patient taking digoxin.

A 79-year-old man has an eight year history of atrial fibrillation.
In spite of the fact that he takes no medication, his resting ventricular rate is about 90/minute. During an annual visit to a clinic
where different physicians have seen him on each occasion, he
reports infrequent episodes of mild angina pectoris, no symptoms
of congestive heart failure, and no awareness of cardiac action.
His 12-Lead ECG, which is unchanged from tracings dating back
eight years (Fig. 22.1) shows atrial fibrillation with a ventricular
rate of about 80/minute, right bundle branch block pattern with
associated ST and T wave abnormalities, and non-diagnostic ST
and T wave abnormalities in the inferior leads. Although the patient is feeling well, and the cardiovascular examination is unremarkable except for the atrial fibrillation, digoxin 0.25 mg orally
daily, is prescribed. When he returns for a followup examination
two months later, his pulse is regular at a rate of about 40 beats
per minute, and the 12-Lead ECG shown in Fig. 22.2 is recorded.

1. Which of the following describe the rhythm?
    a) atrial fibrillation
    b) atrial arrest
    c) sinoventricular conduction
    d) complete AV block
    e) junctional rhythm
    f) fascicular or ventricular rhythm
    g) escape rhythm

ANSWER: (a, d, f, g) The irregular baseline, best seen in Lead V1,
suggests that the atrial rhythm is fibrillation, and the discernible
atrial activity excludes atrial arrest and sinoventricular conduction.
The regular QRS rhythm in the presence of atrial fibrillation suggests
that there is complete AV block, with a QRS rhythm that is independent of atrial activity. The slow QRS rhythm in the presence of
complete AV block qualifies as an escape rhythm. The LBBB configuration of the QRS complexes suggests that ventricular activation
occurs via the right bundle branch. The origin of the QRS rhythm
could be either in the right bundle branch itself (fascicular rhythm)
or in the His bundle (junctional rhythm). Since the patient's previous electrocardiograms have shown a RBBB pattern, impulses
arising in the bundle of His would not be expected to be conducted
via the right bundle branch unless the conduction delay in the right
bundle branch were tachycardia-dependent; in addition, since the
left bundle branch, which previously conducted atrial fibrillatory
impulses, is apparently not conducting at this time, simultaneous
bradycardia-dependent conduction delay in the left bundle branch
would have to be present. This combination of circumstances must
be extremely unlikely. The more likely possibility is that the QRS
rhythm originates in the right bundle branch. Since the right bundle

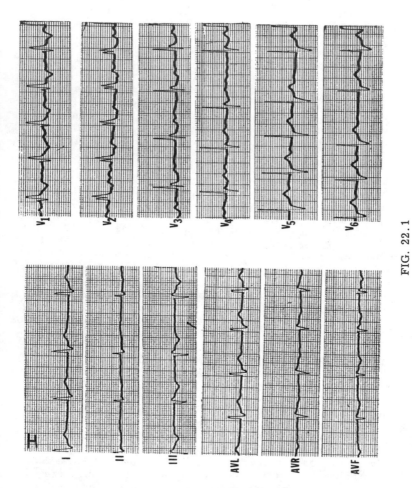

FIG. 22.1

branch has not shown the ability to conduct impulses over the previous eight years and now appears to be generating impulses, the area of impulse formation must lie distal to the area of conduction block. The origin of the QRS rhythm in the right bundle branch indicates that automaticity of the right bundle branch is greater than that of the His bundle. While the reason for this is not clear, it is possible that junctional automaticity is depressed by virtue of concealed discharge of a junctional pacemaker by fibrillatory impulses that reach but are not conducted through the His bundle.

2. Where is the most likely site of AV block in this patient?
   a) AV node
   b) left bundle branch
   c) bundle of His

ANSWER: (a) Since this patient has had evidence of abnormally depressed AV nodal function (demonstrated by the ventricular response of 90/minute in the absence of digoxin or propranolol therapy) and is now receiving digoxin which itself slows AV nodal conduction but has little effect on His bundle or bundle branch conduction, the AV node is the most likely area of block. It might be possible to identify the site of complete AV block by the response of the QRS rhythm to maneuvers and/or medications which alter AV nodal function. Atropine, beta-adrenergic stimulating agents, and the performance of muscular activity facilitate AV nodal conduction, often to the point where complete block in the AV node is overcome. In this patient, isometric handgrip is performed and the three continuous Lead I rhythm strips shown in Fig. 22.3 recorded. In the top strip, QRS complexes with LBBB pattern occur at regular intervals of 1.52 seconds (rate about 40/minute), as in Fig. 22.2. At the arrow, the patient performs the handgrip maneuver, which he maintains for about 15 seconds. During the maneuver, and for the first few seconds following it, all QRS complexes but the fifth have a RBBB pattern. Their occurrence at varying cycle lengths ranging from 0.98 to 1.44 seconds suggests that these RBBB complexes are stimulated by the atrial fibrillatory impulses. Shortly after release of handgrip (bottom strip), the LBBB complexes reappear at their previous cycle lengths. Isometric handgrip, probably both by vagal withdrawal and by sympathetic input has caused transient disappearance of the high-grade AV block. Since conduction block occurring in the bundle of His or the bundle branches would not be expected to decrease during the performance of muscular activity, it is most likely that the AV node is the site of conduction block.

3. Reasonable management of this rhythm disturbance might include:
   a) withholding digoxin and measuring serum digoxin level
   b) temporary right ventricular pacing
   c) intravenous atropine administration
   d) intravenous isoproterenol administration

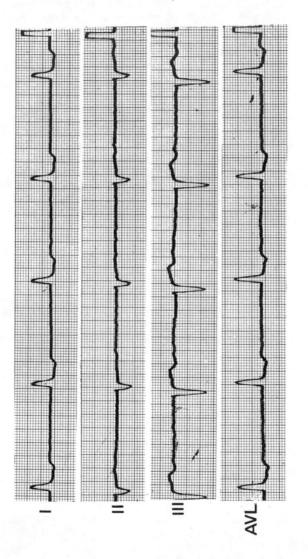

I

II

III

AVL

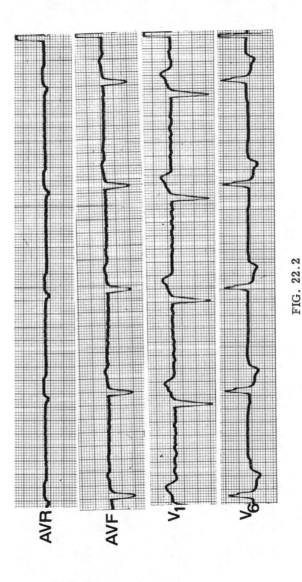

FIG. 22.2

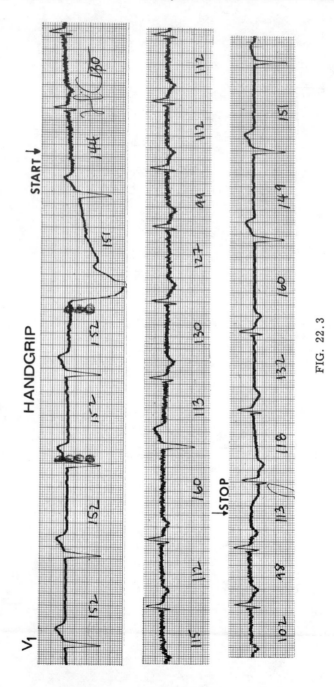

FIG. 22.3

ANSWER: (a, b, c, d) Complete AV block occurring in the presence of atrial fibrillation in a patient receiving digoxin must be attributed to the digoxin until proved otherwise. Withholding digoxin is therefore essential, and measuring serum digoxin level may help assess the sensitivity of the patient's AV node to digoxin. Since the handgrip maneuver has demonstrated that changing autonomic nervous system traffic results in return of conduction through the AV node, it is likely that atropine and isoproterenol administration would be effective in overcoming the AV block, should it become necessary to do so. Pacing from the right ventricle could also be used to increase ventricular rate, but in this stable patient without bradycardia-related tachyarrhythmias it is probably not necessary.

Digoxin is withheld and the patient's cardiac rhythm is monitored. The serum digoxin level on admission is mildly elevated at 2.4 ng/ml. Over the next 48 hours, lessening of AV block is documented by the appearance of more QRS complexes of RBBB pattern, and fewer episodes of LBBB complex escape rhythm; the rate of the escape rhythm has increased from about 40 to about 44/minute. At times, QRS complexes with a normal QRS configuration and duration are observed (Fig. 22.4).

4. How can the appearance of normal QRS complexes be explained in this patient with established RBBB?
   a) supernormal AV conduction
   b) supernormal IV conduction
   c) fusion complex due to depolarization of the ventricles by
      fibrillatory impulses conducted via the left bundle branch
      and ectopic impulses conducted via the right bundle branch

ANSWER: (c) Three QRS complexes with LBBB pattern are followed by a normal-appearing QRS complex occurring at a coupling interval of about 1.35 seconds, about 0.02 seconds before the next RBB ectopic impulse is expected to result in ventricular activation. The fifth QRS complex, having a RBBB pattern and occurring at a much shorter cycle length, is stimulated by fibrillatory impulses. Since the initial 0.02-0.03 vectors of the normal QRS complex are identical to those of the RBBB complex, it is likely that the initial portion of the normal QRS complex is attributable to ventricular activation via the left bundle branch. Since ventricular activation by impulses originating in the right bundle branch would be expected to commence about 0.02 seconds after the initial forces of the normal complex have been inscribed, there would be a normal sequence of ventricular activation via both bundle branches, resulting in a normal QRS complex.

Supernormal conduction of impulses is said to exist when an impulse is conducted more rapidly than expected on the basis of prior electrocardiographic events. Experimentally, periods of supernormal AV or IV conduction occur in early and temporally very limited periods of ventricular repolarization. Most clinical examples have been

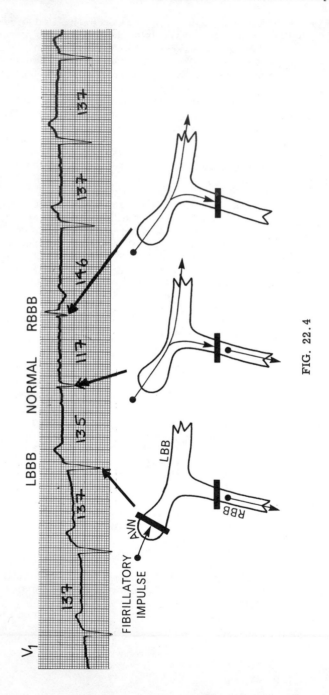

FIG. 22.4

observed in settings of depressed AV or IV conduction. However, the existence of supernormal conduction in humans is still controversial, and most examples can be explained by other more clearly documented mechanisms, such as phase 4 diastolic depolarization, "gap" phenomena, and fusion beats.

Over the next four days, as the serum digoxin level falls, the RBBB complexes continue to occur at irregular but progressively shorter intervals until, when the serum digoxin level is 1.4 ng/ml, no LBBB complexes are present. At this time the ventricular rate is about 60/minute and the patient is discharged from the hospital on no digoxin. When last seen 14 months later his rhythm is atrial fibrillation with RBBB complexes at a rate of about 85/minute at rest.

BIBLIOGRAPHY

Akhtar M, Damato AN, Caracta AR, Batsford WP, Josephson ME, Lau SH: Electrophysiologic effects of atropine on atrioventricular conduction studied by His bundle electrogram. Amer J Cardiol 33:333, 1974.

Dinari G, Aygen MM: Sinoventricular conduction. New Engl J Med 289:1238, 1973.

Fisch C, Greenspan K, Knoebel SB, Feigenbaum H: Effects of digitalis on conduction of the heart. Prog Cardiovasc Dis 6:343, 1964.

Ingelfinger JA, Goldman P: The serum digitalis concentration - Does it diagnose digitalis toxicity? New Engl J Med 294:867, 1976.

Kastor JA, Yurchak PM: Recognition of digitalis intoxication in the presence of atrial fibrillation. Ann Int Med 67:1045, 1967.

Macdonald HR, Sapru RP, Taylor SH, Donald KW: Effect of intravenous propranolol on the systemic circulatory response to sustained handgrip. Amer J Cardiol 18:333, 1966.

Smith TW: The clinical use of serum cardiac glycoside concentration measurements. Amer Heart J 82:833, 1971.

Massumi RA: Bradycardia-dependent bundle branch block. A critique and proposed criteria. Circulation 38:1066, 1968.

Rosenbaum MB, Elizari MV, Lazzari JO, Halpern MS, Nau GJ, Levi RJ: The mechanism of intermittent bundle branch block: relationship to prolonged recovery, hypopolarization and spontaneous diastolic depolarization. Chest 63:666, 1973.

CASE 23: DC cardioversion of atrial flutter in a woman with mitral stenosis.

A 48-year-old woman with mitral stenosis and slow atrial flutter undergoes DC cardioversion with 20 watt-seconds at a time when she is taking digoxin, quinidine sulfate, and propranolol. The continuous tracing of Lead II is shown in Fig. 23.1, on pp. 180, 181.

1. What is the ventricular rhythm which emerges immediately after the cardioversion (middle strip)?
    a) junctional (His bundle)
    b) idioventricular

ANSWER: (a) Following the 20 watt-second electrical discharge the electrocardiographic stylus requires about 7.6 seconds to be able to respond properly. The first visible post-cardioversion beat as well as all subsequent QRS complexes appear to have a configuration similar to those occurring during the atrial flutter. All the QRS complexes, both pre- and post-cardioversion, are therefore probably conducted through the same His-Purkinje system axis. The first five QRS complexes in the middle strip are not preceded by P waves, suggesting that the early post-cardioversion QRS rhythm is a junctional rhythm. The gradually shortening RR intervals demonstrate the "warmup" phenomenon of an emerging, or escaping, pacemaker.

2. What is the atrial rhythm which emerges immediately after the cardioversion (middle strip)?
    a) sinus
    b) ectopic atrial
    c) stimulated in retrograde manner from the AV junction

ANSWER: (a) Atrial activity after cardioversion is first identifiable in the ST segment of the first QRS complex in the middle strip. The P waves are upright in this Lead II, suggesting that they are of sinus origin. They move closer and closer into the QRS complexes, eventually merging into the fifth QRS complex. The subsequent P waves precede the QRS complexes by variable PR intervals until a stable PR interval of 0.22 seconds is achieved beginning with the second beat of the bottom strip. The remaining beats have constant PR intervals, suggesting that sinus impulses are capturing the ventricles. Accurate measurement demonstrates a "warmup" phenomenon in the sinus node, with gradual shortening of the PP intervals from the time of their first appearance (PP = 1.04 sec) to the time of stability of the PP interval at a cycle length of about 0.93 seconds.

3. What are the relationships between the P waves and the QRS complexes in the middle strip? In the bottom strip?
    a) related in a 1:1 fashion, with antegrade conduction

b) related in a 1:1 fashion, with retrograde conduction
c) completely unrelated (dissociated)
d) initially related, then unrelated (dissociated)
e) initially unrelated (dissociated), then related

ANSWER: (c) middle strip; (e) bottom strip. Sinus rhythm with 1:1 AV conduction is achieved in the second beat of the bottom strip. Prior to this, the atrial rhythm is sinus and the ventricular rhythm is junctional; but, as atrial and ventricular rhythms are independent, atrioventricular dissociation is present. AV dissociation in this case can be attributed to independent emergence of atrial (sinus) and ventricular (junctional) rhythms with the junctional pacemaker emerging first. Although the sinus rate actually exceeds the junctional rate slightly at all times, conduction from the atria through to the ventricles can occur only when the P wave precedes the QRS complex by about 0.22 seconds, which in this case does not take place until about 17.4 seconds have elapsed after the electrical discharge. Up to this point, dissocation between atria and ventricles results from a lack of opportunity of the sinus impulse to conduct into ventricular tissue which has already been depolarized by the junctional impulse.

The emergence of independent atrial and ventricular rhythms, resulting in transient AV dissociation due to lack of opportunity for ventricular capture, is a fairly common occurrence after DC cardioversion of atrial arrhythmias.

BIBLIOGRAPHY

Chung EK: Principles of Cardiac Arrhythmias. The Williams & Wilkins Co., Baltimore, pp. 176-242, 1971.

Marriott HJL, Menendez MM: A-V dissociation revisited. Prog Cardiovasc Dis 8:522, 1966.

Miller R, Sharrett RH: Interference dissociation. Circulation 16:803, 1957.

Scherf D, Cohen J: Atrioventricular rhythms. Prog Cardiovasc Dis 8:499, 1966.

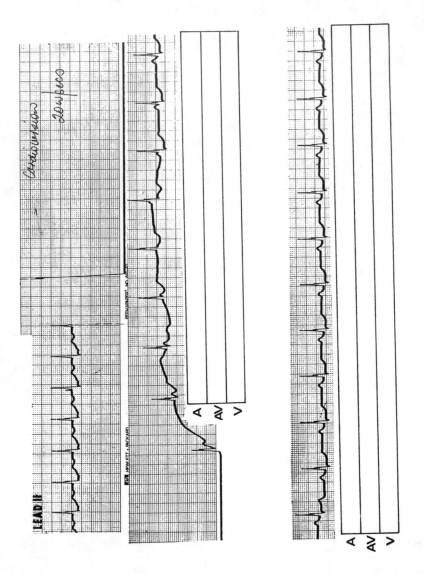

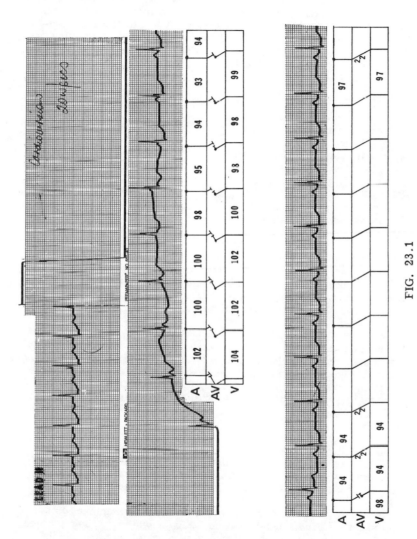

FIG. 23.1

CASE 24: Premature normal-appearing QRS complexes in a patient
with right bundle branch block.

An 80-year-old man with no symptoms of coronary artery disease
is admitted to the hospital for treatment of congestive heart failure.
Physical examination suggests moderately reduced cardiac output,
moderately elevated left- and right-sided filling pressures, generalized cardiomegaly, and no valvular dysfunction. The pulse is
72/minute and somewhat irregular. The blood pressure is 110/88
in the sitting position. The 12-Lead ECG recorded on admission
is shown in Fig. 24.1.

1. What patterns of intraventricular conduction are seen in this
   tracing?
   a) right bundle branch block
   b) left bundle branch block
   c) left anterior fascicle block
   d) left posterior fascicle block

ANSWER: (a, b, c) Most of the QRS complexes preceded by P waves
at a PR interval of about 0.15 seconds are sinus beats conducted
with right bundle branch block, and left axis deviation presumably
due to left anterior fascicle block. The wide QRS complexes not preceded by P waves have a left bundle branch block pattern suggesting
that they are stimulated by impulses arising in the right bundle branch.
Two consecutive sinus beats are seen only in Lead aVF, where the
estimated intersinus interval is about 0.86 seconds; PP intervals in
other Leads range from about 1.70 to 1.90 seconds, suggesting that
the atrial rhythm is sinus arrhythmia with intersinus intervals of
about 0.85-0.95 seconds.

The coupling intervals of the left bundle branch block complexes to
preceding sinus-stimulated QRS complexes range from 0.52 to 0.78
seconds, and the intervals between these complexes (seen in Leads
III, aVL, and V_1) are identical at 1.58 seconds. These features
raise the possibility that the left bundle branch block beats are parasystolic. To confirm this possibility, the continuous Lead V_1 rhythm
strip shown in Fig. 24.2 is recorded.

In Fig. 24.2, the interectopic intervals are all multiples of about
1.47-1.52 seconds, and the coupling intervals to sinus-stimulated
QRS complexes vary between 0.55 and 0.90 seconds. The left bundle branch block rhythm is therefore parasystolic.

2. How can the normal-appearing, narrow QRS complexes in the
   top strip (fifth beat) and bottom strip (seventh beat) be explained?
   a) sinus beats with intermittent supernormal intraventricular
      conduction

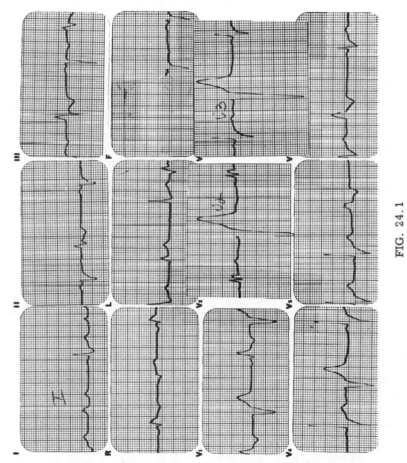

FIG. 24.1

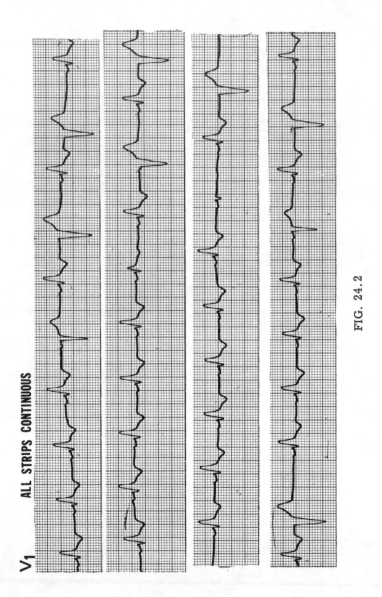

ALL STRIPS CONTINUOUS

V_1

FIG. 24.2

b) sinus beats showing that the right bundle branch block is rate-
dependent

c) fusion beats in which the ventricles are activated by both sinus
and parasystolic impulses

ANSWER: (c) These normal-appearing QRS complexes indicate that
at times the ventricles are activated normally, as occurs if the activating impulses arrive via the right and left bundle branches with
normal temporal relationships (i.e., activation via the right bundle
branch following activation via the left bundle branch by about 0.03-
0.04 seconds). If, fortuitously, the parasystolic impulse arising
in the right bundle branch activates ventricular tissue 0.03-0.04
seconds after the sinus impulse has been conducted via the left bundle branch, the QRS complex would be of normal duration and configuration. Since the intervals between the narrow QRS complexes
and the left bundle branch block complexes which follow them are
1.53 and 1.54 seconds, respectively, and the estimated cycle length
of the parasystolic focus is about 1.47-1.52 seconds (average 1.50
seconds), a parasystolic impulse would be expected to have activated
ventricular tissue shortly (0.03-0.04 seconds) after the sinus impulse had initiated ventricular activation via the left bundle branch
system.

The sixth QRS complex in the second strip, and the seventh QRS complex in the third strip have rSR' and rSr' patterns, respectively, but
their durations (0.12 seconds and 0.08 seconds) are shorter than
those of other sinus beats conducted with right bundle branch block
pattern (0.16 seconds). This suggests that both the sinus impulse
conducted via the left bundle branch and the parasystolic impulse
originating in the right bundle branch contribute to the configuration
and duration of these two QRS complexes. These two QRS complexes
are not of perfectly normal contour because the sinus impulse traveling down the left bundle branch excites part of the ventricles normally activated by the right bundle branch before the parasystolic
impulse can reach and activate the area. Greater degrees of right
bundle branch block pattern indicate greater delay in the time interval between activation of the ventricles by the sinus impulse and by
the parasystolic impulse.

A noteworthy observation in these tracings is that the parasystolic
impulses appear to arise in tissue which is apparently unable to conduct a sinus impulse. For this to occur, the site of impulse formation in the right bundle branch must be distal to the site of conduction
block.

Rate-dependent right bundle branch block as an explanation for the
narrow QRS complexes here is excluded by the finding that sinus
beats following pauses much longer than those terminated by the
narrow QRS complexes are conducted with the same right bundle
branch block pattern (e.g., the third QRS complex in the bottom
strip).

Supernormal conduction is said to occur when an impulse is conducted more rapidly than expected on the basis of prior electrocardiographic events. Experimentally, supernormal intraventricular conduction occurs in an early and temporally very limited period of repolarization. Most clinical examples have been observed in settings of depressed AV or IV conduction. However, the existence of supernormal AV or IV conduction in humans is still controversial, and most examples can be explained by other, more clearly documented mechanisms (fusion beats, "gap" phenomena, phase 4 diastolic depolarization). In this case, normal intraventricular conduction occurs only very late in diastole, much later than the expected supernormal period of the preceding QRS complexes.

BIBLIOGRAPHY

Contro S, Magri G, Natali G: Premature beats overcoming impaired intraventricular conduction. Amer Heart J 5:378, 1956.

Damato AN, Lau SH: Concealed and supernormal atrioventricular conduction. Circulation 43:967, 1971.

Moe GK, Childers RW, Merideth J: An appraisal of supernormal A-V conduction. Circulation 38:5, 1968.

Pick A, Langendorf R, Katz LN: The supernormal phase of atrioventricular conduction. Circulation 26:388, 1962.

Schamroth L, Lewis CM: Normalization of a bundle branch block pattern in early beats. J Electrocardiol 4:199, 1971.

Wit AL, Damato AN, Weiss MB, Steiner C: Phenomenon of gap in atrioventricular conduction in the human heart. Circulation Res 27:679, 1970.

CASE 25: Sudden unexpected death in a seventeen-year-old.

A 17-year-old healthy student, informed two days earlier by her
physician that she is pregnant, suddenly collapses and loses consciousness while talking with her boyfriend. After calling an ambulance he begins cardiopulmonary resuscitation. When the ambulance
arrives her cardiac rhythm is documented to be ventricular fibrillation (Fig. 25.1A). Sinus rhythm is restored by DC defibrillation
and although her pulse and blood pressure become normal within
seconds, she remains in coma. The 12-Lead ECG shown in Fig.
25.1B is recorded on admission to the hospital.

1. Which of the following describe the ECG?
    a) slow sinus arrhythmia
    b) normal for a girl this age
    c) prolonged QT interval
    d) accelerated atrioventricular conduction
    e) junctional rhythm

ANSWER: (a, c, d) All QRS complexes are narrow and of normal
contour, indicating that ventricular activation occurs normally via
the AV junction-His-Purkinje system. The QRS complexes are preceded by normal-appearing P waves which, occurring with mild
irregularity at a rate of about 45/minute, indicate that the atrial
rhythm is slow sinus arrhythmia. The short PR intervals of about
0.11-0.12 seconds indicate accelerated (i.e., unusually rapid) atrioventricular conduction which, in the presence of normal QRS complexes, might occur if the AV node were anatomically short, or if it
conducted impulses more rapidly than usual, or if there were a
rapidly conducting accessory pathway from the atrium to the AV
junction. The QT interval is markedly prolonged at about 0.59-0.64
seconds (expected QT interval at this heart rate in the range of about
0.50 seconds).

Although the PR interval is short, the normal P wave contour would
be most unusual in junctional rhythm. Slow sinus arrhythmia may
occur in healthy young people, but the markedly prolonged QT interval makes this ECG abnormal.

2. Is the prolonged QT interval likely to be of clinical significance
    in this patient?
    a) yes
    b) no

ANSWER: (a) The occurrence of syncopal episodes in association
with a prolonged QT interval constitutes a well-defined syndrome
in which sudden unexpected death occurs commonly. The syncopal
attacks are due to paroxysms of spontaneously terminating ventricular tachycardia, and sudden unexpected death is presumably due to

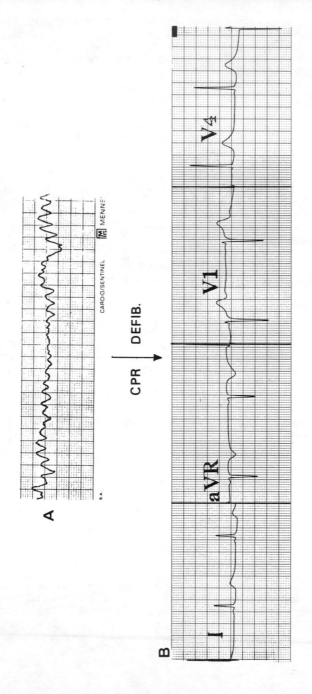

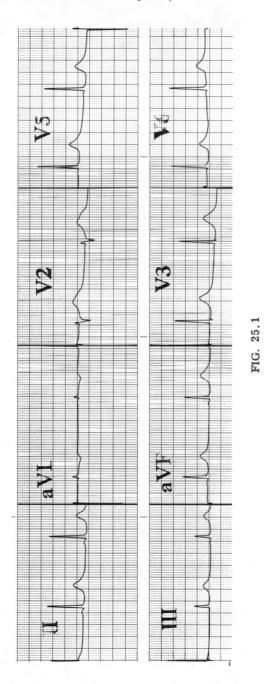

FIG. 25.1

sustained ventricular tachycardia and/or ventricular fibrillation.
These episodes usually occur at times of physical or emotional
stress; in this young woman the pregnancy may have conceivably
constituted such a stress. Occasionally, this syndrome occurs in
families, and it is noteworthy that this patient's mother died suddenly at age 31, after having visited an emergency room on two
occasions in the two years preceding her death with complaints of
"palpitations". Some patients with this syndrome have syncopal
attacks daily while others may have only one or two episodes in a
lifetime. Since the QT interval probably represents the time required for repolarization of Purkinje fibers, prolongation of this
interval suggests abnormally slow repolarization, which is known
to predispose to ventricular arrhythmias. The ventricular tachycardia and ventricular fibrillation in these patients occur when a
ventricular premature beat falls late in diastole near the downslope
or end of the T wave, rather than near the peak of the T wave. The
cause of the long QT interval in these patients is currently ascribed
to relative or absolute increase in sympathetic traffic from the left
stellate ganglion into the ventricles.

3. Is the short PR interval likely to be of clinical significance in
   this patient?
   a) yes
   b) no

ANSWER: (b) A short PR interval may be of clinical significance if
it is associated with a delta wave and a wide QRS complex attributable to ventricular activation occurring partially via an accessory
AV pathway which terminates in ventricular myocardium. Such
anomalous or accessory AV conduction pathways may, by virtue of
their short refractory periods and rapid conduction velocities, be
able to transmit atrial impulses at such rapid rates that syncope due
to fast ventricular rhythms may occur. While patients with short
PR interval and normal-appearing QRS complexes may develop atrial
arrhythmias, most commonly paroxysmal supraventricular tachycardia, these rhythms have to our knowledge neither degenerated
into ventricular tachycardia or fibrillation nor been so rapid as to
result in syncope or sudden death.

4. Administration of which of the following medications might increase the predisposition to ventricular arrhythmias in this
   patient?
   a) quinidine preparations
   b) digoxin
   c) diphenylhydantoin

ANSWER: (a) Administration of a quinidine preparation should be
avoided in the setting of prolonged QT interval, as quinidine itself
generally lengthens this interval and thus might facilitate the appearance of ventricular arrhythmias. In fact, in patients without the
long QT interval syndrome, administration of quinidine preparation

has been documented to result in syncope and sudden death due to paroxysms of ventricular tachycardia and ventricular fibrillation. Since digoxin and diphenylhydantoin may shorten the QT interval, their administration would not be expected to increase the predisposition to ventricular arrhythmias.

The patient is monitored in the Coronary Care Unit. Over the next several days she regains consciousness, and her physical and mental function return to normal. A typical rhythm strip during this period is shown in Fig. 25.2.

5. Which of the following terms describe the rhythm in Fig. 25.2?
   a) sinus arrhythmia
   b) ventricular tachycardia
   c) unifocal ventricular premature beats
   d) multifocal ventricular premature beats

ANSWER: (a, b, d) All narrow QRS complexes are stimulated by the sinus P waves and precede them. The variability in PP intervals indicates sinus arrhythmia. The fourth, sixth, eighth, and tenth QRS complexes - wide, bizarre, and occuring prematurely - are ventricular premature beats. The contours of the fourth, sixth, and eighth premature ventricular beats are different, suggesting that each impulse arises in a different part (focus) of the ventricle. The ventricular premature beats are therefore multifocal in origin. The tenth QRS complex is a ventricular premature beat followed in rapid succession by two wide QRS complexes, the three consecutive beats at this rate (about 176/minute) qualifying as a burst of ventricular tachycardia.

6. Long-term management of this patient might include which of the following?
   a) no therapy
   b) administration of a beta-adrenergic blocking agent
   c) administration of diphenylhydantoin
   d) implantation of a permanent pacemaker
   e) administration of digoxin
   f) left stellate ganglionectomy

ANSWER: (b, c, d, f) Treatment of this patient is strongly advised since about 70% of patients with the syndrome of long QT interval and syncope die if untreated. The chronic administration of beta-adrenergic blocking agents such as propranolol has been shown to substantially reduce the frequency of syncopal episodes and probably also diminishes mortality. Although the numbers of patients treated in this manner are small, beta-blockade appears to be the most successful form of therapy at this time. Its effectiveness might be due to blockade of sympathetic traffic into the ventricles from the left stellate ganglion. In a few patients, diphenylhydantoin has also been reported to prevent syncopal episodes. Digoxin, when administered in conjunction with propranolol, has also been found to be

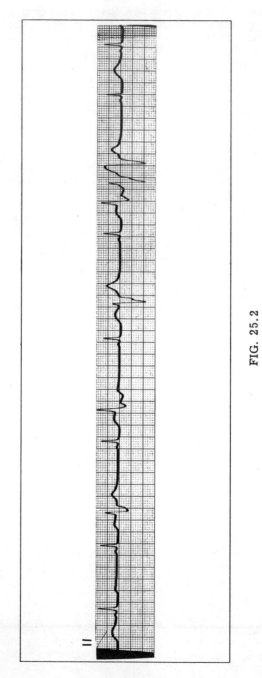

FIG. 25.2

effective although it is not clear that the digoxin itself has a beneficial effect. Since increasing the heart rate may decrease the pre-
position to ventricular arrhythmias and can shorten the QT interval,
it might be reasonable to implant an atrial or ventricular pacemaker
to ensure adequate heart rates in symptomatic patients with slow
resting heart rates. In those patients with life-threatening syncopal episodes not preventable by pharmacologic or pacemaker therapy,
performance of left stellate ganglionectomy has been effective.

The patient is taken to the cardiac catheterization laboratory in an
attempt to establish the presence or absence of anomalous AV conduction pathways, and to initiate and terminate ventricular tachycardia. No evidence of anomalous AV conduction pathway is found
and, despite the introduction of single and pairs of ventricular pacing
stimuli during both spontaneous sinus rhythm and fixed-rate ventricular pacing, sustained ventricular tachycardia cannot be initiated.
The patient is treated with diphenylhydantoin and propranolol orally
in doses which achieve therapeutic plasma levels. However, the
potentially disastrous consequences of the previous cardiac arrest
on the fetus prompts therapeutic abortion. The patient leaves the
hospital feeling well, with no ventricular premature beats and the
QT interval having shortened slightly. Over the next three months
she has no episodes of syncope despite the fact that she takes her
medication irregularly and on occasion plasma concentrations of
the medications are only barely detectable.

BIBLIOGRAPHY

Csanady M, Kiss Z: Heritable Q-T prolongation without congenital
deafness (Romano-Ward syndrome) Chest 64:359, 1973.

Johansson BW, Jorming B: Hereditary prolongation of QT interval.
Brit Heart J 34:744, 1972.

Moothart RW, Pryor R, Hawley RL, Clifford NJ, Blount SG Jr:
The heritable syndrome of prolonged Q-T interval, syncope, and
sudden death. Chest 70:263, 1976.

Moss AJ, McDonald J: Unilateral cervicothoracic sympathetic
ganglionectomy for the treatment of long QT interval syndrome.
New Engl J Med 285:903, 1971.

Roy PR, Emanuel R, Ismail SA, El Tayib MH: Hereditary prolongation of the Q-T interval. Amer J Cardiol 37:237, 1976.

Reynolds EW, Vander Ark CR: Quinidine syncope and the delayed
repolarization syndromes. Mod Concepts Cardiovasc Dis 55:117,
1976.

Phillips J, Ichinose H: Clinical and pathologic studies in the hereditary syndrome of a long Q-T interval, syncopal spells, and sudden death. Chest 58:236, 1970.

Schneider RR, Bahler A, Pincus J, Stimmel B: Asymptomatic idiopathic syndrome of prolonged Q-T interval in a 45-year-old woman.
Chest 71:210, 1977.

Schwartz PJ, Periti M, Malliani A: The long Q-T syndrome. Amer
Heart J 89:378, 1975.

Selzer A, Wray HW: Quinidine syncope: Paroxysmal ventricular
fibrillation occurring during treatment of chronic atrial arrhythmias.
Circulation 30:17, 1964.

Watanabe Y: Purkinje repolarization as a possible cause of the U
wave in the electrocardiogram. Circulation 51:1030, 1975.

Yanowitz BA, Preston JB, Abildskov JA: Functional distribution of
right and left stellate innervation to the ventricles: production of
neurogenic electrocardiographic changes by unilateral alteration of
sympathetic tone. Circulation Res 18:416, 1966.

Mathews EC Jr, Blount AW, Townsend JI: Q-T prolongation and
ventricular arrhythmias, with and without deafness, in the same
family. Amer J Cardiol 29:702, 1972.

Garza LA, Vick RL, Nora JJ, McNamara DG: Heritable Q-T prolongation without deafness. Circulation 41:39, 1970.

Cochran PR, Linnebur AC, Wright W, Matsumoto S: Electrophysiological studies in patients with the long Q-T syndrome. Clin Res
25:88, 1977.

Ratshin RA, Hunt D, Russell RO Jr, Rackley CE: QT-interval prolongation, paroxysmal ventricular arrhythmias, and convulsive syncope. Ann Int Med 75:919, 1971.

CASE 26: Alternation of groups of narrow and wide QRS complexes in a patient with acute myocardial infarction.

A 64-year-old man comes to the Emergency Room complaining of severe oppressive chest pain which occurred while he was eating. His skin is moist and he appears seriously ill. His pulse is 85/ minute and slightly irregular, his blood pressure is 110/70, the jugular venous pressure is normal, and there is no evidence of pulmonary congestion. The three continuous Lead II rhythm strips shown in Fig. 26.1 are recorded in the Emergency Room. The PP intervals (in hundredths of a second) are noted above the baseline, and the RR intervals (also in hundredths of a second) below the baseline.

1. Which terms characterize the tracing in Fig. 26.1?
   a) sinus arrhythmia   e) accelerated ventricular rhythm
   b) AV block   f) fusion beat
   c) ventricular ectopic beat   g) capture beat
   d) junctional rhythm   h) AV dissociation

ANSWER: (a, c, e, f, g, h) Except for the fourth QRS complex in the top strip (X) and the sixth QRS complex in the bottom strip (X), the QRS complexes are of two types: (1) narrow (0.08 seconds) normal-appearing Rs complexes and (2) wide (0.17 seconds) bizarre QS complexes. All Rs complexes are preceded by P waves at intervals of about 0.19 seconds, suggesting that they are stimulated by the P waves; the P waves, having a normal contour in Lead II, are likely sinus in origin. The gradual lengthening and shortening of the PP intervals indicates sinus arrhythmia.

As the QS complexes are wide and bizarre and are temporally unrelated to the sinus P waves, they probably originate in the ventricles. Their uninterrupted occurrence over a period of about 11.3 seconds establishes a ventricular rhythm. Since ventricular rhythms usually occur at rates of 35-45/minute, this rhythm at a rate of 83-88/minute may be called an "accelerated" ventricular rhythm.

Beginning in the top strip, two ventricular beats are followed by a P wave which, occurring about 0.08 seconds before the third QRS complex, is too early to capture the ventricles which have been activated by the on-time ventricular focus. The fourth QRS complex, occurring at an RR interval about equal to the cycle length of the preceding ventricular beats, has an initial contour similar to the ventricular beats. It follows a P wave by about 0.16 seconds, when the PR interval of sinus beats is about 0.19 seconds. Its mid to late contour is similar to the sinus-stimulated QRS complexes and its duration is intermediate between the narrow (0.08 seconds) and wide (0.17 seconds) complexes. It is thus probably a fusion beat, in

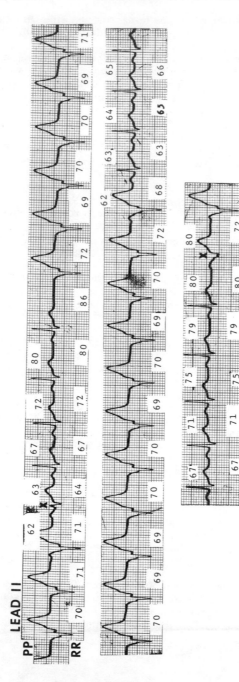

FIG. 26.1

which early ventricular activation results from the ventricular impulse, and later activation from both the ventricular and sinus impulses. The next four beats are sinus in origin, but the intersinus interval lengthens. Following a short pause in QRS rhythm of about 0.86 seconds, a ventricular beat initiates a run of accelerated ventricular rhythm during which P waves cannot clearly be seen, presumably because they are occurring within the wide QRS complexes. During this run there is AV dissociation due to lack of opportunity of the P waves to capture the ventricles which are being activated by the ventricular focus. A P wave is clearly seen preceding the last ventricular beat of the run in the middle strip. The cycle lengths of the emerging P waves rapidly become shorter than the cycle length of the ventricular rhythm such that the P waves stimulate a run of nine QRS complexes. During this run of sinus rhythm, the sinus rate slows, resulting in a short pause in QRS rhythm of about 0.80 seconds. This pause, like that in the top strip, is terminated by a fusion complex. Since at the time of the fusion beat the PP interval of about 0.80 seconds exceeds the cycle length of the accelerated ventricular rhythm (about 0.70 seconds), the fusion beat is followed by a ventricular beat.

Since all P waves falling outside of the QRST complexes stimulate QRS complexes, there is no evidence of AV block.

2. The 12-Lead ECG indicates an acute anterior myocardial infarction. How might this rhythm be managed in this hemodynamically stable patient?
   a) administration of intravenous lidocaine
   b) DC cardioversion
   c) administration of intravenous digoxin
   d) watchful waiting
   e) administration of intravenous atropine

ANSWER: (d, e) Accelerated ventricular rhythm* occurs commonly in the setting of acute myocardial infarction, usually within the first 24-36 hours of the onset of symptoms. Its rate varies from about 60 to 100 beats per minute, and is usually within a few beats per minute of the sinus rate. The occurrence of two rhythms at similar yet varying rates results in several second periods of alternation of ventricular and sinus-stimulated beats, and fusion beats often occurring at the transition between the runs of different complexes.

Accelerated ventricular rhythm may be thought of as an accelerated escape rhythm. The rhythm itself has never to our knowledge been documented to initiate ventricular tachycardia or ventricular fibrillation. Whereas it has been reported that patients with this rhythm

* This rhythm is referred to in the literature as accelerated idioventricular rhythm. Since the term idioventricular has in general been used to describe slow ventricular escape rhythms occurring in the presence of complete AV block, we feel that the use of the term in this setting is not appropriate.

have a lower incidence of ventricular fibrillation than do patients with ventricular tachycardia, other reports indicate that patients with accelerated ventricular rhythm are more likely to develop ventricular tachycardia than are patients without accelerated ventricular rhythm. The rhythm is usually of little hemodynamic consequence, although the loss of atrial contribution to ventricular filling may result in a fall in blood pressure in some patients. Watchful waiting is therefore a reasonable form of management of this hemodynamically and electrically benign arrhythmia. If for some reason suppression of the rhythm is desirable, atropine administration, by increasing the sinus rate and abolishing the variation in PP intervals, will usually result in its disappearance. It has not been established that administration of either lidocaine or digoxin has any effect on accelerated ventricular rhythm. Since the rhythm is terminated every few seconds by sinus beats, DC cardioversion has no place in the treatment of this arrhythmia.

The patient is admitted to the Coronary Care Unit for observation. The accelerated ventricular rhythm disappears within three hours. The patient remains hemodynamically stable and has only occasional ventricular premature beats during the first few hospital days. On the fifth day he is transferred from the Coronary Care Unit to the ward where he completes an uneventful post-infarction hospital course. When last seen two months after his infarction he feels well and has no angina, symptoms of congestive heart failure, or arrhythmias.

BIBLIOGRAPHY

DeSanctis RW, Block P, Hutter AM: Tachyarrhythmias in myocardial infarction. Circulation 40:681, 1972.

de Soyza N, et al.: Association of accelerated idioventricular rhythm and paroxysmal ventricular tachycardia in acute myocardial infarction. Amer J Cardiol 34:667, 1974.

de Soyza N, et al.: Ectopic ventricular prematurity and its relationship to ventricular tachycardia in acute myocardial infarction in man. Circulation 50:529, 1974.

Norris RM, Mercer CJ: Significance of idioventricular rhythms in acute myocardial infarction. Prog Cardiovasc Dis 16:455, 1974.

Gallagher JJ, Damato AN, Lau SH: Electrophysiologic studies during accelerated idioventricular rhythms. Circulation 44:671, 1971.

Rothfeld E, et al.: Idioventricular rhythm (IVR) in acute myocardial infarction (AMI): A reappraisal. Circulation 42 (Suppl. III):192, 1970.

Scherlag BJ, El-Sherif N, Hope R, Lazzara R: Characterization and localization of ventricular arrhythmias resulting from myocardial ischemia and infarction. Circulation Res 35:372, 1974.

Schamroth L: Idioventricular tachycardia. J Electrocardiol 1:205, 1968.

Rothfeld EL, Zucker IR, Parsonnet V, et al.: Idioventricular rhythm in acute myocardial infarction. Circulation 37:203, 1968.

CASE 27: Long-standing arrhythmia in a man with coronary
artery disease.

A 64-year-old man comes to the Emergency Room complaining of
chest discomfort. He has had exertional chest pain intermittently
for two years and is felt to have ischemic heart disease. His cardiovascular examination is normal, and his 12-Lead ECG is shown in
Fig. 27.1. The rhythm is sinus arrhythmia at an average rate of
about 55/minute. The sinus beats have a normal PR interval, normal QRS axis, duration and configuration. The ST segments show
slight sagging in the inferior and lateral precordial leads, and the
T waves are normal. QRS complexes which are not preceded by P
waves occur in every Lead except Lead V2.

1. What might be the origin of these non-sinus-stimulated QRS
   complexes?
   a) His bundle
   b) anterior fascicle of the left bundle branch
   c) Purkinje system
   d) right bundle branch
   e) posterior fascicle of the left bundle branch

ANSWER: (a, b) The non-sinus-stimulated QRS complexes have a
slightly longer duration (0.09 seconds) than sinus-stimulated QRS
complexes (0.07-0.08 seconds) suggesting that they originate in the
His bundle or proximal bundle branches. They have a more rightward axis, and a different contour from the sinus-stimulated beats.
The right axis deviation, the QRS pattern in Lead V1 and the RS
pattern in Lead V6 suggest that they are conducted into the ventricles with delay in the right bundle branch and in the posterior fascicle of the left bundle branch, and that they therefore probably
originate in the area of the anterior fascicle of the left bundle branch.
QRS complexes originating in the more distal Purkinje system would
be abnormally wide and more bizarre in appearance. QRS complexes originating in the right bundle branch would be conducted into
the ventricles with a left bundle block pattern, and QRS complexes
originating in the posterior fascicle of the left bundle branch would
be expected to be conducted with a pattern of right bundle branch
block and left anterior fascicle block.

2. Which term most appropriately describes this non-sinus-stimulated QRS rhythm?
   a) extrasystolic rhythm
   b) parasystolic rhythm
   c) escape rhythm

ANSWER: (b) The coupling intervals of the wider QRS complexes to
preceding sinus-stimulated QRS complexes are highly variable,

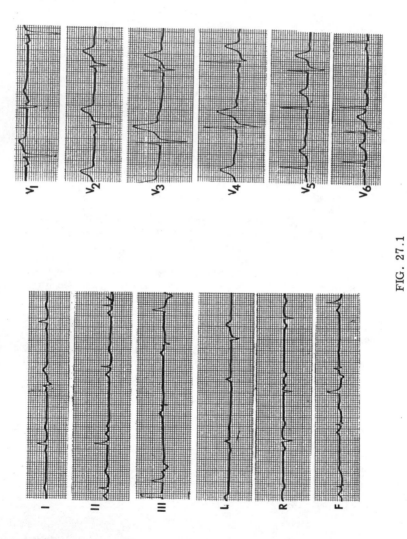

FIG. 27.1

indicating that the rhythm is not dependent upon the basic sinus rhythm and is therefore not extrasystolic. The fact that some non-sinus-stimulated QRS complexes occur at coupling intervals as short as 0.55 seconds (corresponding rate about 102/minute) while the intersinus interval is longer indicates that these beats are not escape beats, and the rhythm not an escape rhythm. The inter-ectopic interval (the interval between two consecutive wider QRS complexes) is about 1.61 seconds in Lead aVF and about 3.08 seconds in Lead III raising the possibility that the interectopic intervals are multiples of a common cycle length. The common cycle length of the non-sinus-stimulated QRS complexes and their variable coupling intervals to preceding sinus-stimulated QRS complexes suggest that the rhythm is parasystolic. The minimum possible manifest cycle length of the parasystolic rhythm in Fig. 27.1 can be estimated from the longest pause following a parasystolic beat, which is seen in Lead II to be 1.39 seconds. If the manifest parasystolic cycle length were less than this, a parasystolic QRS complex would have occurred before the ensuing sinus beat. The interectopic intervals of 1.61 seconds in Lead aVF and 3.08 seconds (2 X 1.54) in Lead III suggest that the parasystolic cycle length is in the range of about 1.5 - 1.6 seconds. A longer rhythm strip, required for more accurate measurement of ecto-pic cycle length, is shown in Fig. 27.2. From this rhythm strip a basic interectopic interval of 1.51 - 1.59 seconds can be measured. That the cycle length is not a fraction of this is suggested by the post-ectopic pause of 1.44 seconds follow-ing the last ectopic beat in the bottom strip, during which time a parasystolic pacemaker with a shorter cycle length would have dis-charged and stimulated a QRS complex. Exit block of parasystolic pacemakers, which has been well-documented in animal experiments, is apparently not common in man. Its presence can be established only by its transient disappearance, which would result in parasys-tolic complexes occurring at shorter interectopic intervals which are a fraction (one-half or one-third) of the more commonly observed interectopic intervals.

3. How might this rhythm be managed in this patient at this time?
    a) lidocaine administration
    b) quinidine administration
    c) digoxin administration
    d) no treatment

ANSWER: (b, d) Since parasystolic rhythms are generally of little or no consequence (only once to our knowledge has a parasystolic rhythm been documented to precipitate ventricular tachycardia), there is little or no need to treat it. The occasional patient who is made uncomfortable by the awareness of irregular cardiac action might be given a quinidine preparation for symptomatic relief. In this patient, review of several electrocardiograms dating back as far as five years always showed the same parasystolic rhythm at about the same basic cycle length.

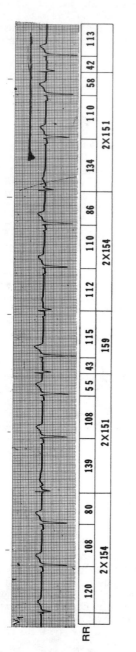

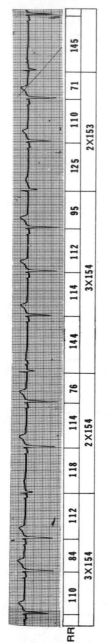

FIG. 27.2

The patient is hospitalized in the Coronary Care Unit, where his chest pain disappears and serial electrocardiograms and serum enzymes fail to document acute myocardial necrosis. He is discharged three days later and when last seen one year after his hospitalization, was still having exertional angina pectoris and no change in his parasystolic rhythm.

BIBLIOGRAPHY

Cohen H, Langendorf R, Pick A: Intermittent parasystole - Mechanism of protection. Circulation 43:761, 1973.

Langendorf R, Pick A: Parasystole with fixed coupling. Circulation 35:304, 1967.

Singer DH, Parameswaran R, Drake FT, Meyers SN, DeBoer AA: Ventricular parasystole and reentry: Clinical-electrophysiological correlations. Amer Heart J 88:79, 1974.

Watanabe Y: Reassessment of parasystole. Amer Heart J 81:451, 1971.

Pick A, Langendorf R: Parasystole and its variants. Med Clin No Amer 60: I-125, 1976.

Arrhythmias of Intermediate Complexity

CASE 28: Syncope in a man with coronary artery disease and progressive widening of the QRS complexes.

A 59-year-old man with no symptoms of cardiovascular disease is
seen for evaluation of hypertension. His 12-Lead ECG is shown in
Fig. 28.1 The QRS complexes occur at essentially regular intervals,
at an average rate of about 75/minute. Each QRS complex is preceded by a P wave at an interval of about 0.18 seconds. The QRS
duration is normal at about 0.09-0.10 seconds. The mean frontal
plane QRS axis is normal at about -25 degrees. The QRS voltage,
ST segments, and T waves are normal.

The patient is treated with Rauwolfia, and later hydrochlorothiazide,
which, over a period of two years, bring his blood pressure down
to normal levels. He continues to have no symptoms of cardiovascular disease, and when he returns for examination 13 years later
at the age of 74, the 12-Lead ECG shown in Fig. 28.2 is recorded.
Compared with the tracing in Fig. 28.1, the PR interval has lengthened from 0.18 to 0.20 seconds, the QRS duration has increased
from 0.09-0.10 to 0.12 seconds, the mean frontal plane QRS axis
has shifted leftward from about -25 degrees to about -60 degrees,
the QRS voltage has decreased somewhat in Leads V5-V6, Q waves
have appeared in Leads V1-V4, and the T waves have become slightly
flat in Leads I and V6, and inverted in Lead aVL.

1. How might the changes between the two ECGs recorded 15 years
apart be explained?

ANSWER: The leftward QRS axis shift and the mild lengthening of intraventricular conduction time are most likely due to the interval development of conduction delay in the anterior fascicle of the left bundle branch (that is, left anterior fascicle block has occurred). Although Q waves might result from the development of left anterior
fascicle block, they are usually of shorter duration and of lesser
magnitude than those seen in Fig. 28.2. The Q waves in the ECG
of Fig. 28.2 are 0.04 seconds in duration and fairly large, suggesting that interval silent anterior myocardial infarction has occurred.
The normal T waves in the precordial leads suggest that the infarction, which was not clinically apparent, is not recent. The left
anterior fascicle block probably occurred as a result of the anterior
infarction. The change in PR interval may be due to the interval development of delayed impulse conduction through the AV node and/or
bundle of His, and/or right bundle branch, and/or the left posterior
fascicle.

The patient does well until four months later, when he has sudden onset of severe chest pain associated with nausea and diaphoresis. He
is admitted to the hospital where serial electrocardiograms and serum

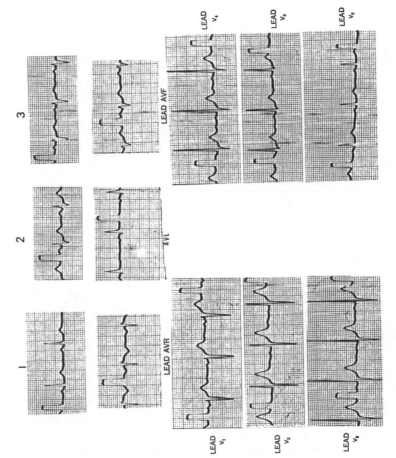

FIG. 28.1

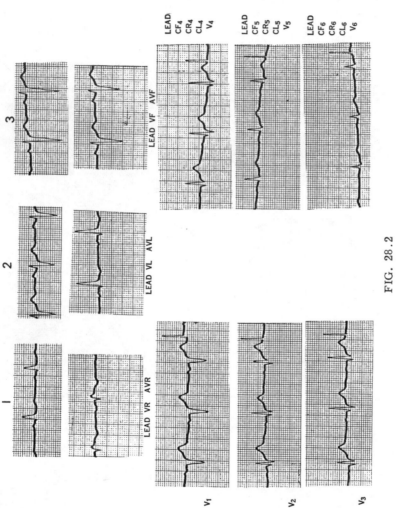

FIG. 28.2

enzyme determinations document acute myocardial infarction. The patient is discharged on digoxin, 0.25 mg orally daily after a four-week hospital stay. His 12-Lead ECG recorded upon discharge is shown in Fig. 28.3.

2. How might the increase in PR interval compared with the ECG recorded four months earlier be explained?

ANSWER: The increase in PR interval could be due to the interval administration of digoxin, to a change in autonomic nervous system traffic into the AV node, or to ischemic damage to the AV node and/or His bundle, and/or the right bundle branch and/or the left posterior fascicle, any or all of which might slow AV conduction.

Over the next eight years the patient continues to take digoxin, 0.25 mg daily, and has no symptoms of angina, congestive heart failure, or arrhythmias. However, at age 82 years, he calls his physician to report that while walking he lost consciousness and fell, suffering a scalp laceration. He is admitted to the hospital, where the ECG shown in Fig. 28.4 is recorded.

3. What is the rhythm?
   a) atrial standstill with junctional rhythm
   b) ventricular rhythm with 1:1 retrograde ventriculoatrial conduction
   c) atrial flutter with 3:1 AV conduction
   d) sinus rhythm with first degree AV block

ANSWER: (d) QRS complexes occur at fairly regular intervals of about 0.70-0.73 seconds (rate of 82-86/minute). While atrial activity is not clearly seen, probable P waves are present in all Leads except V1-V3 as sharp deflections on the downslopes of the T waves. These sharp deflections are upright in Leads I and II, and inverted in Lead aVR, suggesting that the P wave axis is normal and that the P waves are of sinus origin. Their fixed temporal relationship to the QRS complexes suggests that the rhythm is sinus with marked first degree AV block (PR interval about 0.30 seconds). The presence of P waves excludes the diagnosis of atrial standstill, and the normal P wave axis suggests that retrograde ventriculoatrial conduction is not occurring. The isoelectric baseline in inferior Leads suggests that the atrial rhythm is not flutter.

4. How is intraventricular conduction occurring?
   a) via the right bundle branch
   b) via the anterior fascicle of the left bundle branch
   c) via the posterior fascicle of the left bundle branch
   d) via both the left anterior and left posterior fascicles
   e) via the right bundle branch and left posterior fascicle

ANSWER: (c) The QRS complexes have an abnormally leftward mean frontal plane axis of about -60 degrees, attributable to left anterior fascicle block. The QRS duration is prolonged to 0.13 seconds, and

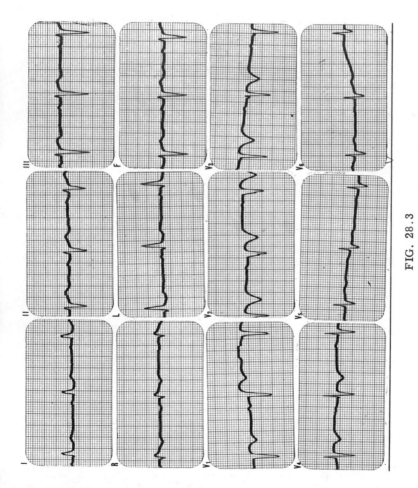

FIG. 28.3

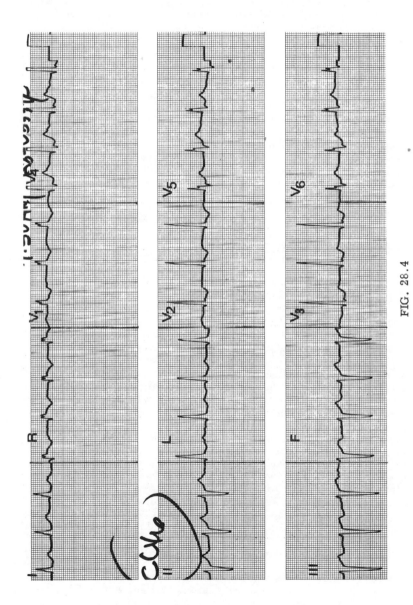

FIG. 28.4

the QRS configuration in Leads aVR and V1 suggests conduction delay in the right bundle branch. In the framework of the trifascicle
conduction system, intraventricular conduction is therefore occurring with delay (or block) in both the right bundle branch and in the
anterior fascicle of the left bundle branch. Activation of the ventricles must be occurring via the posterior fascicle of the left
bundle branch.

5. How might the prolonged PR interval reasonably be explained?

ANSWER: In the presence of conduction delay in two fascicles, it is
likely that associated PR interval prolongation represents conduction
delay in the remaining fascicle, but AV nodal conduction time may also
be prolonged. Precise localization of the area of atrioventricular conduction delay in patients with fascicle disease cannot be accurately inferred from surface electrocardiograms. His bundle recordings could
be utilized to more accurately localize the site of conduction delay to be
in the AV node, His bundle, left posterior fascicle, or any combination
of these.

6. What are the most likely disturbances of cardiac rhythm that
    could account for this patient's episode of syncope?
    a) ventricular tachycardia
    b) ventricular fibrillation
    c) sinus arrest
    d) pauses occasioned by AV nodal Wenckebach periods
    e) transient complete AV block

ANSWER: (a, e) In a patient with coronary artery disease, ventricular
tachycardia is a common cause of syncope, even in the absence of
ischemic heart pain. Transient complete atrioventricular block resulting in bradycardia-induced syncope (Stokes-Adams-Morgagni
attacks) is also a likely cause of syncope in this patient with conduction delays in the right bundle branch, the left anterior fascicle, and
also in the left posterior fascicle and/or AV node and His bundle.
Sinus arrest is a possible cause of syncope in elderly individuals,
but symptomatic sinus node dysfunction seems to be less common
in the presence of extensive His-Purkinje system dysfunction than
in the presence of relatively normal intraventricular conduction.
Atrioventricular Wenckebach periods do not usually cause pauses
in ventricular rhythm long enough to result in syncope unless the
atrial rhythm is unusually slow. Ventricular fibrillation is certainly a common cause of sudden unexpected death in patients with
coronary artery disease, but its spontaneous termination would be
most unlikely unless it were related to quinidine administration.

The patient is admitted to the Coronary Care Unit so that his rhythm
might be monitored. He has no symptoms or signs of either congestive heart failure or myocardial ischemia, and is hemodynamically
stable. A few hours after admission the rhythm strip (MCL$_1$) shown
in Fig. 28.5 is recorded.

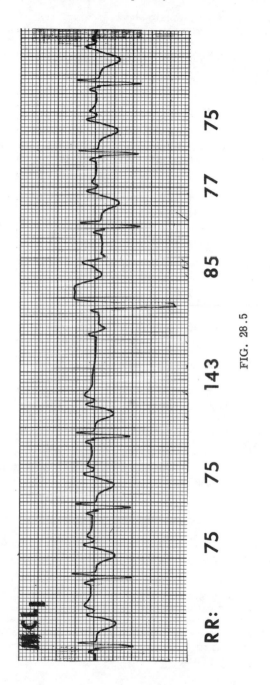

FIG. 28.5

7. What does this rhythm strip show?
   a) junctional rhythm with an episode of 2:1 exit block
   b) sinus rhythm
   c) idioventricular rhythm with an episode of 2:1 exit block
   d) first degree AV block
   e) Mobitz Type II second degree AV block

ANSWER: (b, d, e) Except for the fifth QRS complex, all QRS complexes have the same rSR' configuration, suggesting that intraventricular conduction is occurring with right bundle branch block. The RR intervals between consecutive QRS complexes with the right bundle branch block pattern are identical at about 0.75 seconds (rate of about 80/minute), with the exception of the slightly longer RR interval between the sixth and seventh QRS complexes (0.77 seconds). The only P wave seen in its entirety is the one preceding the fifth (rS) QRS complex. Recognizing this P wave contour, it can be seen that P waves are in fact occurring in the terminal portions of the T waves of all the rSR' complexes, and that the PP intervals are essentially equal at about 0.75 seconds with the exception of that between the sixth and seventh P waves (0.77 seconds). The estimated PR intervals of the second, third, and fourth QRS complexes are equal at about 0.35 seconds, suggesting that the basic rhythm is sinus with first degree AV block and right bundle branch block. Junctional and ventricular rhythms with 1:1 retrograde conduction to the atria would not be likely to have such long PR intervals of about 0.43 seconds.

The P wave following the fourth QRS complex is on time but is not followed by a QRS complex and therefore represents an episode of Mobitz Type II second degree AV block. In this patient with conduction delays (blocks) in the left anterior fascicle and in the right bundle branch, the episode of Mobitz Type II second degree AV block is presumably due to sudden conduction block in the left posterior fascicle. The P wave following the non-conducted P wave, occurring on time, is followed 0.28 seconds later by a QRS complex which, not having a right bundle branch block pattern, is either (1) an escape beat originating in and conducted into the ventricles via the right bundle branch, or (2) a sinus-stimulated beat conducted down the right bundle branch, whose refractory period has been exceeded during the prior pause of 1.43 seconds. Fig. 28.6, recorded shortly after Fig. 28.5, showing consistent 2:1 AV block with underlying first degree AV block (PR interval about 0.28 seconds) and no right bundle branch block suggests that the latter explanation is more likely.

The fifth QRS complex in Fig. 28.5 is of abnormally long duration (0.13 seconds) indicating delayed intraventricular conduction time. Inasmuch as this patient's underlying left anterior fascicle block should not prolong the QRS duration by more than 0.02 seconds it is likely that distal Purkinje conduction delay accounts for the long duration of this fifth QRS complex. The shorter PR interval of 0.28 seconds

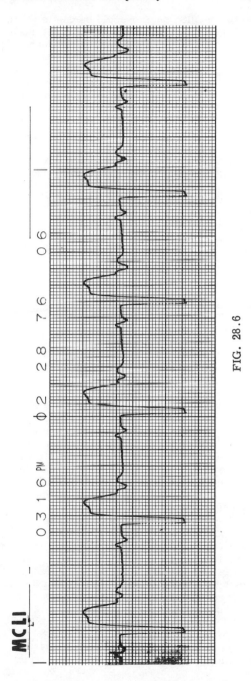

FIG. 28.6

preceding this fifth QRS complex could be due to (1) transient autonomic nervous-system-induced shortening of AV nodal conduction
time resulting from the hemodynamic consequences of the preceding
pause, or (2) the right bundle branch having a greater conduction
velocity, but longer refractory period, than the posterior fascicle
of the left bundle branch. The remaining QRS complexes in Fig.
28.5 are conducted with first degree AV block and right bundle
branch block and are identical to the initial beats in the rhythm
strip.

In view of this evidence of probable trifascicle dysfunction and episodes of Mobitz Type II second degree AV block, the decision is
made to implant a permanent ventricular pacemaker as soon as is
practical. The patient's rhythm continues to be monitored and although he has frequent episodes of Mobitz Type II second degree AV
block with ventricular rates of about 45/minute (Fig. 28.6), he has
neither syncope nor presyncopal symptoms. On the second hospital day, while sitting on the toilet, the patient feels lightheaded and
transiently loses consciousness. His ECG at this time is shown in
Fig. 28.7.

8. What is the rhythm?
   a) ventricular tachycardia
   b) supraventricular tachycardia with aberrant intraventricular
      conduction
   c) ventricular fibrillation
   d) atrial fibrillation with rapid ventricular response
   e) atrial flutter with variable AV conduction

ANSWER: (a) Wide, bizarre QRS complexes at intervals as short as
about 0.24 seconds (rate about 250/minute) are seen clustered to-
gether at the beginning and end of the strip, separated by five beats
of alternating direction. The second and fourth of the less bizarre
QRS complexes (X) are similar in configuration to the more rapidly
occurring QRS complexes suggesting that the focus of origin is similar to that of the clustered beats. Furthermore, the coupling intervals of these two beats to their preceding QRS complexes (0.60 seconds) are identical to the coupling interval of the QRS complex (●)
that initiates the second burst of rapid beats to its preceding QRS
complex. Atrial activity is difficult to identify because of body movement artifact, but probable P waves are visible at the arrows at a
basic rate of about 100/minute. The wide, bizarre QRS complexes
occurring rapidly in a mildly irregular pattern, and the second burst
apparently initiated by a wide QRS complex following a brief run of
bigeminal rhythm, suggest that the bursts of rapid beats represent
paroxysms of ventricular tachycardia.

The rhythm is too well-organized to be ventricular fibrillation.
Supraventricular tachycardia is not usually this rapid, and would
be unlikely to be initiated by a premature ventricular beat following
a run of bigeminal rhythm. Atrial fibrillation would be unlikely to

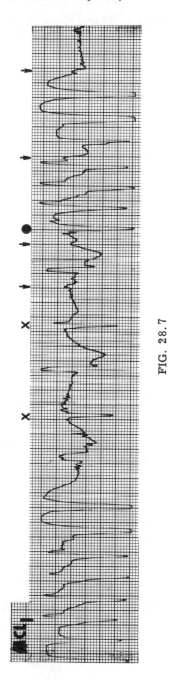

FIG. 28.7

have so rapid a ventricular response interspersed with sudden periods of such slowing of the QRS rhythm, except in the presence of accessory atrioventricular conduction pathways. Atrial flutter with variable AV conduction, including periods of presumed 1:1 AV conduction to account for the rapid ventricular rate, is unusual in a patient of this age, and also would not account for the slower rhythm seen in the center of the strip unless an accessory atrioventricular conduction pathway were present. The identification of discrete P waves at a rate of 100/minute excludes the possibilities of atrial fibrillation and atrial flutter.

9. How might the patient be managed at this time?
   a) lidocaine administration
   b) quinidine administration
   c) procainamide administration
   d) propranolol administration
   e) ventricular pacing

ANSWER: (a, b, c, d, e) The treatment of ventricular tachycardia is aimed at suppression of ventricular premature beats and alteration of intraventricular conduction velocities. Lidocaine, quinidine, procainamide, and propranolol might all aid in achieving these goals, but they might also increase the tendency to ventricular arrhythmias by slowing the heart rate and/or increasing atrioventricular block. Lidocaine is probably least likely, and propranolol most likely, to depress AV conduction. Propranolol might also depress ventricular function with the potential result of congestive failure. Ventricular pacing might decrease the tendency for ventricular ectopy, including ventricular tachycardia, by increasing the heart rate, and would permit administration of antiarrhythmic medications with less concern for their potentially detrimental effects on impulse formation and conduction.

This episode is treated with intravenous lidocaine, 100 mg followed by constant infusion at a dose of 3 mg/minute. Only single and occasional pairs of ventricular premature beats occur and intraventricular conduction continues to alternate between first degree AV block with right bundle branch block, and first degree AV block with periods of 2:1 AV block without right bundle branch block. Twenty-four hours later a permanent demand pacemaker using a right ventricular endocardial electrode is implanted, with the demand rate set for about 72 beats per minute. The lidocaine is then stopped. When last seen seven months after pacemaker implantation the patient feels well, and has no syncope or presyncopal symptoms. His electrocardiograms over this period of time show a paced ventricular rhythm almost all of the time.

BIBLIOGRAPHY

Denes P, Dhingra RC, Wu D, Chuquimia R, Amat-y-Leon F, Wynd-
ham C, Rosen KM: H-V interval in patients with bifascicular block
(Right bundle branch block and left anterior hemiblock). Amer J
Cardiol 35:23, 1975.

DePasquale NP, Bruno MS: Natural history of combined right
bundle branch block and left anterior hemiblock (Bilateral bundle
branch block). Amer J Med 54:297, 1973.

Dhingra RC, Denes P, Wu D, Chuquimia R, Rosen KM: The significance of second degree AV block and right bundle branch block.
Circulation 49:638, 1974.

Dhingra RC, Denes P, Wu D, Chuquimia R, Amat-y-Leon F, Wyndham C, Rosen KM: Syncope in patients with chronic bifascicular
block. Ann Int Med 81:302, 1974.

Dhingra RC, Wyndham C, Amat-y-Leon F, Wu D, Denes P, Towne
WD, Rosen KM: Significance of A-H interval in patients with
chronic bundle branch block. Amer J Cardiol 37:231, 1976.

Levites R, Haft J: Significance of first degree heart block (prolonged
P-R interval) in bifascicular block. Amer J Cardiol 34:259, 1974.

Narula O, Samet P: Right bundle branch block with normal, left, or
right axis deviation. Amer J Med 51:432, 1971.

Rosenbaum MB, Elizari MV, Lazzari JO: The Hemiblocks. Olds-
mar, Florida, Tampa Tracings, 1970.

Scheinman M, Weiss A, Kunkel F: His bundle recordings in patients
with bundle branch block and transient neurologic symptoms. Circulation 48:322, 1973.

CASE 29: Palpitations and syncope in a patient with coronary artery
        disease.

A 52-year-old man is seen in a follow-up visit six months after
undergoing saphenous vein aortocoronary bypass surgery to the
right and left anterior descending coronary arteries for severe
angina pectoris. He has, in addition, trivial aortic regurgitation
and mitral stenosis presumably due to rheumatic heart disease.
He now has no ischemic heart pain and no symptoms of congestive
heart failure, but does complain of frequent "palpitations". His
ECG, shown in Fig. 29.1, reveals sinus rhythm with atrial premature beats. The P wave contour and duration in Leads II and V1
suggests a left atrial abnormality, presumably due to the mitral
valve disease and/or left ventricular dysfunction. He is treated
with quinidine sulfate in doses that achieve a therapeutic serum level,
and has only rare "palpitations" over the next six months. At this
time he begins to experience episodes of lightheadedness and occasional syncope associated with palpitations and chest discomfort.
During one of these episodes he seeks medical assistance at which
time the ECG shown in Fig. 29.2 is recorded.

1. What are the possible rhythms?
   a) ventricular tachycardia
   b) supraventricular tachycardia (SVT)
   c) atrial flutter with 1:1 AV conduction
   d) atrial fibrillation
   e) sinus tachycardia

ANSWER: (b, c) QRS complexes of 0.10 seconds duration are occurring with perfect regularity at a rate of about 226/minute. While
atrial activity is not clearly identifiable, the small deflections on
the upstroke of the T waves, best seen in Lead V6, probably represent atrial complexes. The regularity of the QRS rhythm excludes
the diagnosis of atrial fibrillation and the unusually rapid rate excludes the diagnosis of sinus tachycardia. While ventricular tachycardia may occur with narrow QRS complexes if it originates in the
proximal portion of a fascicle, the rates in the few reported cases
have been in the range of 110-120 beats per minute. Atrial flutter
with 1:1 AV conduction is unusual and when it occurs the atrial rate
is in a somewhat slow range, as is present in this tracing. However, regular tachycardia with rates in this range are unusual, but
when they occur they are almost always SVT.

Since the patient is weak and lightheaded, has chest discomfort and
is hypotensive, DC cardioversion is performed. The rhythm is converted to sinus with a 50 watt-second discharge. A 12-Lead ECG
with the patient in sinus rhythm is similar to that in Fig. 29.1, and
the patient feels well. He is instructed to take his previous dose of
quinidine, and to start propranolol, 20 mg four times daily, which

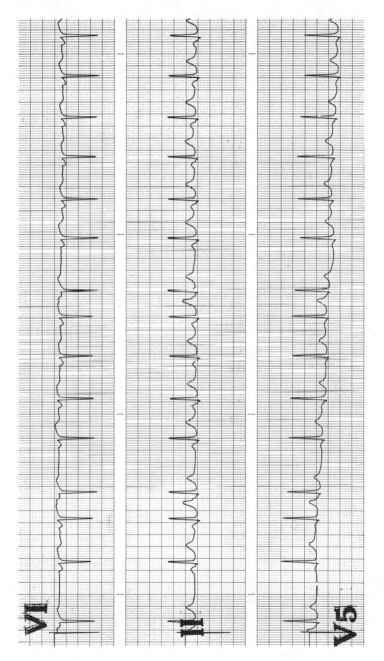

FIG. 29.1

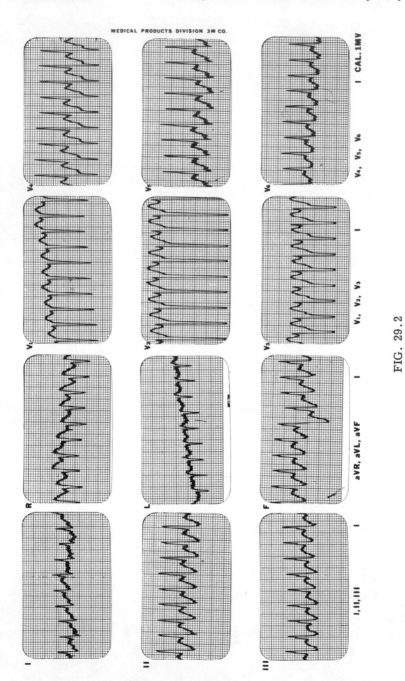

FIG. 29.2

he had tolerated well when it was prescribed for angina pectoris.
He returns to his physician several weeks later, stating that he has
had several syncopal episodes and spells of lightheadedness associated with palpitations and chest discomfort. The ECG recorded
while he has no symptoms is shown in Fig. 29.3.

2. What is the rhythm?
    a) atrial flutter with 2:1 AV conduction
    b) sinus rhythm
    c) junctional rhythm

ANSWER: (a) Narrow QRS complexes occur at regular intervals at
a rate of about 94/minute. In Lead aVL, atrial activity is clearly
identifiable as upright deflections preceding the QRS complexes, and
less clearly identifiable superimposed on the early portion of the T
waves. In Leads II, III, and aVF the atrial activity is identifiable
as predominantly negative deflections preceding the QRS complexes,
and also immediately following the QRS complexes. The atrial rate
appears to be about 188/minute, and the deflections have fixed temporal relationships to the QRS complexes. The regular "sawtooth"
baseline in Leads II, III, and aVF is attributable to flutter waves.
The atrial rhythm is therefore flutter, and there is 2:1 AV conduction.

At this time, coronary and bypass graft angiography, as well as His
bundle electrography are performed. The coronary artery anatomy
is unchanged from the preoperative study and both aortocoronary bypass grafts are patent. His bundle recording reveals a His-Purkinje
system conduction time (HV) time which is just above the upper
limits of normal. For almost twelve hours before and for about
ten hours after the angiographic study the patient receives neither
quinidine nor propranolol. About twenty-two hours following discontinuation of these medications he complains of sudden lightheadedness, palpitations, and chest discomfort, at which time the two continuous ML II rhythm strips shown in Fig. 29.4 are recorded. At
the end of the top strip left carotid sinus massage is performed.

3. What is the tachycardia?
    a) atrial flutter with 1:1 AV conduction
    b) ventricular tachycardia
    c) supraventricular tachycardia (SVT)

ANSWER: (a) All QRS complexes are identical, and occur at a regular rate of about 224/minute until, in the last portion of the bottom
strip, abrupt and variable lengthening of RR intervals occurs. During the increase in QRS cycle length, atrial activity is clearly recognizable as flutter, occurring at a rate of about 224/minute.   The
tachycardia is therefore atrial flutter with 1:1 AV conduction. Ventricular tachycardia with atrial flutter and complete AV block would
not be expected to be effected by carotid sinus massage, and had
ventricular tachycardia terminated fortuitously during carotid massage, the QRS complexes occurring at its termination would be expected to have contours different from those during the tachycardia.

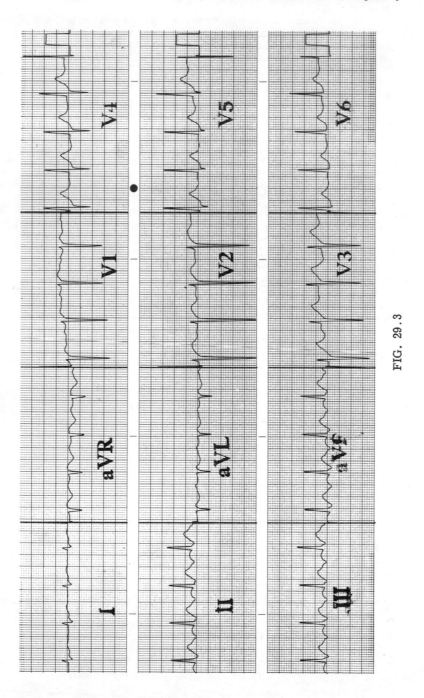

FIG. 29.3

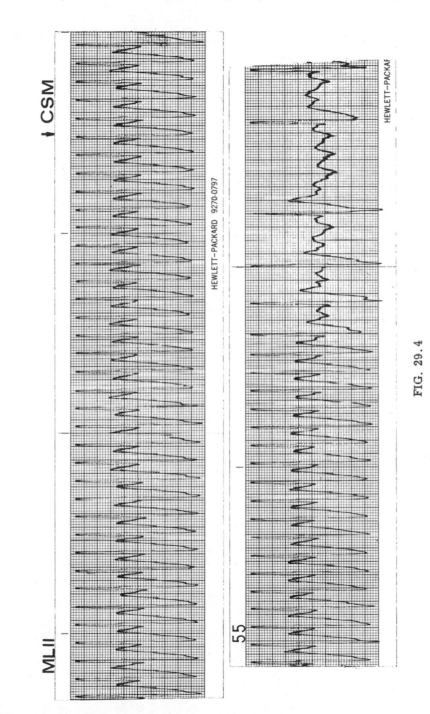

FIG. 29.4

Carotid sinus massage certainly might terminate SVT, following
which there would be a pause in atrial rhythm. This pause is usually
terminated by sinus (but occasionally by ectopic atrial, junctional,
or ventricular) complexes.

Immediately following the carotid sinus massage, the rhythm strip
shown in Fig. 29.5 is recorded. It shows atrial flutter at a rate of
about 230/minute and 2:1 AV conduction. The increase in flutter
rate from about 188/minute in Fig. 29.3 to about 224/minute in
Figs. 29.4 and 29.5, and the change from 2:1 to 1:1 AV conduction
is probably attributable to the withholding of quinidine sulfate and
propranolol in the 22-hour period encompassing the angiographic
study. On the basis of Figs. 29.4 and 29.5, it is likely that the
tachycardia in Fig. 29.2 was atrial flutter with 1:1 AV conduction
rather than SVT.

Propranolol, 40 mg orally every six hours, is administered. The
flutter rate decreases to about 200/minute, and 2:1 AV conduction
is present. However, 48 hours after starting propranolol therapy,
the patient complains of lightheadedness and transiently loses vision.
His rhythm at this time is shown in the two continuous ML II strips
in Fig. 29.6. Throughout the tracing, atrial flutter at a rate of
about 200 per minute is present. In the top strip five QRS complexes
occurring at intervals of about 0.58-0.60 seconds (rate about 100/
minute) are followed by a pause in QRS rhythm of about 8.1 seconds,
following which identical QRS complexes resume at shortening cycle
lengths until an RR interval of about 0.58 seconds (rate about 105/
minute) is reached. Thus, the conduction of atrial flutter impulses
to the ventricles has transiently ceased, causing symptoms of low
cerebral blood flow. Propranolol is withheld, and over the next four
hours the patient has several additional episodes of highgrade AV
block, with periods of ventricular asystole lasting as long as twenty
seconds.

This patient's AV node-His-Purkinje system, which has been capable
of conducting atrial flutter impulses at a rate of 220-230/minute,
suddenly seems incapable of conducting them for a period of about
eight seconds. There are several possible explanations for this
occurrence: (1) propranolol, by decreasing AV nodal conductivity,
might contribute to high-grade AV block; interestingly, when in sinus
rhythm the patient had previously tolerated this medication without
problems in doses higher than he is presently receiving; (2) failure
of impulse conduction could conceivably be due to a disease process
within the His bundle or bundle branches resulting in transient AV
block; the normal intraventricular conduction pattern and the barely
prolonged His-Purkinje system conduction (HV) time documented
two days earlier make this an unlikely possibility; (3) the flutter impulses, penetrating into the AV node to varying depths, could be con-
tinually depolarizing a junctional pacemaker so that an escape beat
or rhythm cannot appear; (4) transient ischemia of the AV node and/or
His bundle in this patient with extensive atherosclerotic disease of

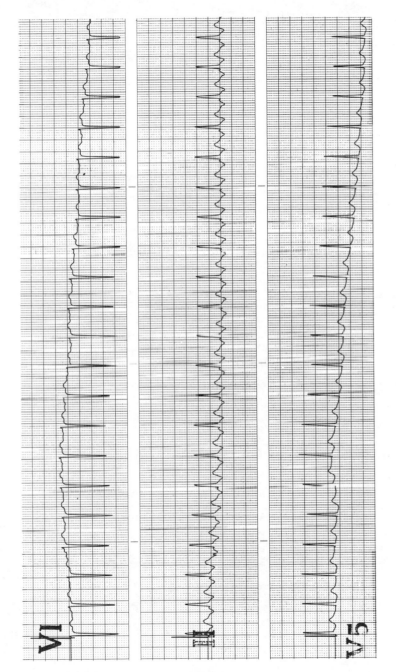

FIG. 29.5

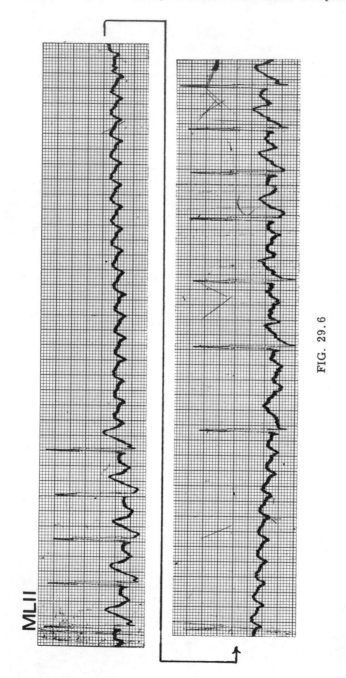

FIG. 29.6

the right coronary artery system, which supplies the AV nodal
artery, could also explain the periods of highgrade AV block.

4. Long-term management of this patient might include:
   a) digoxin administration
   b) propranolol administration
   c) quinidine administration
   d) permanent demand ventricular pacing
   e) DC cardioversion
   f) atropine administration

ANSWER: (a, b, c, d, e) This patient is known to become symptomatic during atrial flutter both because his ventricular rate is very
rapid (in the absence of medications which slow AV conduction,
such as digoxin or propranolol) and also very slow (in the presence
of such medication). It is therefore reasonable to attempt to restore sinus rhythm with DC cardioversion, while prescribing quinidine in the hopes of maintaining it. The patient's abnormal P wave
duration and contour seen in Fig. 29.1, and the previous relapse
from sinus rhythm into atrial flutter despite adequate quinidine administration suggest that long-term maintenance of sinus rhythm
may not be possible. If the atrial flutter is allowed to persist, or
recurs following DC cardioversion, digoxin and/or propranolol will
be required to slow the ventricular rate and to prevent periods of
1:1 AV conduction; these same medications, however, might precipitate periods of highgrade AV block. Permanent demand ventricular pacing will ensure that undue slowing of ventricular rate
will not occur regardless of atrial rhythm, so that propranolol
and/or digoxin might be safely prescribed.

A permanent right ventricular demand endocardial pacemaker is implanted, propranolol 40 mg orally every six hours and quinidine sulfate 300 mg orally every six hours are administered, and DC cardioversion from atrial flutter to sinus rhythm is performed with a 20
watt-second discharge. The post-cardioversion tracing (Fig. 29.7)
shows mild sinus arrhythmia at a rate of about 65/minute, and normal demand pacemaker function. The P waves are abnormally broad,
suggesting an intraatrial conduction abnormality. The PR interval
is prolonged, probably due both to intraatrial conduction delay, and
to AV nodal conduction delay resulting from propranolol administration. The QT interval is prolonged to about 0.52 seconds, probably
due to quinidine administration. The patient is discharged and is
advised to take propranolol 40 mg every six hours and quinidine sulfate 300 mg every six hours.

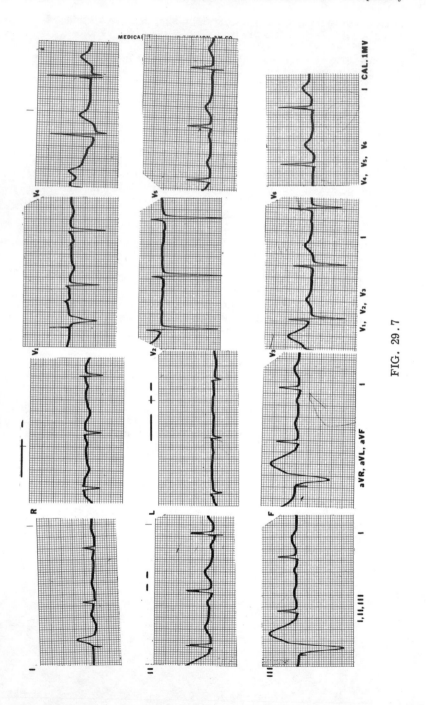

FIG. 29.7

BIBLIOGRAPHY

Pick A: Mechanisms of cardiac arrhythmias: from hypothesis to physiologic fact. Amer Heart J 86:249, 1973.

Damato AN, Lau SH: Concealed and supernormal atrioventricular conduction. Circulation 43:967, 1971.

Bigger JT Jr, Goldreyer BN: The mechanism of supraventricular tachycardia. Circulation 42:673, 1970.

Berkowitz WD, Wit AL, Lau SH, Steiner C, Damato AN: The effects of propranolol on cardiac conduction. Circulation 40:855, 1969.

Arani DT, Carleton RA: The deleterious role of tachycardia in mitral stenosis. Circulation 36:511, 1967.

Childers R: Concealed conduction. In: Symposium on cardiac rhythm disturbances I. Med Clin No Amer 60:149, 1976.

Langendorf R, Pick A: Concealed conduction. Further evaluation of a fundamental aspect of propagation of the cardiac impulse. Circulation 13:381, 1956.

CASE 30: Cardiovascular collapse in a man with acute renal failure complicating hemorrhagic pancreatitis.

A 54-year-old previously healthy man is hospitalized with acute hemorrhagic pancreatitis. During the course of his illness he develops acute renal failure. When he becomes obtunded, with a blood urea nitrogen of 154 mg% and a serum creatinine of 6.4 mg%, dialysis is planned. The two non-continuous tracings shown in Fig. 30.1 are recorded over a 15-minute period as he is being prepared for dialysis.

1. Serial changes in these two tracings are most likely due to which of the following?
    a) hypercalcemia   d) hypokalemia
    b) hypocalcemia   e) uremic pericarditis
    c) hyperkalemia   f) acute myocardial ischemia

ANSWER: (c, f) In the top strip, P wave contour and duration, PR interval, and QRS contour and duration are within normal limits. The T waves, which are somewhat tall and peaked, may be seen in healthy individuals, in the presence of moderate hyperkalemia, and in the earliest stages of acute myocardial ischemia. The short QT interval for this heart rate might occur because of the presence of hypercalcemia, or, possibly, hyperkalemia. In the lower strip of Fig. 30.1, the QRS complexes are wider (0.12 vs. 0.07 seconds), the T waves are taller and now definitely sharply pointed, and the QT interval is longer (0.41 vs. 0.28 seconds) despite no change in heart rate. Such changes, occurring within minutes, could be due to either increases in serum potassium level or to evolution of myocardial ischemia, but in this patient with oliguric renal failure, they are almost certainly due to hyperkalemia. Hypercalcemia would not be expected to prolong the QRS duration or to increase the amplitude of the T waves; hypocalcemia would be expected only to lengthen the QT segment which, in the presence of hyperkalemia might exaggerate the T wave abnormalities; and hypokalemia would be expected to prolong the QT interval by increasing the amplitude of a U wave, and might possibly depress the ST segment. Uremic pericarditis would be expected to elevate the ST segment without altering either the duration of the QRS complex or the QT interval.

2. How might this patient be reasonably managed at this time?
    a) watchful waiting
    b) administration of an ion exchange resin (Kayexalate⊗)
    c) intravenous administration of glucose and insulin
    d) intravenous administration of sodium bicarbonate
    e) intravenous administration of calcium gluconate
    f) intravenous administration of furosemide (Lasix⊗)
    g) performance of peritoneal dialysis or hemodialysis

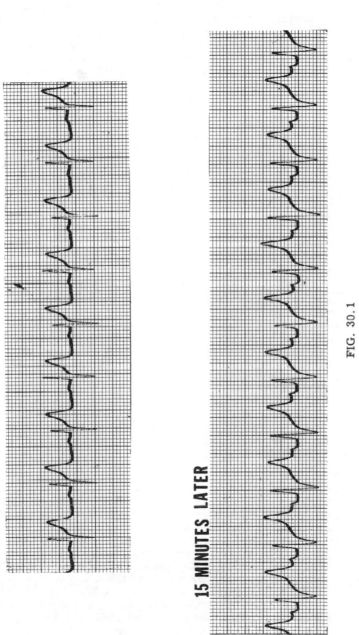

15 MINUTES LATER

FIG. 30.1

ANSWER: (b, c, d, e) Probably the most common cause of death in patients with acute renal failure is hyperkalemia, which may acutely cause serious cardiac arrhythmias and depression of left ventricular performance. Treatment aimed at lowering the serum potassium level as rapidly as possible is therefore in order, and can best be achieved by intravenous administration of sodium bicarbonate, followed by intravenous administration of glucose and insulin, both therapies effecting a shift of potassium from the extracellular to the intracellular fluid. Since the patient's total body potassium content is probably elevated, treatment aimed at removal of potassium from the body is also appropriate. Rectal administration of an ion exchange resin such as Kayexalate ⓡ , and the performance of dialysis will lower total body potassium content, but only over a period of several minutes to hours. While intravenous administration of furosemide may cause significant kaliuresis in patients who are not oliguric, this would not be expected to occur in a patient with oliguric renal failure. Intravenous administration of calcium gluconate does not per se reduce either the serum potassium level or total body potassium content, but may reverse the potentially fatal arrhythmias and conduction abnormalities induced by hyperkalemia.

Within minutes of the recording of the lower strip of Fig. 30.1, the patient develops agonal respirations and diaphoresis, and his peripheral pulses become impalpable. The cardiac rhythm at this time is shown in Fig. 30.2A and B. The patient is immediately given closed chest cardiac compression and artificial ventilation with endotracheal intubation, while intravenous sodium bicarbonate, and glucose and insulin are administered. Tracings 30.2C and 30.2D are recorded within the first five minutes of the start of the resuscitation.

3. Which of the following terms might describe the rhythms in
   Fig. 30.2?
   a) sinoatrial exit block   d) ventricular ectopic beat
   b) atrial arrest   e) group beating
   c) junctional beat

ANSWER: (a, b, c, d, e) It is virtually impossible to accurately analyze in surface electrocardiographic Leads the arrhythmias occurring at the time of hyperkalemia-induced cardiovascular collapse and, because of the emergent nature of the situation, intracardiac recording and pacing have not been used to elucidate the nature of the arrhythmias. Also, the results of experimental studies cannot be directly transposed to the clinical situation in which there are almost always other electrolyte disturbances and acidemia. Despite these limitations, however, certain observations can be made in Fig. 30.2. The last QRS complex in strip A, the sixth in strip B, and the first and last in strip C are similar in contour (but not duration) to the QRS complexes in the lower strip of Fig. 30.1. These complexes are probably stimulated by the P waves which precede them at intervals of 0.14-0.18 seconds, suggesting that they are sinus-stimulated.

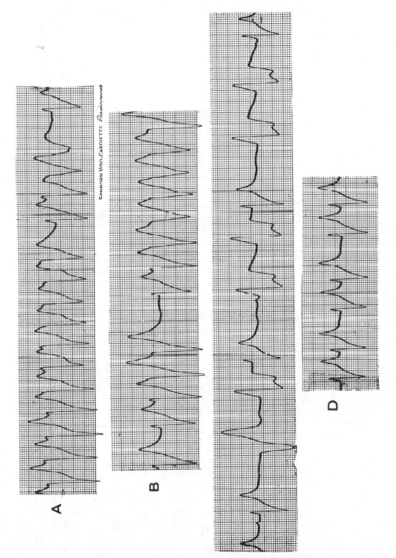

FIG. 30.2

The twelfth QRS complex in Fig. 30.2A and the second in Fig. 30.2B, identical in contour to the sinus-stimulated QRS complexes but not preceded by P waves, are probably junctional in origin. However, one cannot exclude the possibility that these ventricular complexes are stimulated by sinus impulses but that atrial activity (P waves) is not seen because of atrial arrest. This phenomenon has been documented to occur in experimental hyperkalemia and has been termed "sinoventricular conduction". It is possible that the wider and more bizarre QRS complexes that are occurring rapidly and with mild irregularity in Fig. 30.2A and 30.2B are also sinus or junctional in origin. The second QRS complex in Fig. 30.2C, being wide, bizarre, quite different in contour from sinus (or junctional) beats and not preceded by a P wave, is most likely a ventricular ectopic beat. The other wide QRS complexes in Fig. 30.2C (the third, fifth, sixth, eighth, and ninth) may also be ventricular ecto- pic beats but originating in a focus different from the area of origin of the second QRS in Fig. 30.2C. In Fig. 30.2D no P waves are seen but there is group beating in which pairs of identical QRS com- plexes with contours identical to sinus-stimulated QRS complexes are separated by intervals less than twice the intervals between pairs of beats. The group beating could be due to (1) an accelerated junctional rhythm with 3:2 Wenckebach type of exit block from the junctional pacemaker, (2) sinus rhythm with atrial arrest (sinoven- tricular conduction) and 3:2 atrioventricular Wenckebach conduction, or (3) sinus rhythm with 3:2 sinoatrial exit block and atrial arrest, with normal atrioventricular conduction.

Fig. 30.3 displays tracings taken eight, fifteen, and twenty minutes after the onset of treatment, at which time the patient is breathing spontaneously and has an adequate blood pressure. In Fig. 30.3A, seven wide bizarre QRS complexes occur with regularity, and are probably ventricular in origin; they are preceded and followed by runs of supraventricular complexes. This alternation of supraven- tricular and ventricular complexes probably reflects moment-to- moment fluctuation in ionic milieu of the cardiac conduction system. In Fig. 30.3B the rhythm has returned to sinus with normal PR in- terval, prolonged QRS duration, prolonged QT interval for this heart rate, and peaked T waves. Five minutes later (Fig. 30.3C) the PR interval and QRS duration have shortened and the T wave is no longer peaked. These changes toward normal are due to the gradual return of the serum potassium level to normal.

Dialysis is continued for a period of about two weeks, during which time renal function improves and no further cardiac rhythm disturbances occur. However, the patient dies of sepsis.

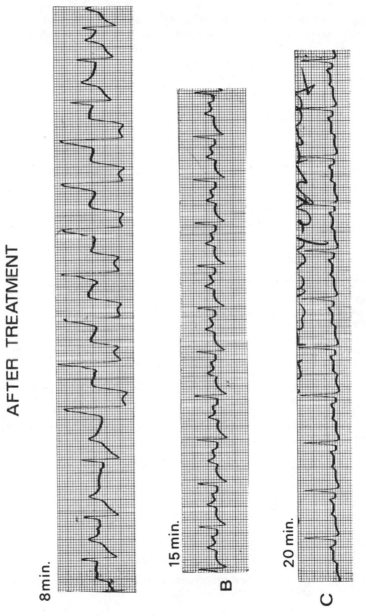

AFTER TREATMENT

8min.

A

15 min.

B

20 min.

C

FIG. 30.3

BIBLIOGRAPHY

Ettinger PO, Regan TJ, Oldewurtel HA, Khan MI: Ventricular conduction delay and asystole during systemic hyperkalemia. Amer J
Cardiol 33:876, 1974.

Bashour T, Hsu I, Gorfinkel HJ, Wickramesekaran R, Rios JC:
Atrioventricular and intraventricular conduction in hyperkalemia.
Amer J Cardiol 35:199, 1975.

Fisch C: Relation of electrolyte disturbances to cardiac arrhythmias. Circulation 47:408, 1973.

Levine HD, Vazifdar JP, Lown B, Merrill JP: "Tent-shaped" T
waves of normal amplitude in potassium intoxication. Amer Heart
J 43:437, 1952.

Merrill JP, Levine HD, Somerville W, Smith S, III: Clinical recognition and treatment of acute potassium intoxication. Ann Int
Med 33:797, 1950.

O'Neil JP, Chung EK: Unusual electrocardiographic finding - Bifascicular block due to hyperkalemia. Amer J Med 61:537, 1976.

Fisch C, Knoebel S, Feigenbaum H, Greenspan L: Potassium and
monophasic action potentials, electrocardiogram, conduction and
arrhythmias. Prog Cardiovasc Dis 8:837, 1966.

VanderArk CR, Ballantyne F, III, Reynolds EW: Electrolytes and
the electrocardiogram. Cardiovasc Clinics 5:270, 1973.

Surawicz B, Lasseter KC: Effect of drugs on the electrocardiogram.
Prog Cardiovasc Dis 13:26, 1970.

Punja MM, Schneebaum R, Cohen J: Bifascicular block induced by
hyperkalemia. J Electrocardiol 6:71, 1973.

Pick A: Arrhythmias and potassium in man. Amer Heart J 72:295,
1966.

Jacobson LB: Sinoventricular conduction during atrial arrest. J
Electrocardiol 5:385, 1972.

Bellet S, Jedlicka J: Sinoventricular conduction and its relation to
sinoatrial conduction. Amer J Cardiol 24:831, 1969.

Sherf L, James TN: A new electrocardiographic concept: Synchronized sinoventricular conduction. Dis Chest 55:127, 1969.

CASE 31: Anterior wall myocardial infarction in a woman with left bundle branch block.

A 72-year-old woman with past history of mild hypertension treated with hydrochlorothiazide comes to the hospital appearing critically ill and complaining of symptoms suggesting acute myocardial infarction. She appears to have low cardiac output despite mild jugular venous distension and scattered rales. There is mild cardiomegaly, abnormal anterior precordial motion, and loud S_3 and S_4 gallops. Except for occasional pauses the pulse is regular at about 110/minute. The blood pressure is 88/60 mmHg in the recumbent position. The 12-Lead ECG, shown in Fig. 31.1A, reveals wide (0.14 seconds) QRS complexes with abnormally leftward mean frontal plane QRS axis of about -45 degrees, and contours suggesting left bundle branch conduction delay. The ST segment elevation in Leads V_2-V_5, much more marked than expected from conduction delay in the left bundle branch, suggests anterior wall ischemic injury. The Lead V_1 rhythm strip is shown in Fig. 31.1B.

1. Which terms describe the rhythm?
   a) sinus tachycardia
   b) non-conducted atrial premature impulses
   c) sinoatrial exit block
   d) Type I second degree AV block
   e) Type II second degree AV block

ANSWER: (a, e) Cycle lengths of the wide QRS complexes are about 0.53-0.56 seconds, and about twice this at 1.06-1.10 seconds. Clearly seen P waves, occurring at regular cycle lengths of about 0.53-0.56 seconds (rate about 107-113 per minute) precede each QRS complex by about 0.17-0.18 seconds, and presumably stimulate them. While accurate determination of P wave axis in Fig. 31.1A is difficult because of the rapid rate, the atrial rhythm is probably sinus. Since P waves which are present in the terminal portions of the T waves of the fifth, sixth, seventh, and twelfth QRS complexes of Fig. 31.1B are on time, neither atrial premature beats nor sinoatrial exit block is present. Thus, the pauses in QRS rhythm are due to block of the sinus impulse within the atrioventricular conduction system. AV block of sinus impulses occurring without variation of the PR intervals of preceding beats is defined as Type II second degree AV block, in contrast to Type I (Wenckebach) second degree AV block, in which beats with varying and often progressively prolonging PR intervals precede the non-conducted on-time sinus impulse.

2. Where is (are) the likely site(s) of AV block of the sinus impulses at this time?
   a) AV node
   b) His-Purkinje system

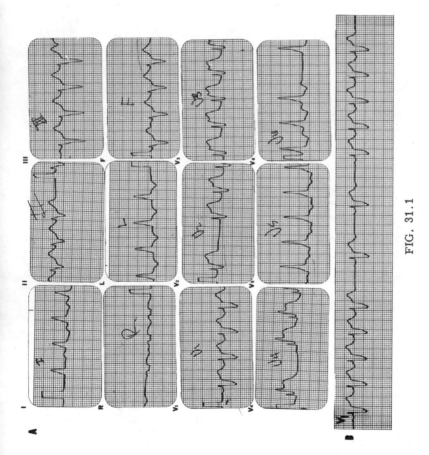

FIG. 31.1

ANSWER: (b) In Type II second degree AV block the atrial impulse
is virtually always blocked within the His-Purkinje system and almost never within the AV node. In the setting of acute anterior wall
myocardial infarction, Type II second degree AV block reflects extensive ischemic injury to the right and left bundle branches, and
perhaps even to the His bundle. The extensive myocardial necrosis
is responsible for the high incidence of cardiogenic shock seen in
this setting. In this patient whose conducted beats show left bundle
branch block, failure of transmission of sinus impulses into the
ventricles suggests conduction block in the His bundle and/or right
bundle branch.

3. How might this rhythm disturbance be reasonably managed?
    a) temporary transvenous right ventricular pacing
    b) atropine administration
    c) isoproterenol administration
    d) corticosteroid administration

ANSWER: (a) Type II second degree AV block in the setting of acute
anterior wall myocardial infarction heralds the occurrence of sudden
complete AV block. Since the resulting bradycardia is often fatal,
its prevention is in order. Temporary transvenous right ventricular endocardial pacing, currently the most effective and reliable
means of preventing bradycardia, should be undertaken as soon as
possible. However, ventricular pacing is felt by some to be a futile
maneuver which does not dramatically alter the 80% mortality of patients with anterior wall myocardial infarction who do develop complete AV block.

The administration of atropine would not be expected to be useful in
this patient, as it has little if any effect on infranodal conduction and
on the rate of infranodal escape pacemakers. Isoproterenol, which
may transiently improve AV conduction and/or increase the rate of
escape pacemakers is ill-advised in acute myocardial infarction
because it increases myocardial oxygen demand and may consequently
increase the extent of myocardial ischemic injury. Corticosteroids,
which may improve AV conduction in the setting of acute inflamma-
tory diseases such as rheumatic fever, have not been documented to
reliably improve AV conduction in acute myocardial infarction.

A temporary transvenous electrode catheter is advanced into the
right ventricle. On three occasions within a five-minute period, it
precipitates ventricular fibrillation which is easily converted to
sinus rhythm with 400 watt-second electrical discharges. Lidocaine,
100 mg, is administered intravenously in an attempt to diminish the
chance of stimulating ventricular fibrillation, and stable right ventricular pacing is achieved.

At this point intravenous diuretics and dopamine are administered
for the treatment of low cardiac output, hypotension, and pulmonary
congestion. Over a period of six hours there is a slight increase in

blood pressure, a slight decrease in heart rate, and there appears
to be a mild increase in cardiac output and a decrease in pulmonary
congestion. A 12-Lead ECG at this time (Fig. 31.2), when compared with the tracing of Fig. 31.1A reveals diminution of the ST
elevation, inversion of the terminal portion of the T waves, and the
appearance of paced ventricular beats (S) terminating the pauses
(of about 1.13 seconds) occasioned by the periods of AV block.

Two hours later the patient complains of a sudden increase in chest
discomfort, and she feels and looks profoundly ill. Now the blood
pressure is 78/50 mmHg, the respirations are labored, and the patient is obtunded. The Lead V_2 rhythm strip shown in Fig. 31.3 is
recorded at this time.

4. Which terms describe the rhythm?
    a) sinus tachycardia
    b) non-conducted atrial premature impulses
    c) Type I second degree AV block
    d) Type II second degree AV block
    e) malfunctioning demand ventricular pacemaker

ANSWER: (a, b) Wide QRS complexes are preceded by P waves at
intervals of 0.18-0.20 seconds, indicating that they are stimulated
by them. However, the P waves falling in the T waves of the third,
fourth, fifth, eighth, ninth, tenth, eleventh, twelfth, and fourteenth
QRS complexes are blocked in the AV conduction system. These
non-conducted P waves are premature, occurring at cycle length
shorter (0.32-0.40 seconds) than the sinus cycle length (measured from the first to second, sixth to seventh, and thirteenth
to fourteenth QRS complexes at about 0.50 seconds). Thus,
the rhythm is sinus tachycardia with frequent atrial premature
impulses which are not conducted to the ventricles, with the
possible exception that the eighth QRS complex is preceded by
a P wave which may be premature. Since all sinus P waves
stimulate QRS complexes, there is no evidence of second degree AV block; only the premature atrial beats are blocked,
because they fall in the refractory period of one or more portions of the AV conduction system.

Since the escape interval of the demand ventricular pacemaker is
about 1.13 seconds, and the longest pause in QRS rhythm is about
1.00 seconds (between the tenth and eleventh QRS complexes), there
is no evidence of pacemaker malfunction.

Over the next several hours there is substantial hemodynamic deterioration, and the patient requires mechanical ventilation. She
begins to pace all QRS complexes, so the pacemaker is temporarily
turned off to see the underlying cardiac rhythm (Fig. 31.4A and B).

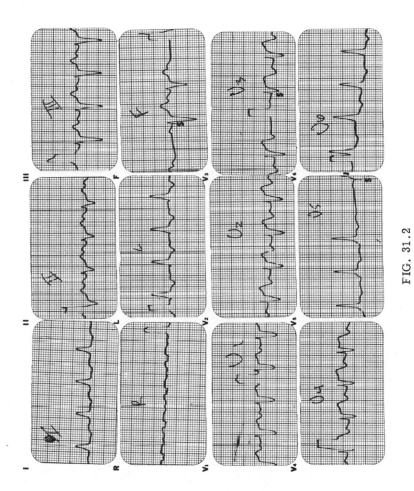

FIG. 31.2

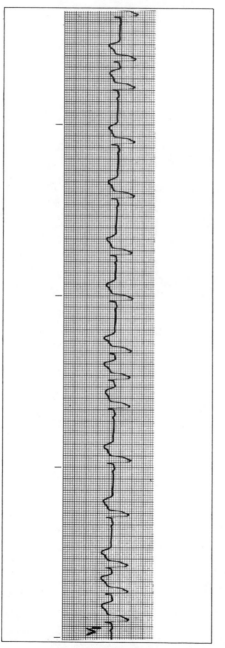

FIG. 31.3

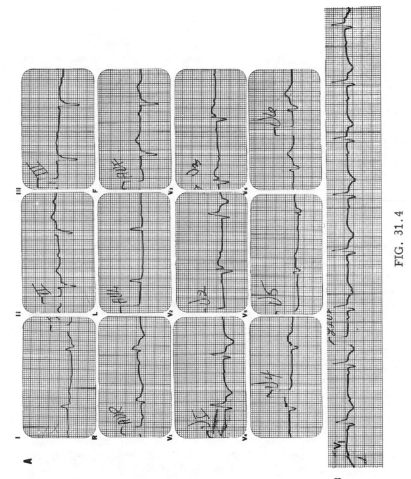

FIG. 31.4

5. Which terms describe the rhythm?
   a) ventriculophasic sinus arrhythmia
   b) complete AV block
   c) Type II second degree AV block
   d) ventricular escape rhythm
   e) junctional escape rhythm
   f) left posterior fascicle escape rhythm

ANSWER: (b, d, f) Wide QRS complexes, occurring at intervals
ranging from 1.07-1.32 seconds (rate about 45-56/minute) show
abnormally leftward mean frontal plane QRS axis of about -75 degrees, suggesting left anterior fascicle block, and contours suggesting right bundle branch block. The QR patterns in Leads V_1-V_4
indicate anterior wall myocardial infarction. In the framework of
the trifascicular intraventricular conduction system composed of
the right bundle branch and the anterior and posterior fascicles of
the left bundle branch, ventricular activation now must be occurring
primarily via the posterior fascicle of the left bundle branch. Atrial
activity, recognized as discrete P waves, is occurring at shorter
cycle length than the QRS complexes. The normal contour, axis,
and duration of the P waves indicate that they are sinus in origin.
Since the P waves and the QRS complexes are temporally unrelated
complete AV block is present. The ventricular rhythm occurring
at a rate of about 45/minute could conceivably be originating in the
left posterior fascicle, or in the AV junction from which it is conducted to the ventricles with block in the right bundle branch and
in the anterior fascicle of the left bundle branch. In this patient,
whose sinus impulses were previously conducted via the right bundle
branch, a junctional rhythm developing below an area of complete
block would be expected to continue to conduct via the right bundle
branch. Here, since the ventricles are activated via the posterior
fascicle of the left bundle branch, the ventricular rhythm most likely
originates in this fascicle, distal to the area of block.

The Lead V_1 rhythm strip clearly shows the first nine P waves occurring at alternating cycle lengths, the remaining eight P waves
occurring at constant cycle length of about 0.58 seconds (rate about
103/minute). The term "ventriculophasic sinus arrhythmia" in the
setting of complete AV block refers to the phenomenon in which two
consecutive P waves which include a QRS complex occur at shorter
cycle length than two consecutive P waves which do not include a
QRS complex. In the rhythm strip shown here the reverse is present; that is, consecutive P waves which include QRS complexes
occur at longer cycle length than those which do not.

Despite ventricular pacing, and pharmacologic and mechanical
maneuvers aimed at supporting the cardiovascular and respiratory
systems, gradual deterioration occurs and the patient dies about
28 hours after the onset of symptoms. Autopsy examination of the
heart reveals a thrombus in the proximal portion of the left anterior
descending coronary artery, and extensive myocardial infarction in-
volving the interventricular septum and the anterior wall of the left
ventricle.

BIBLIOGRAPHY

Atkins JM, Leshin SJ, Blomqvist G, Mullins CB: Ventricular conduction blocks and sudden death in acute myocardial infarction. New
Engl J Med 288:281, 1973.

Bauer GE, Julian DG, Valentine PA: Bundle-branch block in acute
myocardial infarction. Brit Heart J 27:724, 1965.

Godman MJ, Lassers BW, Julian DG: Complete bundle-branch
block complicating acute myocardial infarction. New Engl J Med
282:237, 1970.

Lichstein E, Gupta PK, Chadda KD, Liu H, Sayeed M: Findings of
prognostic value in patients with incomplete bilateral bundle branch
block complicating acute myocardial infarction. Amer J Cardiol
32:913, 1973.

Norris RM, Croxson MS: Bundle branch block in acute myocardial
infarction. Amer Heart J 79:728, 1970.

Ritter WS, Atkins JM, Blomqvist CG, Mullins CB: Permanent
pacing in patients with transient trifascicular block during acute
myocardial infarction. Amer J Cardiol 38:205, 1976.

Waters DD, Mizgala HF: Long-term prognosis of patients with incomplete bilateral bundle branch block complicating acute myocardial
infarction. Role of cardiac pacing. Amer J Cardiol 34:1, 1974.

Killip T: Arrhythmias in myocardial infarction. In: Symposium on
cardiac rhythm disturbances II. Med Clinics of No Amer 60:233,
1975.

Hope RR, Scherlag BJ, El-Sherif N, Lazzara R: Hierarchy of
ventricular pacemakers. Circulation Res 39:883, 1976.

CASE 32: Varying P wave contours in a man with past history
of atrial flutter.

A 70-year-old man with past history of atrial flutter and no evidence
of valvular heart disease has an ECG performed during a routine
follow-up examination, at which time his only medication is digoxin.
Simultaneously recorded Leads V_1 and II are shown in Fig. 32.1.

1. Which of the following are likely to be present in Fig. 32.1?
   a) sinus rhythm
   b) junctional rhythm
   c) atrial premature beat
   d) junctional premature beat
   e) aberrant intraventricular conduction
   f) aberrant intraatrial conduction
   g) normal intraatrial conduction
   h) rhythm of development
   i) ectopic atrial rhythm

ANSWER: (a, c, e, f, g, h) All QRS complexes are of normal duration, indicating that ventricular activation always occurs via the AV
junction-His-Purkinje system. The first eight QRS complexes occur
with reasonable regularity at intervals of about 0.65 seconds (corresponding rate about 92/minute) and are preceded at intervals of about
0.14 seconds by P waves which presumably stimulate them. The
bifid contour of these P waves in Lead II indicates abnormal intraatrial conduction, which might occur if sinus impulses activated
atrial tissue in an abnormal temporal sequence or if an ectopic atrial
pacemaker were initiating atrial activation. The normal PR interval
of 0.14 seconds and the upright P wave in Lead II might occur in
sinus rhythm or in an ectopic atrial rhythm, but would be unusual
in junctional rhythm, in which the PR interval would be expected to
be less than 0.12 seconds and the P wave contour inverted in Lead
II.

The ninth QRS complex (●) occurs prematurely, and its contour,
different from that of all other QRS complexes, indicates that intraventricular activation is slightly altered, or aberrant. This ninth
QRS complex is stimulated by the prematurely occurring P wave
which precedes it by 0.16 seconds and is superimposed upon the T
wave of the eighth QRS complex. The aberrant intraventricular conduction indicates that a portion of the His-Purkinje system is not
fully repolarized (that is, is refractory) when the premature atrial
impulse reaches it; and the PR interval of this beat is longer than
usual (0.16 vs. 0.14 seconds) because AV nodal conduction time is
longer at shorter cycle length.

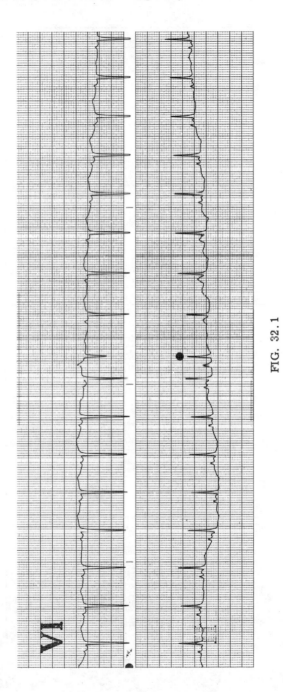

FIG. 32. 1

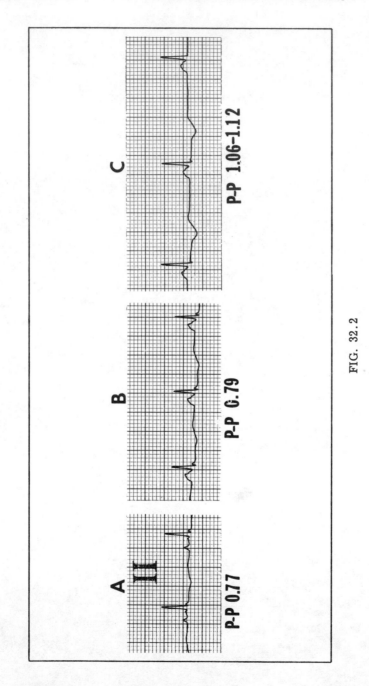

FIG. 32.2

The tenth P wave is of normal contour and duration, suggesting that it is sinus in origin. The P wave following the atrial premature beat occurs after a pause of 0.75 seconds, and then a gradual shortening of PP intervals occurs until, at the thirteenth P wave the previous cycle length of 0.65 seconds is reached. The gradually shortening cycle length of the pacemaker which emerges to terminate the pause occasioned by a premature impulse is referred to as a "rhythm of development" or a "warm-up" phenomenon.

The normal contour of the P wave following the atrial premature beat indicates that intraatrial conduction is normal, and suggests that the emerging atrial rhythm originates in the sinus node. The following two P waves are progressively less normal (that is, more aberrant), and the thirteenth and remaining P waves are clearly aberrant and identical to the first eight P waves. The progressively abnormal intraatrial conduction pattern with shortening cycle length of the presumably sinus pacemaker supports the premise that the basic rhythm is sinus with intraatrial conduction abnormalities that are rate-dependent. In Fig. 32.1, sinus impulses terminating intervals of more than 0.69 seconds have a normal contour because the intraatrial conducting pathways are non-refractory, while sinus impulses terminating intervals of less than 0.69 seconds find some part(s) of the intraatrial conduction pathways refractory and are therefore conducted aberrantly. Similar findings occurred in several other routine tracings from this patient taken some weeks apart (Fig. 32.2, Lead II) in which aberrant intraatrial conduction occurs at the shorter PP intervals of 0.77 seconds; normal intraatrial conduction occurs at the longer PP intervals of 1.06-1.12 seconds; and mildly aberrant conduction occurs at intermediate PP intervals of 0.79 seconds. In this patient, the diagnosis of sinus rhythm, rather than ectopic atrial rhythm, can be established only because of events occurring after the pause occasioned by the atrial premature beat.

Since atrial premature beats have the potential to initiate atrial tachyarrhythmias it is probably appropriate to prescribe medication aimed at suppressing them in this patient with a prior episode of atrial flutter.

BIBLIOGRAPHY

Chung E: Aberrant atrial conduction. Unrecognized electrocardiographic entity. Brit Heart J 34:341, 1972.

James TN, Sherf L: Specialized tissues and preferential conduction in the atria of the heart. Amer J Cardiol 28:414, 1971.

Pick A, Langendorf R, Katz LN: Depression of cardiac pacemakers by premature impulses. Amer Heart J 41:49, 1951.

Sherf L: The atrial conduction system: clinical implications. Amer J Cardiol 37:814, 1976.

CASE 33: Atrial pacing following mitral valve replacement.

A 55-year-old man with atrial fibrillation of several months' duration associated with non-rheumatic mitral regurgitation undergoes
mitral valve replacement in an attempt to alleviate his symptoms
of congestive heart failure. When cardiopulmonary bypass is discontinued, the cardiac rhythm is slow sinus arrhythmia at an average rate of about 45/minute, associated with frequent ventricular
ectopic beats. In order to maintain adequate heart rate, pacing
wires are sewn onto the right ventricle. Despite right ventricular
pacing at rates of 80-100/minute, the patient is slightly hypotensive
notwithstanding an adequate left atrial pressure. In an attempt to
augment left ventricular performance by appropriately timed atrial
systole, pacing wires are sewn onto the right atrium. With atrial
pacing, the blood pressure rises to acceptable levels. The operation is completed and the patient is transferred to the Intensive Care
Unit where over the next several days his course is characterized
by low cardiac output and moderate hypotension. Atrial pacing is
continued and the tracings shown in Fig. 33.1 (two continuous strips
of Lead VI) are recorded at this time.

Except for the sixth QRS complex in the bottom strip, the QRS complexes are narrow, suggesting that the ventricles are being activated
via the normal AV node-His-Purkinje system pathways. The fifth
QRS complex in the bottom strip, being wide and bizarre and premature, is probably a ventricular ectopic beat. There appears to
be group beating of the QRS complexes. Considering the fifth QRS
complex in the top strip as the beginning of a group, every sixth
QRS complex occurs at a much shorter coupling interval to its preceding QRS complex than do the other QRS complexes within a group.

Except for the ventricular ectopic beat, all QRS complexes are preceded by P waves, suggesting that all the narrow QRS complexes
are stimulated by the P waves. The P waves appear to be of three
different contours: deeply inverted, upright, and slightly inverted
and bifid (the sixth and twelfth P waves in the upper strip and probably also the P wave falling in the ST segment of the ventricular
ectopic beat).

1. What are probable mechanisms responsible for the three
    different P waves?
    a) sinus node discharge
    b) atrial pacemaker discharge
    c) fusion of sinus impulses and paced atrial impulses

ANSWER: (a, b, c) The inverted P waves are probably of sinus
origin as they always precede the QRS complexes by about 0.18
seconds and have the expected configuration of sinus P waves in the

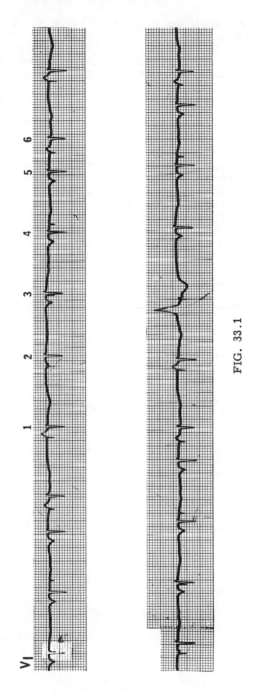

FIG. 33.1

presence of left atrial enlargement. The upright P waves are
initiated by a high frequency deflection, indicating that these are
paced P waves. The slightly inverted, bifid P waves have a pacing
artifact occurring shortly after the onset of an initial negative deflection, suggesting that they are atrial fusion beats, in which the
atria are activated partly via the sinus impulse and partly via the
artificial atrial pacemaker impulse.

The sequence of group beating is as follows: the first three P waves
in the top strip are sinus, occurring at intervals of about 0.91
seconds. The fourth P wave is a paced beat occurring about 0.53
seconds after the preceding sinus P wave. There then follows a
pause of 1.07 seconds which is terminated by another paced P wave.
The failure of a sinus P wave to occur during this pause, which exceeds the previous sinus cycle length, suggests that the first paced
P wave has effected sinus node function and caused a change in its
automatic rate and/or in the conduction of its impulses into atrial
tissue. The sixth P wave, occurring 1.05 seconds later, is a fusion beat in which atrial tissue is depolarized by both a sinus impulse
and a pacemaker-stimulated impulse. The seventh P wave, occurring about 0.91 seconds later, is a sinus beat, indicating that the
previous sinus automatic rate has been reestablished. There follow
two sinus P waves at the same 0.91 second interval. Then a paced
P wave occurring about 0.50 seconds later completes the group.

2. What accounts for the group beating?
   a) sinoatrial Wenckebach periods
   b) pacemaker-induced atrial parasystole

ANSWER: (b) Pacemaker artifacts are occurring with regularity at
intervals of about 1.07 seconds (corresponding rate about 56/minute),
independent of other electrocardiographic events. Thus, the atrial
pacemaker is acting as a parasystolic focus, and the resulting paced
rhythm is an atrial parasystole. The sinus impulses, which are
reasonably constant at a somewhat shorter interval of 0.91-0.92
seconds (corresponding rate about 66/minute), show a slight pause
only after the first paced P wave in each group. The sinus node and
the artificial atrial pacemaker, each discharging essentially independently and at different rates, accounts for the group beating.
There is no systematic shortening of the sinus cycle lengths (PP intervals) to suggest sinoatrial Wenckebach periods.

3. What is the refractory period of atrial tissue surrounding the
   pacemaker as estimated from these two rhythm strips?
   a) 0.20 seconds
   b) 0.30 seconds
   c) 0.40 seconds
   d) 0.50 seconds
   e) cannot accurately be measured but is in the range of 0.39-
      0.49 seconds

ANSWER: (e) The refractory period of atrial tissue surrounding the (parasystolic) paced atrial focus can be defined as the longest interval after a spontaneous P wave when a pacing artifact cannot capture the atrium and stimulate a P wave. It can be estimated here by measuring the longest sinus P-to-pacemaker spike interval which is not followed by a P wave (about 0.39 seconds following the second beat in the top strip). Since pacemaker artifacts falling about 0.49 seconds after a sinus P wave (as in the next to last beat in the bottom strip) do capture the atria, the atrial refractory period is greater than 0.39 seconds and less than 0.49 seconds. For more accurate analysis, longer tracings containing more sinus P-to-pacemaker artifact intervals would be required.

This patient's hemodynamic and cardiac rhythm status stabilized over a period of several days, and his epicardial pacing wires were removed. He was discharged from the hospital and when last seen about five months after discharge was in sinus rhythm with occasional ventricular premature beats. His mitral valve prosthesis appeared to be functioning well, but he was still bothered by symptoms of heart failure on moderate exertion.

BIBLIOGRAPHY

Chung EK: Parasystole. In: Principles of Cardiac Arrhythmias, Baltimore, The Williams and Wilkins Company, 1971.

Chung EK, Walsh TJ, Massie E: Atrial parasystole. Amer J Cardiol.14:255, 1964.

Chung EK, Walsh TJ, Massie E: Combined atrial and ventricular parasystole. Amer J Cardiol. 16:462, 1965.

Fisch C, Chevalier RB: Intermittent atrial parasystole. Circulation 22:1149, 1960.

Langendorf R, Lesser ME, Plotkin P, Levin BD: Atrial parasystole with interpolation; observations on prolonged sinoatrial conduction. Amer Heart J. 63:649, 1962.

Eliakim M: Atrial parasystole, Effect of carotid sinus stimulation, Valsalva maneuver and exercise. Amer J Cardiol. 16:457, 1965.

CASE 34: Rapidly increasing heart rate during acute pulmonary edema.

A 72-year-old woman is hospitalized with an acute myocardial infarction. Her hospital course is complicated initially by congestive heart failure, for which digoxin, furosemide, and isosorbide dinitrate are administered, and later by pericarditis, pleuritis, and fever, for which prednisone is administered. A 12-Lead ECG recorded about two weeks after admission (Fig. 34.1) when she is hemodynamically stable, shows sinus rhythm at a rate of about 98/minute, normal PR interval, left atrial abnormality, normal QRS duration, and abnormalities suggesting extensive anterior wall myocardial infarction. On the twentieth post-infarction day she complains of chest discomfort, and within minutes diaphoresis, hypotension, and tachycardia appear. Morphine sulfate is administered intravenously and the patient is transferred to a monitoring area where her cardiac rhythm is sinus tachycardia at a rate of about 122/minute (Fig. 34.2A). Over a period of about 30 minutes she develops florid pulmonary edema for which she is treated with supplemental inspired oxygen, and intravenous furosemide, aminophylline, and additional morphine sulfate. During treatment, the heart rate increases to 154/minute and the cardiac rhythm, shown in Fig. 34.2B, still appears to be sinus tachycardia. Shortly thereafter the heart rate is noted to be about 190/minute, at which time the rhythm strip shown in Fig. 34.2C is recorded.

1. Which of the following rhythm(s) is (are) likely to be present in Fig. 34.2C?
   a) sinus tachycardia
   b) atrial flutter
   c) ectopic atrial tachycardia
   d) supraventricular tachycardia (SVT)

ANSWER: (c, d) Narrow, normal-appearing QRS complexes, occurring at intervals of about 0.31-0.32 seconds (rate about 187-193/minute) are supraventricular in origin. Atrial activity, detectable as sharp deflections in the ST segments and T waves, occurs in 1:1 relationship to the QRS complexes, but the superimposition of the atrial deflections on the ST segments and T waves precludes accurate analysis of P wave contour and PR intervals. A supraventricular rhythm at this rate is most likely to be SVT or ectopic atrial tachycardia. It is not likely that sinus rhythm would reach this rate in an elderly person, even if critically ill with signs of pronounced sympathetic tone. Atrial flutter is unlikely because the atrial rate of about 190/minute would be unusually slow if 1:1 AV conduction were occurring and 380/minute unusually rapid if 2:1 AV conduction were occurring.

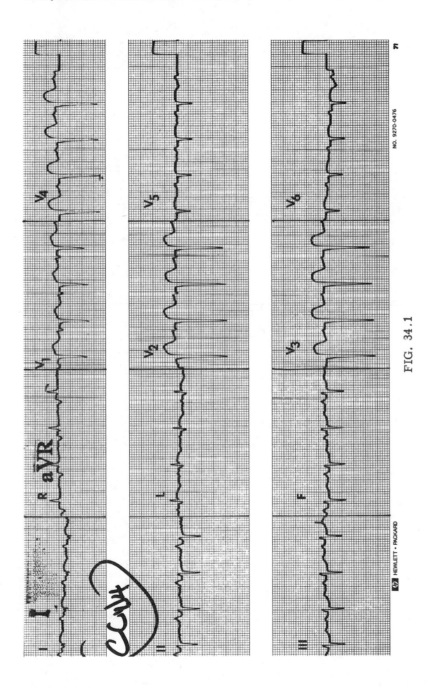

NO. 9270-0476

HEWLETT · PACKARD

FIG. 34.1

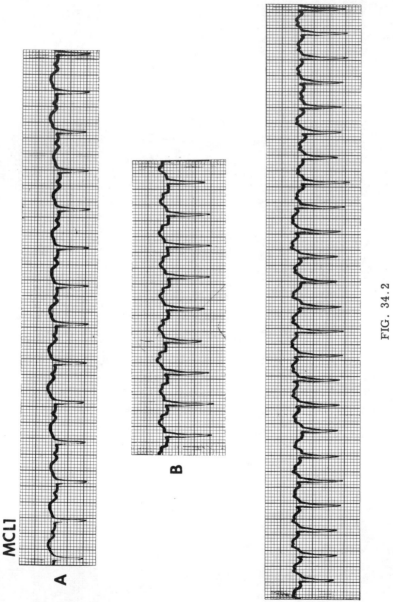

MCL1

A

B

C

FIG. 34.2

The rhythm shown in Fig. 34.2C persists unchanged for approximately thirty minutes, at which time the two continuous rhythm strips in Fig. 34.3 are recorded.

2. In light of the rhythm in Fig. 34.3, what was the rhythm in Fig. 34.2C likely to have been?
    a) ectopic atrial tachycardia
    b) SVT

ANSWER: (a) Throughout Fig. 34.3 atrial activity is occurring with regularity at intervals of 0.31-0.32 seconds (rate about 187-193/ minute). While most RR intervals are equal to the atrial cycle length, some (labeled X) are exactly twice the atrial cycle length, and some (labeled Z) are slightly less than twice the atrial cycle length. The constant P-QRS relationship during the longest RR intervals (X) indicates 2:1 AV conduction (or block) at these times. The pair of QRS complexes (W) following the period of 2:1 AV conduction qualifies as a 3:2 AV Wenckebach period. The PR intervals of the conducted beats at the time of 2:1 AV conduction are slightly shorter than the estimated PR intervals during 1:1 AV conduction, reflecting slower AV nodal conduction at shorter cycle length. This phenomenon is also responsible for the occurrence of the progressively longer PR intervals during the 3:2 AV Wenckebach sequence. The RR intervals labeled Z are 0.04 seconds shorter than twice the atrial cycle length because the PR intervals of the beats terminating them, occurring at longer cycle lengths than the preceding beats, are 0.04 seconds shorter than the PR intervals during 1:1 AV conduction. The occurrence of 1:1, 2:1, and 3:2 AV conduction ratios is typical of ectopic atrial tachycardia in which an independent atrial rhythm stimulates the ventricular rhythm, but is almost unheard of in SVT, in which both atrial and ventricular rhythms result from the same (reentrant) impulse.

3. How might this rhythm be managed in this patient who is profoundly ill with congestive heart failure?
    a) administration of digoxin
    b) withholding of digoxin
    c) administration of propranolol
    d) administration of potassium chloride
    e) watchful waiting with careful observation
    f) DC cardioversion
    g) administration of diphenylhydantoin intravenously

ANSWER: (a, b, d, e, g) In this critically ill patient with post-infarction congestive heart failure and possibly a new ischemic event, left ventricular performance is undoubtedly depressed, and cardiac output is dependent primarily on heart rate. As a heart rate of 190 beats per minute is far too rapid to be optimum, however, slowing of heart rate is desirable. This could be achieved either by depressing AV conduction (increasing AV block) or by converting the rhythm to sinus. Administration of digoxin to patients with atrial

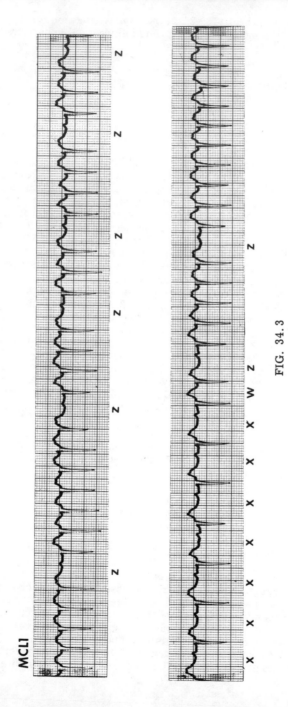

FIG. 34.3

tachycardia with 1:1 AV conduction, whether or not digitalis-induced, may effectively slow the ventricular rate and does not appear to be particularly risky. However, in the presence of digitalis-induced atrial tachycardia with 2:1 AV conduction, digoxin should be withheld as it is unlikely to achieve any hemodynamic improvement in the presence of a ventricular rate of about 95/minute, and has been observed to cause more serious, commonly fatal, arrhythmias. While administration of propranolol, by increasing AV block and slowing ventricular rate in ectopic atrial tachycardia, might conceivably improve congestive heart failure if it were due to tachycardia per se, its beta-blocking effect makes its use in this patient with severely depressed ventricular performance very risky. Although administration of potassium chloride may result in conversion of digitalis-induced atrial tachycardia with 2:1 AV block to sinus rhythm, prior to conversion it almost invariably results in 1:1 AV conduction, which may cause further hemodynamic deterioration in critically ill patients. Since the 1:1 AV conduction occurs concomitantly with a slight decrease in atrial rate, the enhanced AV conduction may be due more to the slower atrial rate, at which the AV node can conduct each atrial impulse, than to facilitation of AV conduction by the potassium chloride per se. Since this patient has atrial tachycardia with 1:1 AV conduction already, administration of potassium chloride at this time does not carry the risk of increasing the ventricular rate. However, potassium chloride should always be used with caution in critically ill patients who, by virtue of having frequent changes in fluid compartments, electrolyte levels, and pH may rapidly develop fatal hyperkalemia. Intravenous administration of diphenylhydantoin may convert this rhythm to sinus, but it should be administered at a rate of no more than 50 mg/min to avoid hypotension. DC cardioversion may successfully restore sinus rhythm, but may also precipitate serious ventricular arrhythmias if the rhythm being cardioverted is digitalis-induced. Since the congestive heart failure probably played a role in the development and persistence of the atrial tachycardia, sinus rhythm may not be maintained until an improved hemodynamic state is achieved. Careful observation of the rhythm, while vigorous treatment of the congestive failure is continued, is also reasonable.

The patient continues to receive intensive treatment for her pulmonary edema, and over a five-hour period she recovers to return to her previous hemodynamic state. As atrial tachycardia with 1:1 AV conduction persists, blood is drawn for serum digoxin level measurement, and digoxin 0.125 mg is administered intravenously. About one hour later the 12-Lead ECG shown in Fig. 34.4 is recorded. Note that the limb leads are recorded at double standard and the precordial leads at normal standard.

4. Which of the following support the diagnosis of ectopic atrial tachycardia?
    a) P wave contour   c) P wave duration
    b) P wave axis   d) the isoelectric baseline

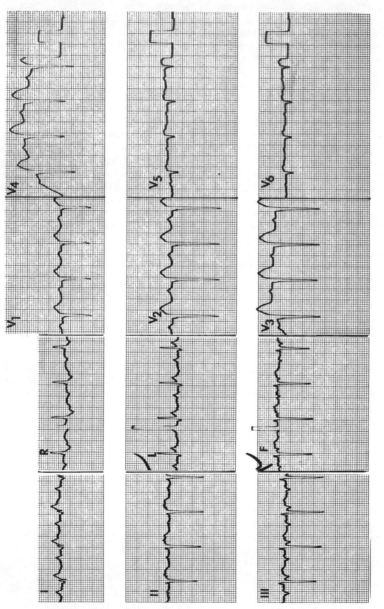

FIG. 34.4

ANSWER: (a, d) The intravenous administration of 0.125 mg of digoxin has not altered the atrial rate but, presumably by slowing AV nodal conduction, has resulted in 2:1 AV block, which allows more accurate analysis of atrial activity. The P waves in Fig. 34.4 have different contour, axis, and duration from the sinus P waves in Fig. 34.1, lending further support to the diagnosis of atrial, rather than sinus, tachycardia. The isoelectric baseline in the inferior Leads also supports the diagnosis of atrial tachy- cardia and excludes the diagnosis of atrial flutter. The sharp con- tours of the P waves are typical of P waves in ectopic atrial tachy- cardia. While neither P wave axis nor duration in atrial tachycardia arc adequately discussed in the literature, the majority of patients are said to have predominantly upright P waves in Lead II, and P duration in many examples does not appear very different from that in sinus rhythm. In this patient P wave duration is about 0.10 sec- onds during both sinus rhythm and atrial tachycardia. The mildly abnormal P wave axis of -10 degrees occurs in a minority of in- stances of ectopic atrial tachycardia.

The patient's atrial tachycardia with 2:1 AV conduction persists for about six hours, when 1:1 AV conduction recurs. Another 0.125 mg of digoxin is administered intravenously and about twenty minutes later 2:1 AV conduction is again present. The serum digoxin level drawn prior to the administration of the first dose of intravenous digoxin, is determined to be elevated at 2.5 ng/ml, so further di- goxin is withheld. The atrial tachycardia, with predominant 2:1 AV conduction and occasional periods of 1:1 AV conduction, persists for another thirty-six hours, at which time it spontaneously ter- minates, resulting in sinus rhythm. A serum digoxin level at this time is normal at 1.2 ng/ml and the atrial tachycardia was there- fore most likely digitalis-induced. After conversion to sinus rhythm, the 12-Lead ECG is identical to the previous tracing of Fig. 34.1. When last seen six weeks after the episode of atrial tachycardia, the patient continues to have evidence of depressed left ventricular per- formance, but has no new arrhythmias.

BIBLIOGRAPHY

Fisch C: Relation of electrolyte disturbances to cardiac arrhyth- mias. Circulation 47:408, 1973.

Fisch C, Knoebel SB: Recognition and therapy of digitalis toxicity. Prog Cardiovasc Dis 13:71, 1970.

Conn RD: Diphenylhydantoin sodium in cardiac arrhythmias. New Engl J Med 272:277,1965.

Karliner JS: Intravenous diphenylhydantoin sodium (Dilantin) in cardiac arrhythmias. Dis Chest 51:256, 1967.

Goldschlager AW, Karliner JS: Ventricular standstill after intravenous diphenylhydantoin. Amer Heart J 74:410, 1967.

Lesser L: Atrial tachycardia in acute myocardial infarction. Ann Int Med 86:582, 1977.

Lown B, Levine HD: Atrial arrhythmias, digitalis, and potassium. Landsberger Medical Books, Inc., New York, 1958.

Lown B, Wyatt NF, Levine HD: Paroxysmal atrial tachycardia with block. Circulation 21:129, 1960.

Mason DT, Zelis R, Lee G, Hughes JL, Spann JF, Amsterdam EA: Current concepts and treatment of digitalis toxicity. Amer J Cardiol 27:547, 1971.

Lown B, Marcus F, Levine HD: Digitalis and atrial tachycardia with block. New Engl J Med 260:301, 1959.

Chung EK: Digitalis-induced cardiac arrhythmias. In: Principles of Cardiac Arrhythmias, Williams and Wilkins Company, Baltimore, 1971.

Bernstein RB, Stanzler RM: PAT with latent block. Arch Int Med 118:154, 1966.

El-Sherif N: Supraventricular tachycardia with atrioventricular block. Brit Heart J 32:46, 1970.

Reynolds EW: The use of potassium in the treatment of heart disease. Amer Heart J 70:1, 1965.

Fisch C, Martz BL, Priebe FH: Enhancement of potassium-induced atrioventricular block by toxic doses of digitalis drugs. J Clin Invest 39:1885, 1960.

Zimmerman HB, Gentsch KW, Gale AH: The action of potassium on the atrioventricular node in digitalized patients. Dis Chest 43: 377, 1963.

Storstein O, Rasmussen K: Digitalis and atrial tachycardia with block. Brit Heart J 36:171, 1974.

Damato AN: Diphenylhydantoin: Pharmacological and clinical use. Prog Cardiovasc Dis 12:1, 1969.

Damato AN, Berkowitz WD, Patton RD, Lau SH: The effect of diphenylhydantoin on atrioventricular and intraventricular conduction in man. Amer Heart J 79:51, 1970.

CASE 35: Tachyarrhythmias occurring in the first hours of acute
myocardial infarction.

A 48-year-old man is hospitalized and treated with anticoagulants
for deep vein thrombophlebitis which has resulted in pulmonary
embolism with signs of pulmonary hypertension. While smoking
in bed after breakfast, he has the sudden onset of severe oppressive
chest pain accompanied by diaphoresis, weakness, and lightheadedness. An electrocardiogram recorded at this time shows sinus
rhythm at a rate of about 80/minute, first degree AV block, and ST
segment elevation in the inferolateral leads consistent with acute
inferior myocardial injury. Within minutes he develops complete
AV block with a junctional rhythm at a rate of about 45/minute.
The blood pressure falls to 80 mmHg systolic, and the patient becomes disoriented. Intravenous atropine, 0.6 mg, given twice in
a three-minute period, results in an increase in the sinus rate to
about 95/minute, an increase in the junctional rate to about 60/
minute, but complete AV block persists. The decision is then made
to insert a temporary transvenous right ventricular demand pacemaker. When the patient arrives in the cardiac catheterization
laboratory ten minutes later the sinus rate is about 100/minute and
there is 1:1 AV conduction with a normal PR interval, the blood
pressure is 120/80, and the patient looks and feels much better.
Suddenly, wide bizarre QRS complexes are noted on the monitor
oscilloscope and the continuous Lead MCL_1 rhythm strip shown in
Fig. 35.1 is recorded.

1. Which terms characterize the rhythm?
    a) accelerated ventricular rhythm
    b) ventricular tachycardia
    c) AV dissociation with capture beats
    d) junctional tachycardia with aberrant intraventricular conduction
    e) sinus arrhythmia
    f) fusion beats
    g) ventricular parasystole

ANSWER: (a, c, e, f) In the top strip there is alternation of two
kinds of QRS complexes: normal-appearing rSr' complexes of normal duration, and bizarre qRS complexes of abnormally long duration. The rSr' complexes are preceded by negatively directed P
waves at intervals of about 0.13 seconds, suggesting that they are
sinus-stimulated complexes. The variability in PP intervals indicates sinus arrhythmia. P waves are not always seen because they
are intermittently occurring simultaneously with the wide QRS complexes. The wide qRS complexes, occurring at relatively constant
cycle length of 0.58-0.61 seconds, and completely unrelated to sinus
P waves, are probably ventricular in origin.

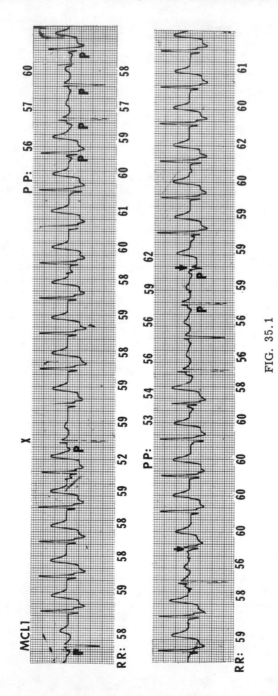

FIG. 35.1

Junctional complexes would not be expected to have contours and durations so different from sinus-stimulated complexes occurring at about the same rate.

In the top strip a sinus-stimulated QRS complex is followed about 0.58 seconds later by a ventricular beat which initiates a run of five ventricular beats. This run is interrupted by a sinus capture beat occurring at cycle length shorter than the cycle length of the ventricular rhythm (0.52 vs. 0.58-0.61 seconds). The ensuing pause of 0.59 seconds is terminated by a ventricular beat which initiates a run of eight ventricular beats, which is in turn interrupted by a sinus capture beat occurring at cycle length shorter than the cycle length of the ventricular rhythm at this time (0.59 vs. 0.60 seconds). Then gradual lengthening of PP intervals to 0.60 seconds allows the emergence of a ventricular beat. Since the interval between the two ventricular beats which enclose a single sinus beat (X) (1.11 seconds) is less than twice the cycle length of the ventricular rhythm (2 X 0.58-0.60 = 1.16-1.20 seconds), the sinus beat has altered the ventricular rhythm. Thus, the focus in which this ventricular rhythm originates is not protected from depolarization by other impulses and is therefore not a parasystolic focus.

The same phenomenon of QRS alternation occurs in the bottom strip, except that the fourth and twelfth QRS complexes (arrows) have contours different from the two predominant complexes and from each other. The twelfth QRS complex, following a P wave at an interval of about 0.13 seconds (about the PR interval of conducted sinus beats) and occurring at an interval of 0.59 seconds (about the cycle length of the ventricular rhythm) is probably a fusion beat in which impulses from both the ventricular focus and sinus node activate the ventricles. The fourth QRS complex is probably a fusion beat also, but baseline artifact precludes more accurate analysis of its contour.

The ventricular rhythm, emerging at a rate of 100-102 per minute during the slow phase of sinus arrhythmia at about the same rate, and capable of being terminated by sinus beats, is an accelerated ventricular rhythm (this has been given the name "accelerated idioventricular rhythm"). It usually occurs within the first 24-36 hours of acute myocardial infarction, its rate varying from about 60 to 100 beats per minute, within a few beats per minute of the sinus rate. The occurrence of two rhythms at similar but slightly varying rates results in transient AV dissociation, of which the onset and offset are often characterized by fusion beats. Accelerated ventricular rhythm is felt to be different from parasystolic rhythm in that its focus of origin is not protected from depolarization by other impulses. Accelerated ventricular rhythm is distinguished from ventricular tachycardia in that 1) its rate is slower and is usually close to the prevailing sinus rate, 2) its onset occurs at relatively long cycle lengths, and 3) it has never been known to degenerate into ventricular fibrillation. Since this rhythm is almost always hemodynamically and electrically benign, no specific therapy is indicated at this time.

As the patient is now hemodynamically stable and since 1:1 AV conduction is now present, the decision is made not to insert a temporary transvenous right ventricular pacemaker. However, since
he has had pre-existing pulmonary hypertension due to pulmonary
embolism, measurement of intracardiac pressures is felt to be
advisable at this time. In an attempt to pass a Swan-Ganz catheter
into the pulmonary artery the catheter becomes coiled in the right
ventricle and the rhythm shown in Fig. 35.2 occurs.

2. How might this rhythm reasonably be managed?
   a) DC defibrillation
   b) DC cardioversion
   c) intravenous lidocaine administration
   d) withdrawal of the Swan-Ganz catheter from the right ventricle
   e) closed chest cardiac massage
   f) endotracheal intubation

ANSWER: (a, d, e) The coarse rapid irregular rhythm is ventricular fibrillation. Since the ventricular fibrillation was probably induced by the Swan-Ganz catheter, it should be immediately removed
from the right ventricle. In a cardiac catheterization laboratory
where a DC defibrillator is present, immediate defibrillation is
essential. Should there be a delay in performing DC defibrillation,
closed chest cardiac massage should be employed as a temporizing
maneuver. While endotracheal intubation is important in managing
cardiopulmonary arrest, it is of lower priority than rapidly performed defibrillation which, reestablishing adequate circulation,
will result in return of adequate respiratory function. Whereas intravenous lidocaine administration may prevent ventricular ectopy
and may terminate ventricular tachycardia, it would not be expected
to terminate ventricular fibrillation. The advantage of DC cardioversion is the introduction of an electrical discharge synchronized
to the QRS complex such that the chance of the electrical discharge
initiating ventricular fibrillation is minimized. Since ventricular
fibrillation is already present, synchronization of the DC impulse
offers no advantage. Of critical importance, however, is the fact
that during ventricular fibrillation the QRS voltage may not be great
enough to be detected by the sensing device of a DC cardioverter
which therefore may not discharge.

DC defibrillation is achieved with a 400 watt-second electrical discharge, following which the rhythm shown in Fig. 35.1 reappears.
The Swan-Ganz catheter is now successfully and uneventfully passed
into the pulmonary artery and the patient transferred to the Coronary Care Unit. He is treated with morphine sulfate for his chest
discomfort,which disappears over a period of 12 hours. Serial
electrocardiograms document the evolution of an inferior wall myocardial infarction. The patient's remaining hospital course is uneventful and he is discharged 20 days later. His only discharge
medication is coumadin, administered for treatment of the thrombophlebitis and pulmonary embolism.

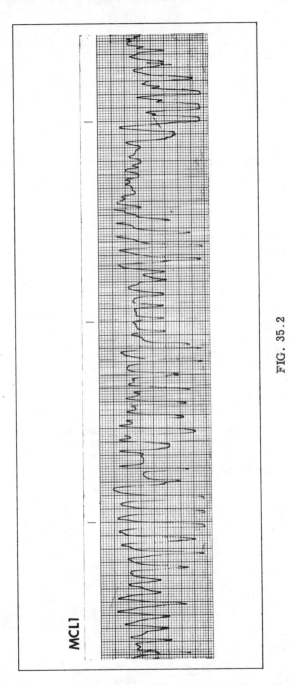

FIG. 35.2

BIBLIOGRAPHY

DeSanctis RW, Block P, Hutter AM: Tachyarrhythmias in myocardial infarction. Circulation 40:681, 1972.

deSoyza N, Bissett JK, Kane JJ, Murphy ML, Doherty JE: Association of accelerated idioventricular rhythm and paroxysmal ventricular tachycardia in acute myocardial infarction. Amer J Cardiol 34:667, 1974.

Norris RM, Mercer CJ: Significance of idioventricular rhythms in acute myocardial infarction. Prog Cardiovasc Dis 16:455, 1974.

Gallagher JJ, Damato AN, Lau SH: Electrophysiologic studies during accelerated idioventricular rhythms. Circulation 44:671, 1971.

Massumi RA, Ertem GE, Vera Z: Aberrancy of junctional escape beats. Amer J Cardiol 29:351, 1972.

Walsh TJ: Ventricular aberration of A-V nodal escape beats. Comments concerning the mechanism of aberration. Amer J Cardiol 10:217, 1962.

Ryan NJ, Cayler GG: Ventricular fibrillation during cardiac catheterization successfully treated with external defibrillation and closed chest cardiac massage. Amer J Cardiol 10:120, 1962.

Swan HJC, Ganz W, Forrester J, Marcus H, Diamond G, Chonette D: Catheterization of the heart in man with use of a flow-directed balloon-tipped catheter. New Engl J Med 283:447, 1970.

Braunwald E, Swan HJC (Eds): Cooperative Study on Cardiac Catheterization. Circulation 37:1 (Suppl 3), 1968.

Schamroth L: Idioventricular tachycardia. J Electrocardiol. 1:205, 1968.

Rothfeld EL, Zucker IR, Parsonnet V et al.: Idioventricular rhythm in acute myocardial infarction. Circulation 37:203, 1968.

CASE 36: Wide QRS tachycardia in a woman with Wolff-Parkinson-White syndrome.

A 67-year-old woman with a past history of Wolff-Parkinson-White syndrome and tachycardias is currently being treated with digoxin 0.25 mg daily, and propranolol, 40 mg four times daily. She now states that she is having another tachycardia of sudden onset. She states further that she is allergic to quinidine and has had severe arthralgias as a result of procainamide administration. She has no history of angina or congestive heart failure. She looks and feels moderately weak, the blood pressure is 85/60 in the supine position, the skin is somewhat pale and the extremities somewhat cool. The 12-Lead ECG is shown in Fig. 36.1.

1. Which of the following terms describe the rhythm in Fig. 36.1?
   a) supraventricular tachycardia (SVT)
   b) ventricular tachycardia with 1:1 ventriculoatrial conduction
   c) atrial flutter with 2:1 AV conduction
   d) aberrant intraventricular conduction

ANSWER: (a, d) Wide QRS complexes having a left bundle branch block pattern occur with regularity at a rate of about 167/minute. While P waves are not unequivocally identifiable, they may account for the sharp negative deflections on the T waves in Lead III and for the sharp upward deflections on the T waves in Lead aVL; in both Leads these deflections precede the QRS complex by about 0.14 seconds. The P waves are not seen with sufficient clarity to measure their frontal plane axis, determination of which might be helpful in assessing whether atrial activation occurs in antegrade or retrograde manner. The isoelectric segments in Leads II, III, and aVF suggests that atrial flutter waves are not present.

Patients with Wolff-Parkinson-White syndrome commonly have supraventricular arrhythmias but only very rarely have ventricular tachycardia. Thus, while the ECG is compatible with SVT and with ventricular tachycardia with 1:1 retrograde VA conduction, the most likely rhythm is SVT. The absence of a delta wave suggests that antegrade AV conduction does not occur via an accessory AV conduction pathway, but the left bundle branch block pattern indicates that ventricular activation occurs predominantly, if not exclusively, via the right bundle branch system. In the majority of instances of SVT in the Wolff-Parkinson-White syndrome, antegrade AV conduction occurs via the normal AV junction-His-Purkinje system, and retrograde VA conduction via the anomalous pathway, as is presumably the case here.

The reason for the aberrant (left bundle branch block type) intraventricular conduction is uncertain. It may be due simply to a rate-dependent conduction delay in the left bundle branch. An alternative

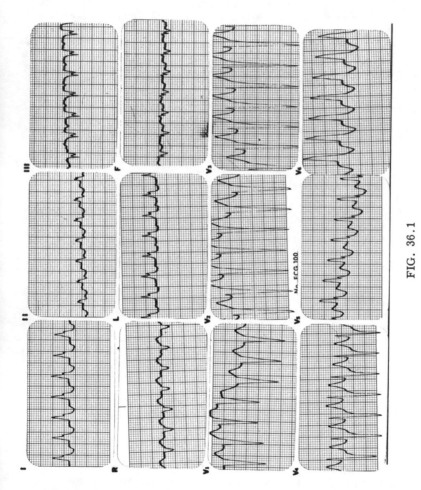

FIG. 36.1

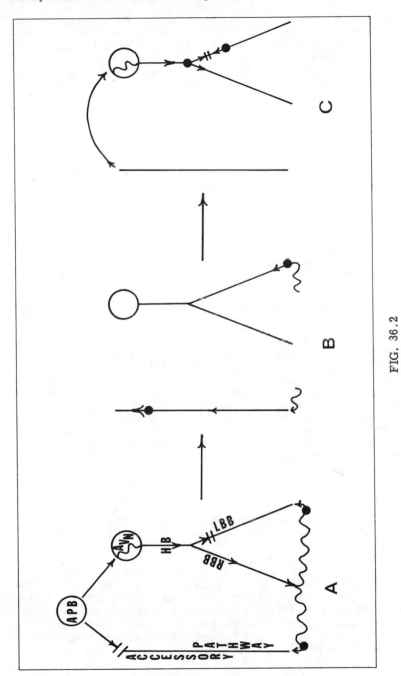

FIG. 36.2

possibility, shown in Fig. 36.2A, is that the atrial premature beat (APB) that presumably initiates the SVT blocks in the accessory AV conduction pathway and in the left bundle branch (LBB) which are still refractory, but initiates ventricular activation via the right bundle branch (RBB). Persistence of the left bundle branch conduction delay might then be due to repeated retrograde depolarization of the left bundle branch (Fig. 36.2B) such that it is in a refractory state when the antegradely returning impulse reaches it (Fig. 36.2C).

2. How might this patient reasonably be managed at this time?
   a) intravenous Tensilon Ⓡ administration
   b) carotid sinus massage
   c) intravenous Vasoxyl Ⓡ administration
   d) intravenous Aramine Ⓡ administration
   e) intravenous Neosynephrine Ⓡ administration
   f) watchful waiting
   g) DC cardioversion

ANSWER: (a, b, c, d, e, g) Treatment of SVT in patients with Wolff-Parkinson-White syndrome requires interruption of the circus movement of impulses into the ventricles via the AV node-His-Purkinje system, and from the ventricles into the atria via the accessory AV conduction pathway. Since abrupt changes in autonomic nervous system traffic into the AV node may terminate SVT, possibly, effective therapeutic interventions include carotid sinus massage, intravenous administration of Tensilon Ⓡ and use of agents with alpha-adrenergic stimulating properties (Aramine Ⓡ , Vasoxyl Ⓡ , Neosynephrine Ⓡ). There is no unquestionably superior therapy in this situation, but if the patient is at the point of cardiovascular collapse, DC cardioversion should be performed immediately. While carotid sinus massage is not likely to terminate SVT in a hypotensive patient, it takes only a few seconds and is not likely to cause serious problems. However, increasing the blood pressure to 160-170 mmHg systolic with alpha-adrenergic stimulating agents and then performing carotid sinus massage, or administering Tensilon Ⓡ intravenously, is more likely to cause termination of the arrhythmia.

The patient is initially given carotid sinus massage without effect, so Aramine Ⓡ solution (50 mg in 250 ml of 5% dextrose in water) is administered by continuous intravenous infusion. When a blood pressure of 160/80 is achieved, right carotid sinus massage (CSM) is repeated while the Lead II rhythm strip shown in Fig. 36.3 is recorded. It shows termination of the tachycardia, and a gradual appearance of sinus P waves which stimulate wide, bizarre QRS complexes. The 12-Lead ECG obtained shortly after conversion to sinus rhythm shows a PR interval of about 0.12 seconds, delta waves, and QRS complexes of about 0.13 seconds duration, establishing the diagnosis of ventricular preexcitation (Fig. 36.4). An atrial premature beat is seen in Lead V1, and ventricular premature beats in Leads III and V1.

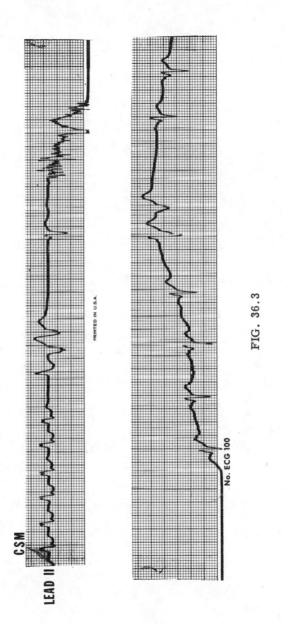

FIG. 36.3

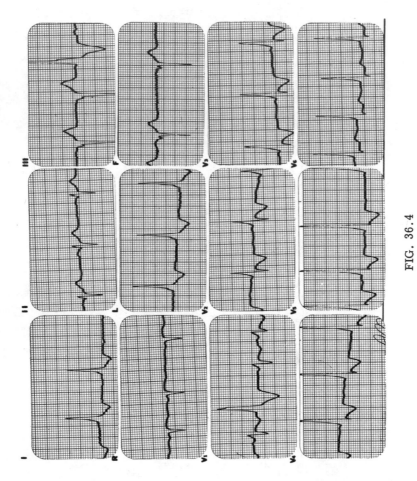

FIG. 36.4

BIBLIOGRAPHY

Durrer D, Schoo L, Schuilenburg RM, Wellens HJJ: The role of premature beats in the initiation and the termination of supraventricular tachycardia in the Wolff-Parkinson-White syndrome. Circulation 36:644, 1967.

James TN: The Wolff-Parkinson-White syndrome: evolving concepts of its pathogenesis. Prog Cardiovasc Dis 13:159, 1970.

Moss AJ, Aledort LM: Use of Edrophonium (Tensilon) in the evaluation of supraventricular tachycardias. Amer J Cardiol 17:58, 1966.

Narula OS: Wolff-Parkinson-White syndrome. A review. Circulation 47:872, 1973.

Wellens HJJ, Durrer D: Effect of procainamide, quinidine, and ajmaline in the Wolff-Parkinson-White syndrome. Circulation 50:114, 1970.

Wellens HJJ, Durrer D: Effects of digitalis on atrioventricular conduction and circus-movement tachycardias in patients with Wolff-Parkinson-White syndrome. Circulation 47:1221, 1973.

Wellens HJJ, Durrer D: Supraventricular tachycardia with left aberrant conduction due to retrograde invasion into the left bundle branch. Circulation 38:474, 1968.

CASE 37: Paroxysms of profound weakness two months after
aortocoronary bypass graft surgery.

A 48-year-old man with no past history of cardiovascular disease
is admitted to the hospital with symptoms suggesting acute myocardial ischemia. The patient is anxious and diaphoretic, but the
physical examination is otherwise within normal limits. The 12-
Lead ECG recorded immediately after the examination is shown in
Fig. 37.1.

1. Which of the following is (are) present in Fig. 37.1?
    a) left bundle branch block
    b) right bundle branch block
    c) left anterior fascicle block
    d) inferior wall myocardial infarction

ANSWER: (b) The normal 1:1 P-QRST relationship with normal P
waves and normal PR intervals indicates sinus rhythm. The abnormally prolonged QRS duration of 0.13-0.14 seconds indicates delayed intraventricular conduction, and the QRS contours in the precordial Leads suggesting right bundle branch block indicate that the
delayed intraventricular conduction is due to ventricular activation
occurring predominantly via the left bundle branch system. While
accurate measurement of mean frontal plane QRS axis in a 12-Lead
ECG showing right bundle branch block is sometimes difficult, the
large positive forces in Lead aVF indicate that abnormal leftward
axis deviation (and thus left anterior fascicle block) is not present.

Although there are q waves in Leads, II, III, and aVF, neither their
duration (0.02-0.03 seconds) nor their magnitude (less than one-
fourth the magnitude of the R wave) are great enough to qualify as
pathologic or indicative of myocardial infarction. A vectorcardiogram (Fig. 37.2) shows that the mean frontal plane QRS axis is normal at about +60 degrees, and criteria for inferior wall myocardial
infarction are not met.

The patient is admitted to the hospital, where he has no enzyme
or electrocardiographic evidence of acute myocardial necrosis.
However, over a period of about one week he has several episodes
of ischemic heart pain at rest, so cardiac catheterization with left
ventricular and selective coronary angiography are performed.
These studies reveal normal left ventricular function and high-grade
proximal stenoses in otherwise large, normal-appearing right and
left anterior descending coronary arteries. Double saphenous vein
aortocoronary bypass graft surgery is performed, the immediate
postoperative course is uncomplicated, and neither serum enzymes
nor radioisotopic scans indicate perioperative myocardial infarction.
The patient is discharged on the twelfth postoperative day, at which
time the 12-Lead ECG shown in Fig. 37.3 is recorded.

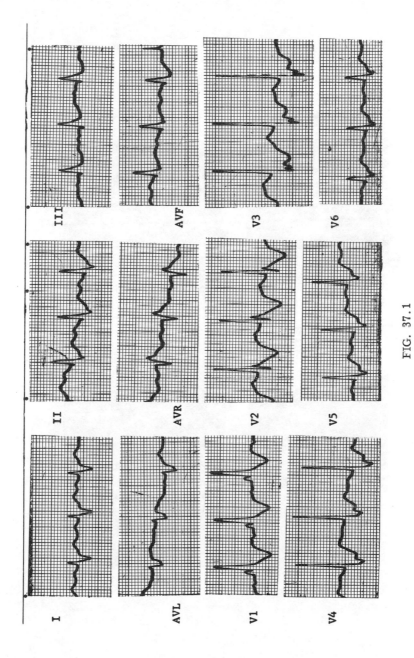

FIG. 37.1

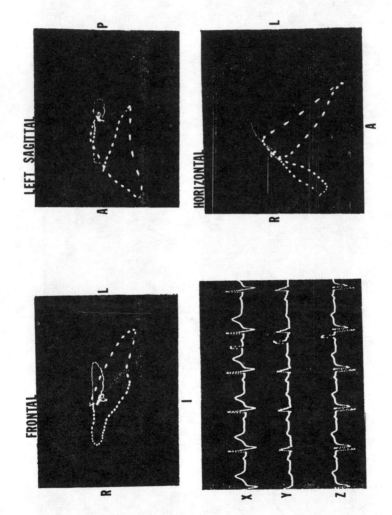

FIG. 37.2

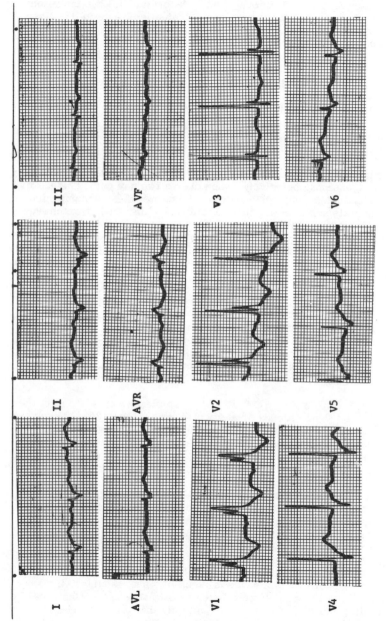

FIG. 37.3

In comparison with the tracing recorded on admission (Fig. 37.1) the rate, rhythm, PR interval, and precordial QRS configurations are unchanged, but there has been a dramatic change in the QRS contours in Lead aVF which, previously having a qRs configuration, now has an RS configuration. Since there has been no interval myocardial infarction, the changes in QRS contour likely represent changes in intraventricular conduction. Once again, the right bundle branch block pattern precludes accurate measurement of mean frontal plane QRS axis so the presence of a specific intraventricular conduction abnormality such as left anterior fascicle block or left posterior fascicle block cannot be established with certainty. A vectorcardiogram is not performed at this time.

The patient continues his convalescence at home and feels well until eight weeks postoperatively, when over a two day period he has five transient unheralded episodes of profound weakness accompanied by diaphoresis and a feeling that he is about to die - all of which suggest a sudden fall in cardiac output and/or blood pressure. The episodes are unrelated to activity, last five to thirty minutes, and disappear spontaneously, leaving the patient feeling fatigued. He then visits his physician who, finding a normal postoperative physical examination, records the ECG shown in Fig. 37.4.

2. Which of the following account(s) for the pauses in QRS rhythm?
   a) sinus arrest
   b) non-conducted atrial premature beats
   c) Type I (Wenckebach) second degree AV block
   d) Type II second degree AV block
   e) pseudo AV block due to non-propagated premature His bundle depolarizations

ANSWER: (d) In Fig. 37.4, the QRS complexes occur at intervals of about 0.63-0.64 seconds or at about twice this at 1.26-1.29 seconds. Throughout the tracing normal-appearing sinus P waves occur with regularity at intervals of about 0.63-0.64 seconds, excluding the diagnoses of atrial premature beats and sinus arrest. All QRS complexes are preceded by P waves which presumably stimulate them, but since some on-time P waves are not followed by QRS complexes, second degree AV block is present. The constant PR intervals (about 0.18 seconds) of the conducted beats that precede the blocked P waves establish the diagnosis of Type II second degree AV block, and exclude the diagnosis of Type I (Wenckebach) second degree AV block, in which the PR intervals of conducted beats preceding the non-conducted P waves show a pattern of generally progressive prolongation. Although non-propagated His bundle premature impulses cannot be excluded as a cause of block of sinus impulses, the absence of premature QRS complexes in fifty seconds of electrocardiographic recording makes it most unlikely that this rare phenomenon, called "pseudo AV block", is causing failure of conduction of the on-time sinus impulse.

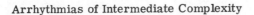

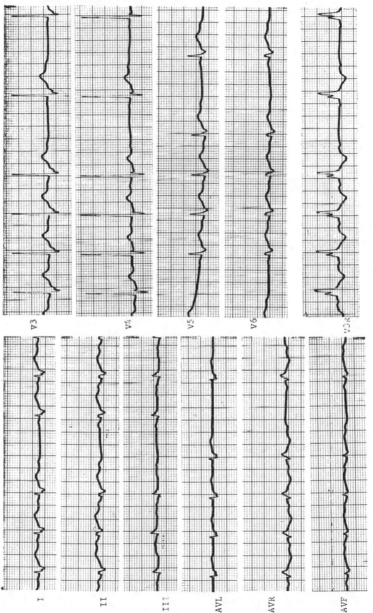

FIG. 37.4

3. How might this patient be reasonably managed at this time?
   a) recommend implantation of a permanent ventricular demand
      pacemaker
   b) reassure him that the transient episodes which suggest low
      cardiac output are not likely to be related to cardiac rhythm
      disturbances
   c) perform ambulatory outpatient monitoring in an attempt to
      document the rhythm at the time of these episodes
   d) perform a His bundle electrographic study before deciding
      on appropriate therapy
   e) teach him to take his pulse so he can measure it during and
      after these episodes

ANSWER: (a) In Type II second degree AV block, which most often
occurs in the presence of extensive disease of the right and left
bundle branch systems, failure of AV conduction is almost invariably due to transient block in conduction tissue below the His bundle.
Patients with Type II second degree AV block commonly develop
transient or complete AV block, at the onset of and during which
syncope, seizure, and sudden death may occur. These potentially
catastrophic events reflect a sudden severe decrease in cardiac output due to the long escape interval, slow automatic rate, and instability of pacemakers which originate below the His bundle. The
transient symptoms of low cardiac output experienced by this patient
in the two days preceding the ECG in Fig. 37.4 were most likely due
to periods of complete AV block with an escape rhythm too slow to
maintain adequate cardiac output. Thus, it is not reasonable to reassure the patient that his recent symptoms are not likely to be due
to cardiac rhythm disturbances. Also, since the occurrence of complete AV block in patients with Type II second degree AV block is
so well-documented, and since its onset is so unpredictable and may
be fatal, it seems most reasonable at this time to recommend insertion of a permanent demand ventricular pacemaker, which is the
only safe, effective, and reliable means of preventing bradycardia-
related symptoms in this setting. To send the patient home while
attempting to document the cardiac rhythm and rate at the time of
these episodes with ambulatory ECG monitoring and pulse counting
may expose the patient to unnecessary risks and therefore is not
reasonable.

His-Purkinje system conduction (HV) time is reported to be abnormally long in patients with fascicle blocks and Type II second degree
AV block who have periods of transient complete AV block. However, the severity of symptoms in this setting is dependent upon the
behavior of an escape pacemaker rather than on the degree of His-
Purkinje system dysfunction as estimated by HV time. Therefore,
the results of a His bundle electrographic study should not alter the
strong recommendation for permanent ventricular demand pacemaker implantation.

The patient is advised to directly enter the hospital for permanent demand ventricular pacemaker implantation. While crossing the street from the physician's office to the hospital he suddenly feels weak, nauseated and lightheaded, and turns pale. He is assisted into the hospital emergency room where his pulse is found to be regular at a rate of about 40/minute and his blood pressure 90/40. The ECG shown in Fig. 37.5 is recorded at this time.

4. Which of the following is (are) likely to be present in the ECG of Fig. 37.5?
   a) Type I (Wenckebach) second degree AV block
   b) Type II second degree AV block
   c) complete AV block
   d) AV dissociation
   e) idioventricular rhythm
   f) junctional rhythm

ANSWER: (c, d, e) QRS complexes almost identical to those during sinus rhythm in Fig. 37.1 occur with regularity at intervals of about 1.57 seconds (rate about 38/minute). P waves also occur with regularity at much shorter intervals of about 0.55 seconds (rate about 110/minute). The regularity of P and QRS rhythms, and the marked variability in PR intervals indicate that the atrial and ventricular rhythms are occurring independently; thus, there is AV dissociation. Since the AV dissociation is present despite P waves occurring outside of the presumed refractory period of the AV conduction system (i.e., outside the QRST complex), complete AV block is the most likely underlying mechanism. The independent ventricular rhythm, often referred to as an "idioventricular" rhythm, has a pattern of right bundle branch block and a mean frontal plane QRS axis identical to that occurring during sinus rhythm, indicating that ventricular activation occurs via impulses entering the ventricles in the same manner as during sinus rhythm. This might occur if the automatic focus were located in the AV junction (i.e., His bundle) or in the left bundle branch system which previously conducted sinus impulses to the ventricles. In patients whose AV conduction disturbances progress from Type II second degree AV block to complete AV block, the area of complete AV block is usually distal to, but occasionally occurs within, the His bundle. In this patient, therefore, the escape rhythm more likely originates in the left bundle branch system than in the AV junction. Recording of the His bundle electrogram might allow identification of the area of origin of the escape pacemaker.

5. How might this rhythm be reasonably managed in this patient while arrangements are being made to implant the permanent ventricular demand pacemaker?
   a) intravenous administration of atropine
   b) intravenous administration of isoproterenol
   c) placement of a temporary transvenous right ventricular endocardial pacemaker
   d) close observation without specific therapy

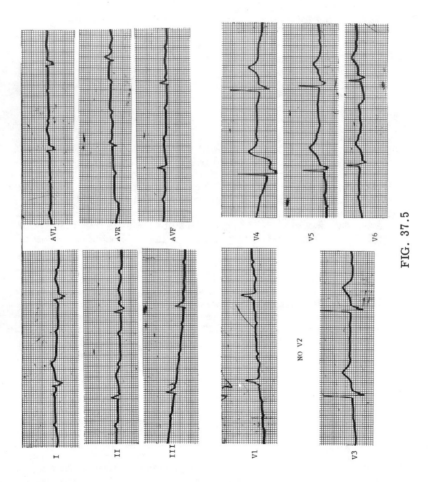

FIG. 37.5

ANSWER: (b, c) Although AV conduction may spontaneously return
within minutes to hours, treatment aimed at increasing the ventricular rate is now in order. As this patient already has signs and symptoms of low cardiac output which are attributable to bradycardia, and
infra-Hisian pacemakers are often unstable and may suddenly cease
to fire, it is not reasonable to simply observe him. The careful intravenous infusion of isoproterenol has proved to be an extremely
effective, safe, and reliable means of increasing ventricular rate in
this setting and may on occasion alter conduction velocity and/or refractory periods such that some degree of AV conduction returns.
Since conduction velocity and automaticity of infra-Hisian tissue is
not generally affected by parasympathetic nervous system traffic,
atropine is not likely to be effective in improving AV conduction or
in increasing the rate of the escape pacemaker in this patient. Since
ventricular pacing is the most reliable way of preventing bradycardia-
related symptoms it is reasonable to insert a temporary transvenous
right ventricular endocardial pacemaker to ensure an adequate hemodynamic state until permanent demand ventricular pacing can be
established.

Isoproterenol is administered continuously by vein until the ventricular rate increases to about 50/minute. The patient is then transferred to the cardiac catheterization laboratory where a pacing catheter is inserted into the right femoral vein, and passed into the right
ventricle. The isoproterenol infusion is discontinued and within
minutes the ventricular rate drops to about 40/minute. Fig. 37.6
displays simultaneously recorded Leads Y, X, and Z of the Frank
orthogonal Lead system*, and a His bundle electrogram (HBE)prior
to positioning to catheter in the right ventricular apex.

6. On the basis of the tracing in Fig. 37.6, in which portion of the
    cardiac conduction system in the ventricular rhythm originating?
    a) AV junction (i.e., His bundle)
    b) left bundle branch system
    c) right bundle branch system

ANSWER: (b) Atrial activity is occurring at intervals of about 0.55
seconds (corresponding rate about 110/minute), ventricular activity
at intervals of about 1.55 seconds (corresponding rate about 39/min-
ute), and AV dissociation due to underlying complete heart block is
still present. Following each atrial deflection (A) at an interval of
about 105 msec in a His bundle deflection (H), indicating that the
area of AV block lies below the His bundle in the bundle branch system.

* In the Frank orthogonal Lead system, Lead X is similar to a Lead
  I, Lead Y to a Lead aVF, and a Lead Z to an inverted Lead V_1 of
  the standard 12-Lead electrocardiogram.

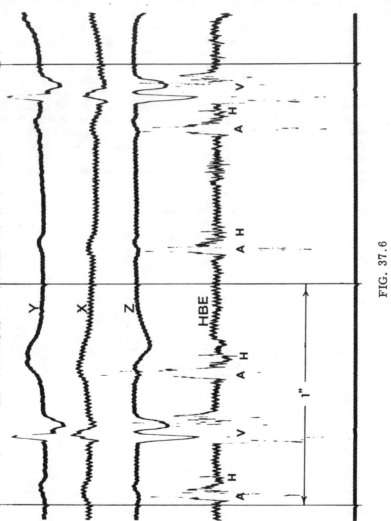

FIG. 37.6

The intracardiac ventricular deflections (V) are not preceded by His deflections, indicating that their origin lies in the bundle branch system distal to the area of block, and the surface Leads showing right bundle branch block suggest that the ventricular rhythm originates in the left bundle branch system. The AH time is normal, indicating normal AV nodal conduction at this time.

The electrode catheter is then positioned into the right ventricular apex, stable demand pacing instituted, and the patient transferred to the Coronary Care Unit. When the pacemaker is turned off, complete AV block is seen to persist. After two days, when serially determined serum enzyme measurements and radioisotopic scans have failed to document acute or recent myocardial necrosis, a permanent demand ventricular pacemaker is implanted. One day later the rhythm shown in Fig. 37. 7 is noted.

7. On the basis of the tracing in Fig. 37. 7, which of the following may be said?
    a) AV conduction has returned and is consistently normal
    b) AV conduction has returned, but periods of AV block still occur
    c) permanent ventricular demand pacing was not necessary and the recent episode could have been managed solely by temporary pacing
    d) the ventricular pacemaker is adequately preventing pauses in ventricular rhythm occasioned by AV block

ANSWER: (b, d) Throughout this monitor Lead, P waves occur with regularity at a rate of about 90/minute. Most are followed at intervals of about 0. 16 seconds by QRS complexes which they stimulate, so AV conduction is now present. However, following the twelfth P wave (●) there is a pause in ventricular rhythm, indicating that AV conduction is not consistently normal, and that periods of AV block are present. The pause of about 0. 85 seconds in ventricular rhythm occasioned by block of this twelfth P wave is terminated by a paced ventricular beat, demonstrating that the bradycardia is prevented. However, the paced beat precludes accurate assessment of the degree (second or third) of AV block. The return of AV conduction in patients with complete AV block below the His bundle is not unusual, but since it is the transition from AV conduction to complete AV block that accounts for Stokes-Adams-Morgagni attacks, it is most unlikely that this patient would do well without permanent ventricular pacing.

The patient is followed for a period of two and one-half years after permanent ventricular pacemaker implantation, during which time he has no symptoms of bradycardia and his pacemaker continues to function normally. At no time during about twenty one-minute rhythm strips recorded during this two and one-half year period is AV conduction ever observed.

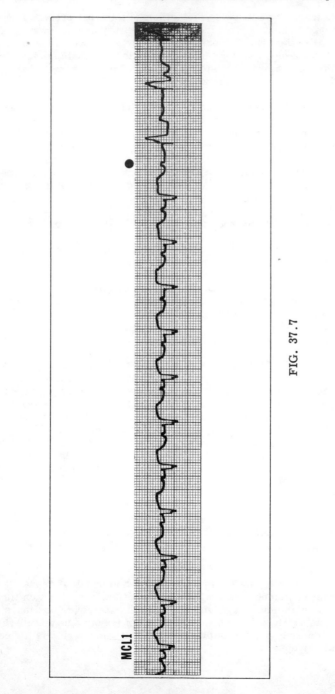

FIG. 37.7

BIBLIOGRAPHY

Dhingra RC, Denes P, Wu D, Chuquimia R, Amat-y-Leon F, Wyndham C, Rosen KM: Syncope in patients with chronic bifascicular block. Significance, causative mechanisms, and clinical implications. Ann Int Med 81:302, 1974.

Dhingra RC, Denes P, Wu D, Chuquimia R, Rosen KM: The significance of second degree atrioventricular block and bundle branch block. Observations regarding site and type of block. Circulation 49:638, 1974.

Dhurandhar RW, Valen FJ, Phillips J: Pseudo second degree atrioventricular block with bradycardia. Successful treatment with quinidine. Brit Heart J 38:1363, 1976.

Dreifus LS, Watanabe Y, Haiat R, Kimbiris D: Atrioventricular block. Amer J Cardiol 28:371, 1971.

Kastor JA: Atrioventricular block. New Engl J Med 292:462, 1975.

Langendorf R, Pick A: Atrioventricular block, Type II (Mobitz) - its nature and clinical significance. Circulation 38:819, 1968.

Narula OS, Samet P: Wenckebach and Mobitz Type II A-V block due to block within the His bundle and bundle branches. Circulation 41:947, 1970.

Narula OS, Scherlag BJ, Samet P, Javier RP: Atrioventricular block: localization and classification by His bundle recordings. Amer J Med 50:146, 1971.

Ranganathan N, Dhurandhar R, Phillips JH, Wigle ED: His bundle electrogram in bundle branch block. Circulation 45:282, 1972.

Rosen KM, Rahimtoola SH, Gunnar RM: Pseudo A-V block secondary to premature nonpropagated His bundle depolarizations. Circulation 42:367, 1970.

Steiner C, Lau SH, Stein E, Wit AL, Weiss MB, Damato AN, Haft JI, Weinstock M, Gupta P: Electrophysiologic documentation of trifascicular block as the common cause of complete heart block. Amer J Cardiol 28:436, 1971.

Langendorf R, Mehlmann JS: Blocked (non-conducted) A-V nodal premature systoles imitating first and second degree A-V block. Amer Heart J 34:500, 1947.

Vera Z, Mason DT, Fletcher RD, Awan NA, Massumi RA: Prolonged His-Q interval in chronic bifascicular block. Relation to impending complete heart block. Circulation 53:46, 1976.

CASE 38: Slow irregular pulse in a woman taking digoxin.

A 50-year-old woman with interstitial pulmonary disease of recent onset and moderately severe longstanding hypertension is admitted to the hospital for evaluation of nausea, weight-loss, inanition, and shortness of breath. She has been taking digoxin 0.25 mg daily, and furosemide 40 mg daily for the shortness of breath which has been thought to be due to congestive heart failure. Physical examination reveals a cachectic woman with blood pressure of 190/115 mmHg, pulse about 60 per minute and irregular, and rapid shallow respirations. There is evidence of left ventricular hypertrophy, right ventricular hypertrophy, and pulmonary hypertension. The serum electrolytes are within normal limits, the blood urea nitrogen is 65 mg%, and the creatinine is 3.2 mg%. The chest x-ray shows generalized cardiomegaly, prominent proximal pulmonary arteries, and a parenchymal pattern consistent with interstitial pulmonary disease. The 12-Lead ECG is compatible with left and right ventricular hypertrophy; two continuous Lead II rhythm strips are shown in Fig. 38.1.

1. Which of the following terms describe the rhythm?
    a) sinus rhythm
    b) ventriculophasic sinus arrhythmia
    c) AV dissociation
    d) first degree AV block
    e) second degree AV block
    f) junctional escape beats
    g) fusion beats

ANSWER: (a, c, d, e, f) All QRS complexes are narrow and of normal contour, suggesting that ventricular activation occurs normally. While RR intervals vary from about 0.90 seconds to about 1.28 seconds, eight of seventeen are in the range of 1.24 to 1.28 seconds (corresponding rate about 47-48/minute). Normal-appearing P waves occur with reasonable regularity at intervals of about 0.66 seconds (corresponding rate about 91/minute, establishing the presence of sinus rhythm. QRS complexes terminating long pauses (occurring at cycle length of ≧1.24 seconds) are junctional (escape) beats, for they are preceded by P waves at intervals either too short (≦0.10 seconds) or too long (0.65-0.66 seconds) to have stimulated them. Thus, AV dissociation is present when junctional complexes are preceded by P waves at intervals ≦0.10 seconds.

All other QRS complexes, preceded by sinus P waves at intervals of 0.14-0.47 seconds, are probably stimulated by the P waves. Longer PR intervals follow shorter RP intervals, reflecting the phenomenon that conduction velocity of impulses through the AV node is slower shortly after AV nodal depolarization because the tissue is not fully repolarized (i.e., is in a relative refractory period).

In the top strip, the second QRS complex is stimulated by the P wave preceding it at an interval of about 0.38 seconds, indicating first degree AV block. The next P wave (P4) is on time but is not followed by a QRS complex, as it is blocked within the AV conduction system; second degree AV block is therefore also present. The following sinus impulse (P5) is conducted with mild first degree AV block and stimulates a QRS complex, indicating that the AV conduction ratio is 2:1. P6 does not stimulate a QRS complex, and P7 probably reaches the AV junction just after the junctional pacemaker has discharged to stimulate a QRS complex. Transient AV dissociation then continues because of both second degree AV block and lack of opportunity for a sinus impulse to capture the AV junction, whose escape interval (1.24-1.28 seconds) is slightly less than twice the sinus cycle length (2 X 0.66 = 1.32 seconds). If the escape interval of the AV junctional pacemaker were greater than twice the sinus cycle length, junctional escape beats would not occur, and the rhythm would be sinus with 2:1 second degree AV block. The sinus P wave at the arrow stimulates a QRS complex by depolarizing (capturing) the AV junction before it discharges spontaneously. The sequences of AV dissociation with intermittent capture occur throughout both rhythm strips.

Ventriculophasic sinus arrhythmia, in which the interval between P waves enclosing a QRS complex is shorter than the interval between P waves not enclosing a QRS complex, is excluded in these rhythm strips as the PP intervals are essentially constant. Fusion beats, which occur when atrial or ventricular activation results from two impulses, are recognized by their contours being intermediate between complexes stimulated by each of the impulses separately. Fusion beats are not present in Fig. 38.1, as all P waves and all QRS complexes are identical.

2. How might this rhythm be reasonably managed in this patient?
   a) measure serum digoxin level
   b) discontinue digoxin
   c) continue digoxin
   d) administer atropine intravenously
   e) administer isoproterenol intravenously
   f) place a temporary transvenous right ventricular endocardial pacemaker

ANSWER: (a, b) This rhythm, consisting of first and second degree AV block in a patient taking digoxin, is almost certainly contributed to, if not caused by, this medication. The digoxin should be discontinued, and a serum digoxin level could be measured. An elevated level would support the impression of digitalis-induced arrhythmia. While the occurrence of junctional escape beats does not allow for accurate diagnosis of the type of second degree AV block, the presence of narrow QRS complexes makes infra-His AV block (Type II) unlikely. Atropine, by blocking parasympathetic input to the AV node, and isoproterenol, by increasing sympathetic input to the AV node, might improve AV conduction and/or increase the escape rate of the junctional pacemaker. However, since the patient is hemodynamically stable, there is little indication for their use at this time.

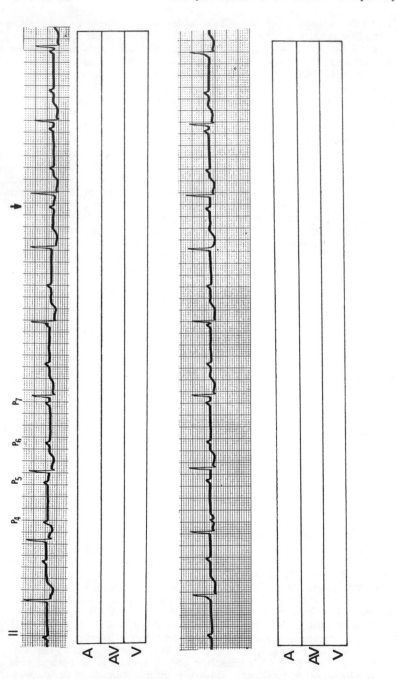

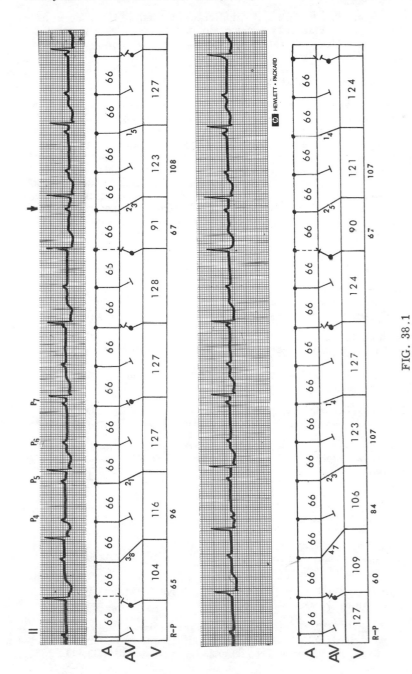

FIG. 38.1

In the event that the clinical situation warranted an increase in ventricular rate, temporary transvenous pacing could be performed if the pharmacologic therapies did not achieve the desired effect. Simply withdrawing digoxin will allow AV conduction to gradually improve such that 1:1 AV conduction with normal PR interval will appear, unless intrinsic AV nodal disease is present.

Digoxin is withheld and the serum digoxin level is determined to be elevated at 3.4 ng/ml, probably because the digoxin dosage of 0.25 mg daily is excessive for this cachectic patient with impaired renal function. Over the next three days AV conduction improves and pari passu the junctional escape beats disappear. Sinus rhythm at a rate of about 81/minute, with 1:1 AV conduction and normal PR interval appear. Over the next two weeks the patient undergoes extensive diagnostic studies aimed at elucidating the nature of her systemic illness but a specific diagnosis cannot be established. Shortly thereafter she has a sudden unexpected cardiopulmonary arrest which she does not survive. Autopsy examination discloses extensive, diffuse, healed vasculitis.

BIBLIOGRAPHY

Dreifus L, Watanabe Y: Effect of digitalis on A-V transmission. In: Dreifus L (Ed): Mechanism and Therapy of Cardiac Arrhythmias. Grune & Stratton, Inc., New York, p. 373, 1966.

Fisch C, Greenspan K, Knoebel S, Feigenbaum H: Effect of digitalis on conduction of the heart. Prog Cardiovasc Dis 6:343, 1964.

Friedberg CK, Donoso E: Arrhythmias and conduction disturbances due to digitalis. Prog Cardiovasc Dis 2:408, 1960.

Kosowsky BD, Haft JI, Lau SH, Stein E, Damato AN: The effects of digitalis on atrioventricular conduction in man. Amer Heart J 75:736, 1968.

Lister JW, Stein E, Kosowsky BD, Lau SH, Damato AN: Atrioventricular conduction in man. Effect of rate, exercise, isoproterenol, and atropine on the P-R interval. Amer J Cardiol 76:516, 1965.

Rios JC, Dziok CA, Ali NA: Digitalis-induced arrhythmias: Recognition and management. Cardiovasc Clinics 2:262, 1970.

Chung EK: Digitalis-induced cardiac arrhythmias. In: Chung EK: Principles of Cardiac Arrhythmias. Williams & Wilkins Co., Baltimore, p. 464, 1971.

Dreifus LS, Watanabe Y, Haiat R, Kimbiris D: Atrioventricular block. Amer J Cardiol 28:371, 1971.

Langendorf R, Cohen H, Gozo EG: Observations on second degree atrioventricular block, including new criteria for the differential diagnosis between Type I and Type II block. Amer J Cardiol 29:111, 1972.

III. COMPLEX ARRHYTHMIAS

CASE 39: Rapid irregular rhythm in a man with cardiomyopathy and severe congestive heart failure.

A 50-year-old man with idiopathic cardiomyopathy, critically ill with signs and symptoms of elevated pulmonary venous pressure and low cardiac output, is admitted to the hospital. He speaks no English and is unaware of the names of the medications he has been taking. His pulse feels somewhat rapid and irregular. A 12-Lead ECG shows abnormalities suggestive of left ventricular hypertrophy, and a Lead V_1 rhythm strip is shown in Fig. 39.1A.

1. Which of the following may be present in Fig. 39.1A?
   a) sinus rhythm
   b) atrial premature beats
   c) ventricular premature beats
   d) aberrant intraventricular conduction
   e) atrial tachycardia
   f) group beating
   g) atrial flutter
   h) multifocal atrial tachycardia
   i) supraventricular tachycardia (SVT)

ANSWER: (a, b, d, e, f) The QRS rhythm occurs in a bigeminal pattern, with alternating long and short RR intervals, with the exception of the ninth QRS complex which occurs at long cycle length, transiently interrupting the group beating. The longer RR intervals range from 0.54 to 0.61 seconds, and the shorter RR intervals from 0.38 to 0.42 seconds. P waves precede all QRS complexes at intervals of 0.13-0.28 seconds, suggesting that the QRS complexes are stimulated by them. The QRS complexes terminating longer cycle lengths are of normal contour and duration, indicating normal intraventricular conduction, while those terminating shorter cycle lengths are of different contour and generally longer duration, indicating aberrant intraventricular conduction. The aberrant intraventricular conduction is attributable to the refractory period of some portions of the His-Purkinje system being longer at this time than the cycle length at which these complexes occur. The longer PR intervals of QRS complexes terminating shorter cycles probably reflect the lengthening of AV nodal conduction time with shortening cycle length, although a contribution to the longer PR interval from longer His-Purkinje system conduction time cannot be excluded.

The atrial rhythm consists of clearly seen P waves occurring at variable intervals. However, the majority (14 of 22) of the PP intervals are in the range of 0.32 to 0.36 seconds, or about twice this at 0.64-0.68 seconds, thus raising the possibility that the basic atrial cycle length is the shorter interval. During each longer PP interval, a P wave would be occurring on time, but is not seen because it is buried within a wide QRS complex, and it does not stimulate

295

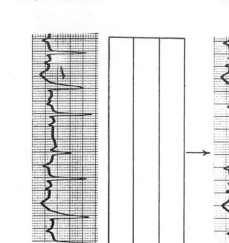

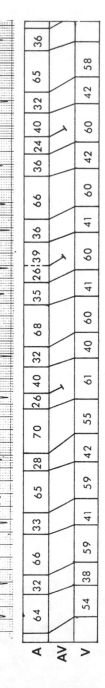

FIG. 39.1A

a QRS complex itself because it falls in the refractory period of the
AV conduction system. The very short PP intervals of 0.28, 0.26,
0.26, and 0.24 seconds are followed by P waves at intervals of 0.70,
0.40, 0.39, and 0.40 seconds. As the sums of the two consecutive
PP intervals of these pairs of beats are 0.98, 0.66, 0.65, and 0.64
seconds (all multiples of 0.32-0.33 seconds), the very early P waves
do not alter the underlying atrial rhythm.   These observations
suggest that the basic atrial rhythm is ectopic atrial tachycardia at
cycle length of 0.32-0.33 seconds (rate about 167-187/minute). The
group beating may therefore represent 3:2 AV Wenckebach periods.
While variability of PP intervals by as much as 0.12 seconds is reported to occur in atrial tachycardia, and would explain the very
short PP intervals in this tracing, it is possible that atrial premature
beats are occurring intermittently, without interrupting the atrial
tachycardia mechanism.

Atrial flutter is excluded by the variability in PP intervals. Also,
an atrial rate of 190/minute would be unusually slow (but not unheard
of) in atrial flutter. Multifocal atrial tachycardia, which may occur
in this clinical setting of profound heart failure, is characterized by
marked variability in both P wave contour and PP intervals.   The
similar if not identical contours of the P waves and the regular group
beating suggest that multifocal atrial tachycardia is not present here.
Whereas sinus rhythm at cycle length of 0.64-0.70 seconds with
atrial premature beats which do not depolarize the sinus node might
account for the group beating, it would not account for the P waves
occurring at cycle length of 0.39 and 0.40 seconds following what
would have to be considered the second of a pair of atrial premature
beats (arrow). However, it is conceivable that the deflections indicated by the arrows are parts of a QRS complex rather than a P
wave, in which case the diagnosis of sinus rhythm with atrial bigeminy is possible, but still less likely than ectopic atrial tachycardia.
The marked variability in PP intervals and the absence of a 1:1 relationship between atrial and ventricular activity precludes the diagnosis of SVT. Since all the wide QRS complexes are reasonably explained as aberrantly conducted atrial impulses, there are no ventricular premature beats in this tracing.

2. Which of the following maneuvers might be safely used to more
    clearly define the arrhythmia in this patient?
    a) recording of an intraatrial electrogram
    b) carotid sinus massage
    c) intravenous administration of atropine
    d) intravenous administration of propranolol
    e) intravenous administration of Tensilon®

ANSWER: (a, b, e) Accurate diagnosis of the rhythm depends on
accurate analysis of atrial activity. Recording of a right atrial
electrogram would define whether or not P waves are occurring within the wider QRS complexes and therefore whether or not the diagnosis
of ectopic atrial tachycardia with variable AV block is tenable.

Carotid sinus massage, by transiently slowing AV nodal conduction
and thereby increasing AV block, would allow atrial activity to be
more clearly seen, an effect which could also be achieved pharmaco-
logically by administration of the cholinesterase inhibitor Tensilon®.
Both carotid sinus massage and Tensilon® administration might also
transiently slow the atrial rhythm if it were sinus, but it is not
known whether either maneuver would affect atrial rate in ectopic
atrial tachycardia. While intravenous administration of propranolol
would also be expected to increase AV block and allow more accurate P wave analysis, it could result in florid pulmonary edema in
this patient with severely depressed cardiac performance. Intravenous administration of atropine would be expected to enhance AV
conduction, and might permit 1:1 AV conduction, thereby allowing
accurate diagnosis of the atrial rhythm. However, during 1:1 AV
conduction the resulting QRS complex might be so wide and bizarre
that atrial activity might be more difficult to identify, and the rapid
ventricular rate would certainly be detrimental to this patient.

The patient is given intravenous Tensilon® as a 2 mg "test dose",
which has no noticeable effect, followed by a 10 mg bolus which
results in the transient appearance of the rhythm shown in Fig.
39.1B.

3. Which of the following terms describes the rhythm in Fig. 39.1B?
   a) atrial tachycardia with 2:1 AV conduction
   b) aberrant intraventricular conduction
   c) ventricular ectopic beat
   d) concealed conduction
   e) retrograde P waves

ANSWER: (a, c, d) The effect of Tensilon® has been to increase the
AV block such that there is a 2:1 AV conduction ratio and atrial
activity can be clearly seen. The identical P waves occurring at
slightly variable intervals of about 0.32-0.36 seconds (rate 167-187/
minute) confirms the previously considered diagnosis of atrial tachycardia, and while Tensilon® has not altered the basic atrial rate it
appears to have made the PP intervals less variable. The wide,
bizarre fifth-from-last (●) QRS complex is more likely a ventricular ectopic beat than an aberrantly conducted atrial beat, for it
follows a P wave by an interval of about 0.08 seconds, too short to
have been stimulated by it. Since the P wave falling in the ST segment of the ventricular ectopic beat occurs when the next atrial impulse is expected and, like the other P waves, has a predominantly
upright deflection, it is not likely to be a retrograde P wave.

The QRS complex which follows the ventricular ectopic beat is stimulated by a P wave at a PR interval much longer (0.35 vs. 0.17 seconds) than other QRS complexes. This longer PR interval reflects
retrograde depolarization of the AV node by the ventricular ectopic
beat such that antegrade AV conduction of the P wave which falls in
the T wave of this beat is unusually slow. Depolarization of the AV

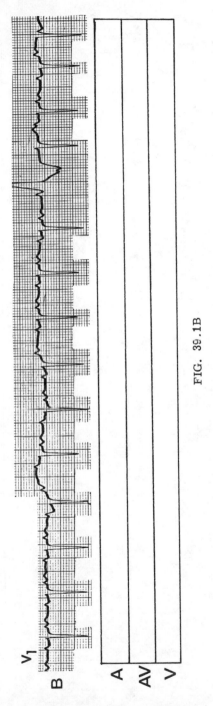

FIG. 39.1B

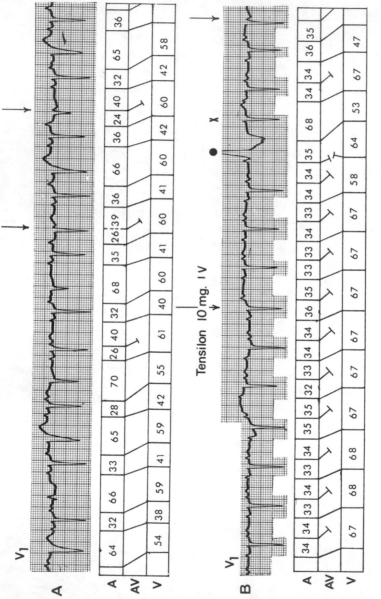

FIG. 39.2

node by the ventricular ectopic beat, an electrocardiographically
silent event, is hypothesized to have occurred on the basis of subsequent events, a phenomenon referred to as "concealed conduction"
of an impulse into the AV node.

Observation of the events following the ventricular ectopic beat
supports other aspects of the discussion of Fig. 39.1A as shown in
the ladder diagram of Fig. 39.2B. The interval of 0.68 seconds
between the P waves clearly seen to precede and to follow the QRS
complex (X) following the ventricular beat is exactly twice the atrial
cycle length, illustrating that a P wave can indeed be completely sub-
merged within a QRS complex. Further, the sharp upstroke on the
last QRS complex (arrow) indeed does represent atrial activity.

4. How might this rhythm be reasonably managed in this patient
    at this time?
    a) measure serum digoxin level
    b) administer potassium chloride
    c) DC cardioversion
    d) careful observation while the congestive heart failure is being
       treated
    e) administer digoxin

ANSWER: (a, d, e) The aim of therapy in this patient with severe
congestive heart failure is to improve cardiovascular performance.
Since neither the atrial tachycardia itself nor the resultant ventricular rate of about 120/minute is likely to be playing a major detrimental role, there is little need for urgent treatment of the arrhythmia itself. Since treatment of the congestive heart failure per se
may result in conversion of the atrial tachycardia to sinus rhythm,
careful observation of the rhythm while treating the heart failure is
reasonable. While administration of potassium chloride may convert the atrial tachycardia to sinus rhythm, prior to conversion the
atrial rhythm usually slows somewhat and 1:1 AV conduction occurs,
resulting in rapid ventricular rates that may have serious hemodynamic consequences. In addition, the administration of potassium
chloride to critically ill patients is somewhat risky as it may result
in fatal hyperkalemia. Digoxin administration may have a beneficial
hemodynamic effect if, by increasing AV block, it results in 2:1 AV
conduction, which would slow the ventricular rate. However, if the
atrial tachycardia is digitalis-induced, digoxin should probably not
be given when 2:1 AV conduction is present, as it may result in
serious ventricular arrhythmias. In order to evaluate the possibility that this rhythm is digitalis-induced, blood should be drawn
for a serum digoxin level measurement before digoxin is administered. Since DC cardioversion of digitalis-induced atrial tachycardia
may be followed by serious arrhythmias, it is prudent to avoid this
therapeutic intervention until the possibility of digitalis intoxication
is excluded.

A serum digoxin level is obtained, and the patient is treated with
supplemental inspired oxygen, diuretics, salt restriction, and bed
rest, and his serum potassium is maintained within the normal
range. The rhythm remains atrial tachycardia with predominantly
3:2 AV conduction, but occasional periods of 1:1 AV conduction
occur. When the serum digoxin measurement fails to detect the
presence of digitalis, the patient is treated with intravenous digoxin,
which results in 2:1 AV conduction occurring almost all of the time,
and about 28 hours after initiation of digitalis therapy, the rhythm
converts to sinus at a rate of 96/minute, with normal PR interval.
Over a period of three weeks the heart failure improves and no new
arrhythmias occur. The patient is discharged and is subsequently
lost to follow-up.

BIBLIOGRAPHY

Fisch C, Knoebel SB: Recognition and therapy of digitalis toxicity.
Prog Cardiovasc Dis 13:71, 1970.

Lown B, Levine HD: Atrial arrhythmias, digitalis, and potassium.
Landsberger Medical Books, Inc., New York, 1958.

Lown B, Wyatt NF, Levine HD: Paroxysmal atrial tachycardia with
block. Circulation 21:129, 1960.

Lown B, Marcus F, Levine HD: Digitalis and atrial tachycardia
with block. New Engl J Med 260:301, 1959.

Storstein O, Rasmussen K: Digitalis and atrial tachycardia with
block. Brit Heart J 36:171, 1974.

Zimmerman HB, Gentsch KW, Gale AH: The action of potassium
on the atrioventricular node in digitalized patients. Dis Chest
43:377, 1963.

Pick A, Igarashi M: Mechanisms, Differential Diagnosis and
Clinical Significance of Digitalis-induced Arrhythmias. In: Digitalis.
Fisch C, and Surawicz B, Eds., Grune and Stratton, New York,
pp. 148-161, 1969.

Dreifus LS, McNight EH, Katz M, Likoff W: Digitalis intolerance.
Geriatrics 18:494, 1963.

CASE 40: A change in pulse from regular to irregular in an elderly
man treated for aspiration pneumonia and heart failure.

An 89-year-old man with no past history of heart disease has a
stroke which results in obtundation and the development of aspiration pneumonia. His 12-Lead ECG shows sinus rhythm at a rate of
about 90/minute, with PR interval of 0.30 seconds as the only abnormality. The house officer, attributing the clinical state and
chest x-ray findings to congestive heart failure superimposed on
pneumonia, prescribes digoxin. After a total dose of 1.75 mg digoxin intravenously in a 24-hour period, a nurse observes that the
patient's pulse is now somewhat irregular at an average rate of
about 90/minute, with frequent pauses.

1. Which of the following are likely causes of the change in rhythm
   from regular to irregular in this patient at this time?
   a) atrial premature beats occurring during sinus rhythm
   b) ventricular premature beats occurring during sinus rhythm
   c) atrial fibrillation
   d) atrioventricular Wenckebach periods
   e) multifocal atrial tachycardia

ANSWER: (a, b, c, d, e) Both atrial and ventricular premature
beats occurring during sinus rhythm are common causes of pauses,
and would not be unusual in an elderly person who has pneumonia.
Ventricular premature beats might also be related to the digoxin administration. However, a more regular pulse rate would be expected
in sinus rhythm with atrial or ventricular premature beats unless
marked sinus arrhythmia were present. Atrial fibrillation, and multifocal atrial tachycardia which is easily confused clinically with atrial
fibrillation, are both frequently observed rhythm disturbances in patients with pneumonia, although in both instances the pulse rate is
usually more rapid. Sinus rhythm with atrioventricular Wenckebach
periods commonly accounts for irregularity of the pulse as well as
pauses, and could in this patient be a manifestation of digoxin excess.

The nurse summons the house officer, who then records the continuous Lead V1 rhythm strip shown in Fig. 40.1.

2. What does the rhythm show?
   a) atrial premature beats
   b) ventricular premature beats
   c) multifocal atrial tachycardia
   d) sinus rhythm with atrioventricular Wenckebach periods
   e) sinus rhythm with atrioventricular dissociation and junctional
      rhythm
   f) group beating

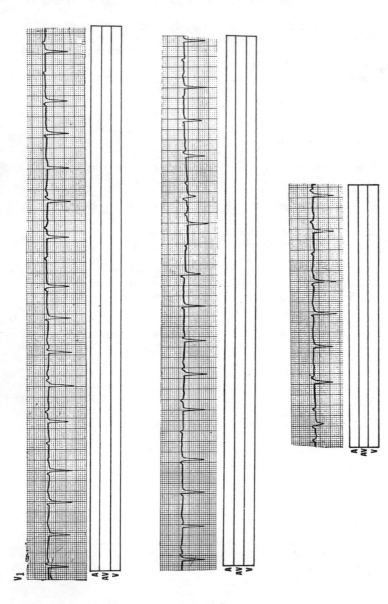

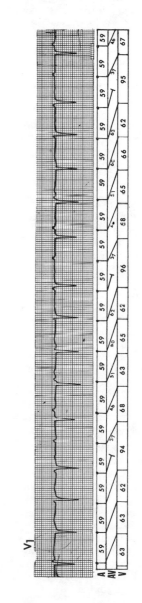
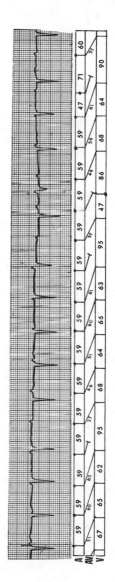
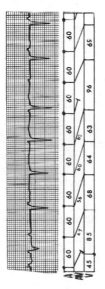

FIG. 40.1

306/ Case 40   Complex Arrhythmias

ANSWER: (a, b, d, f) Except for the 11th QRS complex in the
middle strip and the first QRS complex in the bottom strip, all QRS
complexes are narrow and of identical contour, suggesting that they
are conducted into the ventricles normally via the AV junction-His-
Purkinje.system pathways. The narrow QRS complexes appear to
occur in groups separated by pauses ("group beating"). The wide
QRS complexes in the middle and lower strips occur at coupling intervals of 0.47 and 0.45 seconds, shorter than any RR intervals
between narrow QRS complexes, and are therefore premature.
These are most likely ventricular premature beats.

P waves occur at regular intervals of 0.59-0.60 seconds, except for
the next to last P wave in the middle strip, which, occurring at a PP
interval of 0.47 seconds, is premature and has a contour slightly
different from the remaining P waves. This beat is therefore an
atrial premature beat.

The PR interval of all beats terminating the pauses is 0.37 seconds,
suggesting that these sinus beats are conducted through the AV node
with marked delay. The PR intervals of the subsequent QRS complexes in each group are progressively longer, and are essentially
identical when one group is compared with another. There are six
P waves for every five QRS complexes; in each group, the P wave
that is not conducted into the ventricles, probably because it is
blocked within the AV node, can be seen just prior to the inscription
of the QRS complex preceding the pause. This suggests that the
basic rhythm is sinus with 6:5 Wenckebach type of second degree
atrioventricular block.

3. Can the rhythm be considered to show atrioventricular Wencke-
    bach periodicity despite the fact that the RR intervals do not get
    progressively shorter, but rather the next to last cycle length
    is longer than the RR interval preceding it?

ANSWER: (Yes) In an AV Wenckebach period during regular sinus
rhythm, unequal RR intervals reflect variation in PR intervals. In
the so-called "typical" AV Wenckebach period, the greatest increment in PR interval occurs between the first and second beats of a
sequence, with each succeeding increment in PR interval being less.
The shortening of RR intervals prior to the dropped beat reflects the
progressively smaller increments in PR intervals. The so-called
"atypical" AV Wenckebach period is characterized by occasional increases in PR interval increments, resulting in minimal change or
in an actual lengthening of RR intervals. This phenomenon, if present, usually occurs near the end of an AV Wenckebach period. However, since "typical" AV Wenckebach sequences may well occur less
frequently than "atypical" sequences when the AV conduction ratio is
5:4 and above, these adjectives should probably be avoided.

In Fig. 40.1, the atrioventricular Wenckebach periods begin with a
PR interval of 0.37 seconds. The next PR interval is about 0.46

seconds, the increment in PR interval (the PR interval of the second
beat minus the PR interval of the first beat) being 0.09 seconds. The
third PR interval is 0.51 seconds, an increment of 0.05 seconds, and
the fourth PR interval of 0.60 seconds, an increment of 0.09 seconds,
greater than the preceding PR interval increment. The increased increment of this PR interval results in an RR interval of 0.66 seconds,
0.02 seconds longer than the previous RR interval of 0.64 seconds.
The final PR intervals in the AV Wenckebach periods are 0.61-0.63
seconds, reflecting increments of 0.01-0.03 seconds, and the RR interval prior to the dropped beat is the shortest in the group, about
0.63 seconds.

The common finding in atrioventricular Wenckebach periodicity, that
of progressive increase in atrioventricular nodal conduction time, is
the same whether or not the increase in AV nodal conduction time in-
crementally decreases (resulting in shortening RR intervals) or in-
crementally increases for one or two beats (resulting in no change
or lengthening of RR intervals).

4. What are the effects of the ventricular premature beats in the
    middle and lower strips on subsequent sinus impulse conduction
    and how are these effects explained?

ANSWER: The P waves preceding the ventricular premature beats
are not conducted to the ventricles because, with the unusually long
AV nodal conduction time of the first beat of the AV Wenckebach
sequence as evidenced by the long PR interval, the His-Purkinje
system (and possibly the AV node) will have recently been depolarized by the premature beat and will be refractory at the time these
sinus impulses arrive there. The P waves following the premature
ventricular beats are conducted with PR intervals somewhat shorter
(0.49 seconds in the middle strip, 0.47 seconds in the bottom strip)
than those expected in the third beats of the AV Wenckebach periods
(0.51 seconds in the AV Wenckebach periods not interrupted by a
premature ventricular beat). The likely explanation for these shorter PR intervals is that the ventricular premature beats have already
depolarized the AV node in a retrograde manner before it would have
been depolarized antegradely by the preceding P waves, so it has had
a longer time to recover and can more rapidly conduct the sinus impulse which follows the premature beat. This explanation is supported
by the observation that the ventricular premature beat in the bottom
strip, occurring at a coupling interval shorter than the ventricular
premature beat in the middle strip (0.45 vs. 0.47 seconds), is
followed by a conducted sinus beat with a P̄R interval shorter than
that following the premature ventricular beat in the middle strip
(0.47 vs. 0.49 seconds).

5. What is the effect of the atrial premature beat in the middle strip
    on impulse formation and conduction?

ANSWER: The atrial premature beat, occurring at a coupling interval of 0.47 seconds, is followed 0.71 seconds later by a sinus P wave. Since the sum of 0.47 + 0.71 = 1.28 seconds is equal to twice the intersinus interval, the atrial premature beat has not affected sinus node rhythm or rate, and was therefore probably not conducted into the sinus node itself. Neither is the atrial premature beat conducted into the ventricles, because probably it arrives in the AV node during its refractory period.

6. How might this rhythm disturbance reasonably be managed in this patient?
   a) hold further digoxin
   b) administer additional digoxin
   c) maintain adequate respiratory function
   d) maintain adequate fluid and electrolyte status
   e) administer atropine
   f) administer diphenylhydantoin

ANSWER: (a, c, d, e) The maintenance of adequate respiratory function and fluid and electrolyte status is essential in the management of patients with all forms of illness. Since the AV Wenckebach periods and, perhaps, even the premature ventricular beats are likely to be manifestations of digoxin excess, withholding further digoxin seems advisable. This is especially true in view of the questionable indication for its initial administration. It is often extremely difficult to establish by clinical and radiographic evidence that a patient with pneumonia does indeed have superimposed congestive heart failure. Rapid shallow respirations, rales, gallop rhythms, and radiologic signs of pulmonary congestion can all be due to the pneumonic process itself. Since the administration of digoxin in the setting of hypoxemia and shifts in arterial pH due to pulmonary dysfunction may increase the tendency to arrhythmias, the diagnosis of congestive failure should be clearly established before digoxin is prescribed. The currently available bedside catheterization techniques for measuring hemodynamic parameters allow accurate determination of right and left heart filling pressures, so that therapeutic decisions in complicated medical problems can be based on more definitive information.

Atropine might improve atrioventricular conduction, but since the AV conduction abnormality is not responsible for any hemodynamic problem, there is little reason to treat it specifically. It is also possible that atropine may make mobilization of pulmonary secretions more difficult. Diphenylhydantoin might also improve atrioventricular conduction, but its effects on AV nodal conduction are variable and its use in patients with atrioventricular conduction delay due to digitalis not widely documented. The intravenous administration of diphenylhydantoin might cause the additional problem of hypotension.

7. What can be said about the dose of intravenous digoxin administered to this patient?
a) probably inadequate
b) probably adequate
c) probably excessive

ANSWER: (c) In recent years, the concept of the "digitalizing dose"
has been replaced by the need to tailor the digitalis dosage to suit
the needs and problems of the individual patient. In an elderly man
whose renal clearance of digoxin might very well be low, and who,
because of pneumonia, is likely to be hypoxemic and have electrolyte
and pH abnormalities, digoxin should be administered in small doses
with frequent reevaluation for its continued need.

BIBLIOGRAPHY

Caracta AR, Damato AN, Josephson ME, Riciutti MA, Gallagher JJ,
Lau SH: Electrophysiologic properties of diphenylhydantoin.
Circulation 47:1234, 1973.

Chesler E, Schamroth L: The Wenckebach phenomenon associated
with sialorrhea. Brit Heart J 19:577, 1957.

Chung EK: Digitalis-induced cardiac arrhythmias. In: Principles
of Cardiac Arrhythmias. Williams and Wilkins Co., Baltimore,
1971.

Dreifus LS, Watanabe Y, Haiat R, Kimbiris D: Atrioventricular
block. Amer J Cardiol 28:371, 1971.

Irons GV, Jr, Orgain ES: Digitalis-induced arrhythmias and their
management. Prog Cardiovasc Dis 8:539, 1966.

Katz LN, Pick A: Clinical Electrocardiography. Part 1. The
Arrhythmias. Lea and Febiger, Philadelphia, 1956.

Schwartz LS, Schwartz SP: The effect of digitalis bodies on patients
with heart block and congestive heart failure. Prog Cardiovasc Dis
6:366, 1964.

Somylo AP: The toxicology of digitalis. Amer J Cardiol 5:523,
1960.

Jelliffe RW, Brooker G: A nomogram for digoxin therapy. Amer
J Med 57:63, 1974.

CASE 41: Regular tachycardias beginning thirteen years after
acute myocardial infarction.

A 78-year-old man with a past history of anterior wall myocardial
infarction at age 65, and no angina, symptoms of heart failure, or
prior episodes of tachycardia, now complains of rapid heart action
which began abruptly several hours earlier while he was sitting
quietly. He now feels generally weak but has no chest discomfort.
He takes no medications. Physical examination reveals a pale,
moderately ill-appearing man with a regular pulse of 150/minute,
blood pressure of 110/70 in the recumbent position, mild neck vein
distension, and a clear chest. Cardiac examination reveals abnormal size and motion of the anterior portion of the heart. The ECG
is shown in Fig. 41.1.

1. Which of the following rhythm disturbances might explain this
   electrocardiogram?
   a) atrial flutter with 2:1 AV conduction
   b) supraventricular tachycardia with aberrant intraventricular
      conduction
   c) ventricular tachycardia
   d) atrial fibrillation with rapid ventricular rate
   e) sinus tachycardia with prolonged AV conduction and left
      bundle branch conduction delay

ANSWER: (b, c, e) Wide QRS complexes occur regularly at a rate
of about 150/minute. Although an atrial rhythm cannot be accurately
identified, there is a possibility that atrial activity is seen on the
downslope of the QRS complex in Lead II. If these are indeed atrial
deflections, they occur in a fixed 1:1 temporal relationship to the
QRS complexes. Supraventricular tachycardia with aberrant intraventricular conduction, ventricular tachycardia, and sinus tachycardia with first degree AV block and aberrant intraventricular conduction are all possibilities to explain the rhythm. The isoelectric
baseline in Lead II suggest that atrial flutter is not present,
and, in the absence of digitalis intoxication, the regularity of
the QRS complexes makes atrial fibrillation extremely unlikely.
The abrupt onset of rapid regular heart action at this rate makes
sinus tachycardia an unlikely possibility, and the occurrence of
supraventricular tachycardia for the first time at age 78 is most
unusual. Ventricular tachycardia is therefore the most likely rhythm,
especially in view of the patient's past history of myocardial infarction
and the physical examination suggestive of ventricular aneurysm.

2. What diagnostic and therapeutic interventions might be helpful at
   this time?
   a) intravenous lidocaine   d) Tensilon®
   b) carotid sinus massage   e) digitalis
   c) DC cardioversion

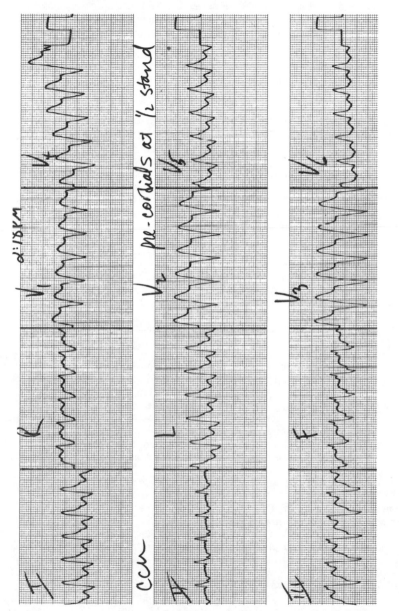

FIG. 41.1

ANSWER: (a, b, c, d) Carotid sinus massage could be performed
(with caution in older patients because of possible underlying carotid arterial disease) in order to attempt to distinguish between supraventricular tachycardia and ventricular tachycardia.

Carotid sinus massage in supraventricular tachycardia could either
terminate the rhythm or slow its rate slightly, but would not alter
the relationship between atria and ventricles. Carotid sinus massage
would be most effective in terminating supraventricular tachycardia
after raising the blood pressure to 160-180 mmHg systolic with
catecholamines having alpha adrenergic properties. Tensilon® , given
in a 2 mg intravenous test dose followed by a 10 mg intravenous bolus
might accomplish termination of supraventricular tachycardia, but
it may cause transient hypotension, bronchospasm, and nausea and
vomiting. Digitalis administration might facilitate the termination
of supraventricular tachycardia but its effect may not be seen for
minutes to hours; moreover, its use might predispose to the appearance of arrhythmias following DC cardioversion, should this be required to terminate the tachycardia.

Carotid sinus massage in ventricular tachycardia would have no effect
on the ventricular rate or rhythm but might, by decreasing conduction
velocity in the AV node, alter ventriculoatrial conduction such that
the 1:1 VA conduction relationship would transiently change. Intravenous Tensilon® could have similar effects. Lidocaine might terminate ventricular tachycardia, and, in intravenous doses of 50-150
mg, its administration generally does not result in serious compli-
cations.

Carotid sinus massage is performed without noticeable effect on
either the QRS or atrial rhythm or rate. Two 50 mg boluses of intravenous lidocaine are then administered, also without effect on
either rate or rhythm, so DC cardioversion to sinus rhythm is
achieved with 10 watt-seconds. The resulting ECG, shown in Fig.
41.2, reveals slow sinus rhythm (rate about 43/minute), an abnormally superior QRS axis probably due to conduction delay in the
anterosuperior "division" of the left bundle branch (left anterior
fascicle block), and an anterior wall myocardial infarction with ST
and T wave abnormalities suggesting anterior wall dyssynergy. The
QRS-T abnormalities are essentially unchanged from tracings obtained over the previous 13 years, dating to the time shortly after
the acute myocardial infarction.

Serial electrocardiograms and CK determinations obtained over a
three-day period fail to document acute myocardial necrosis, and
the patient feels well. His rhythm continues to be sinus bradycardia
with frequent premature ventricular beats.

3. What medications might be administered at this time?
    a) quinidine   d) digitalis
    b) procainamide   e) atropine
    c) diphenylhydantoin   f) none

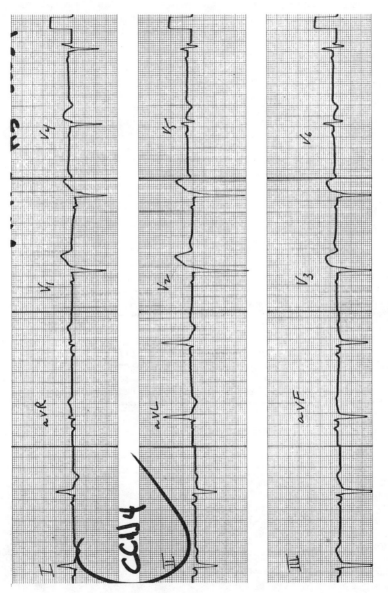

FIG. 41.2

ANSWER: (a, b, e, f) Since the tachycardia is most likely ventricular in origin and is related to a left ventricular aneurysm, medication aimed at suppressing ventricular ectopic activity is justifiable.
A quinidine preparation, or procainamide, would be the agents
more likely to suppress ventricular premature beats. Atropine administration might increase sinus rate and in so doing suppress
ectopic ventricular activity, but its use in older patients is often
complicated by urinary retention, dry mouth, and blurred vision.
The beneficial effect of diphenylhydantoin in this clinical setting is
not widely documented. Digitalis preparations would probably not
be effective in suppressing ventricular ectopy in the absence of congestive heart failure. Withholding medication at this time, for the
purpose of monitoring the patient's rhythm to see if, when, and how
the tachycardia recurs could also be defended, as the tachycardia
does not appear to be life-threatening.

Quinidine sulfate, 300 mg every six hours, is administered orally,
and therapeutic serum levels of 5 mg/L are achieved. ECG monitoring by telemetry reveals a sinus rate of 40-50/minute, and rare
atrial and ventricular premature beats. Two days later, while
washing, the patient has another episode of rapid heart action, and
is found to have an ECG identical to that in Fig. 41.1. At this time
the sensitivity of the monitored Lead II is increased to double standard, and probable P waves are identified (Fig. 41.3A); for more
accurate identification of atrial activity, an electrode catheter is
introduced into a left arm vein and passed into the right atrium,
where the right atrial electrogram (RAE) shown in Fig. 41.3B is
recorded.

4. When considered in conjunction with the 12-Lead ECG in Fig.
    41.1, what rhythm does the atrial electrogram suggest?
    a) atrial flutter with 2:1 AV conduction
    b) ventricular tachycardia with 1:1 retrograde conduction
    c) supraventricular tachycardia with aberrant ventricular
       conduction
    d) accurate diagnosis cannot be made

ANSWER: (d) The right atrial electrogram shows much more clearly
than the surface ECG a 1:1 relationship between atrial (A) and ventricular (V) activity, thereby excluding the diagnosis of atrial flutter
with 2:1 AV conduction. The differential diagnosis between supraventricular tachycardia with aberrant ventricular conduction and
ventricular tachycardia cannot be made on the basis of this electrogram, as the electrogram does not show whether or not the ventricles
stimulate the atria.

During recording of the atrial electrogram, carotid sinus massage
(CSM) is applied, and the electrogram shown in Fig. 41.4 is recorded.
The two continuous strips demonstrate that during carotid sinus massage, the ventricular rate and rhythm are unchanged and that the interval between atrial deflections is intermittently about twice the

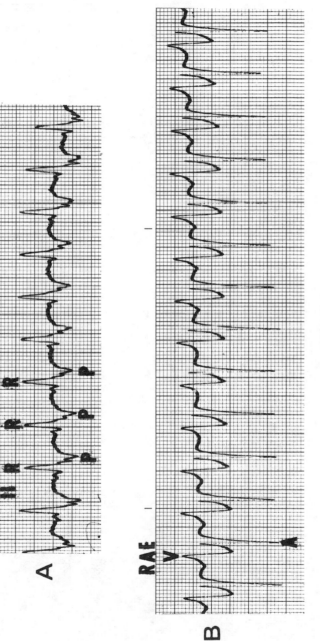

FIG. 41.3

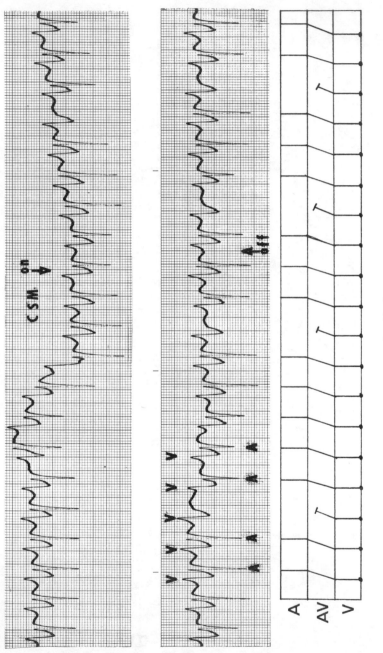

FIG. 41.4

usual AA interval.   The change in the relationship between ventricular and atrial deflections during carotid sinus massage suggests
that the basic rhythm is ventricular tachycardia with 1:1 ventriculoatrial conduction, and that carotid sinus massage has prolonged
ventriculoatrial conduction, such that some ventricular depolarizations are not transmitted through the AV node into the atria.

Near the end of the lower strip in Fig. 41.4, 4:3 VA periodicity
appears. Since during regular ventricular rhythms failure of VA
conduction almost always occurs within the AV node rather than
within the His bundle, the 4:3 VA sequence may represent a VA
Wenckebach period. Had this rhythm been supraventricular tachycardia with prolonged AV conduction, carotid sinus massage should
have resulted in (1) cessation of the tachycardia, (2) transient slowing of the tachycardia rate without alteration of atrial and ventricular relationships, or (3) no change at all in atrial or ventricular
rate or rhythm.

5. At this time the patient is hemodynamically stable. Therapy
    at this point might include:
    a) atrial pacing at a rate exceeding the rate of the tachycardia,
       with sudden cessation of pacing
    b) ventricular pacing at a rate exceeding the rate of the tachy-
       cardia, with sudden cessation of pacing
    c) introduction of single, or pairs of, paced atrial or ventricu-
       lar beats at varying coupling intervals to the tachycardia
       complexes
    d) intravenous lidocaine administration
    e) DC cardioversion

ANSWER: (a, b, c, d, e) Pacing the atrium at a rate above that of
the tachycardia might allow the paced atrial depolarizations to be
transmitted to the ventricles, resulting in capture of the ventricles;
the ventricles might then remain under control of the paced atrial
rhythm. If the reentry circuit or ectopic focus* responsible for the
ventricular tachycardia were depolarized and thereby rendered in-
active by QRS complexes stimulated by the paced atrial impulses,
ventricular tachycardia would be abolished and sinus rhythm would
resume on termination of atrial pacing. If, on the other hand, the
reentry circuit or ectopic focus responsible for the ventricular
tachycardia were not inactivated by paced atrial impulses, ventricular tachycardia would be present on cessation of pacing.

* Since at the present time the distinction between a reentry circuit
  and ectopic focus cannot be established with certainty in man, it
  will not be further discussed. The interested reader is referred
  to the Bibliography for thorough discussion of the subject.

Fig. 41.5 shows the onset of atrial pacing at a rate of about 150/ minute (stimulus interval about 0.40 seconds), when the tachycardia rate is about 130/minute (RR interval 0.46 seconds). The pacing artifacts (s̄) first appear during the ventricular tachycardia; the ninth artifact is followed by a QRS complex that differs from those occurring during the tachycardia, but resembles those QRS complexes in Lead II during sinus rhythm (Fig. 41.2). This beat (CB) is probably a ventricular capture beat, due to depolarization of the ventricles by the paced atrial beat. Throughout the period of atrial pacing, a 1:1 stimulus-to-QRS relationship is present, indicating that all the predominantly negative QRS complexes are stimulated by paced atrial beats.

The ventricular tachycardia reappears immediately following the QRS complex resulting from the final atrial stimulus (fs). The first QRS complex (●) of the returning ventricular tachycardia is coupled to the preceding QRS complex by an interval shorter (0.40 seconds) than its subsequent cycle length (about 0.46 seconds), suggesting that the tachycardia circuit or ectopic focus was not inactivated during atrial pacing.

It has been shown that the location of the pacing site relative to the site of reentry or ectopic impulse formation is an important factor in both inducing and terminating ventricular and supraventricular tachycardias. So, the electrode catheter was advanced from the right atrium into the right ventricle in order to introduce paced ventricular depolarizations in greater proximity to the reentry circuit or ectopic focus than atrial-stimulated QRS complexes could achieve, in the hope of terminating the ventricular tachycardia. Right ventricular pacing at a rate of about 150/minute (pacing interval 0.40 seconds) was attempted at a time when the rate of the tachycardia was about 133/minute (RR interval 0.45 seconds) (Fig. 41.6)

The first pacing stimulus (s_1) results in a QRS complex which has a contour quite different from the tachycardia QRS complexes, probably due to ventricular depolarization originating in a location different from that during the tachycardia. A total of seven serially paced QRS complexes occur. On cessation of pacing, a QRS complex (VEB) of similar contour to the paced QRS complexes occurs at coupling interval of 0.44 seconds, 0.04 seconds longer than the pacing interval, suggesting that this beat is a catheter-induced (mechanically stimulated) ventricular ectopic beat. Following this ventricular ectopic beat two tachycardia QRS complexes occur, the first at a coupling interval shorter than the preceding tachycardia cycle length (0.42 vs. 0.45 seconds), and the second at the expected coupling interval of 0.45 seconds. Then a second, probably mechanically stimulated ventricular ectopic beat occurs at a coupling interval of 0.42 seconds, and is followed by five tachycardia QRS complexes, all of which occur at the usual tachycardia cycle length. Thus, right ventricular pacing at a rate of 150/minute for two

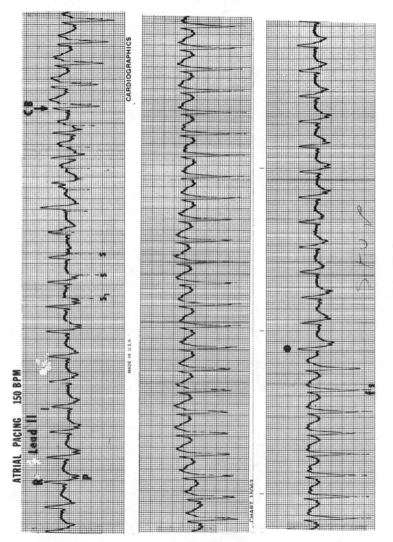

FIG. 41.5

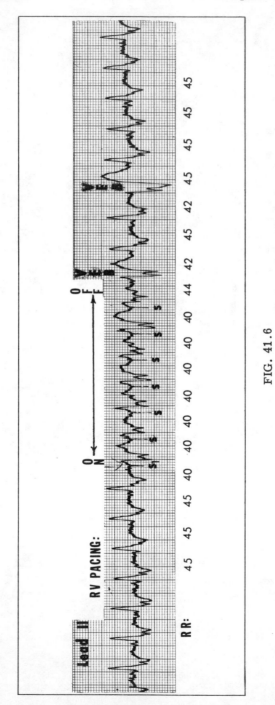

FIG. 41.6

seconds, and single right ventricular ectopic beats at coupling intervals of 0.44 and 0.42 seconds do not inactivate the mechanism responsible for the ventricular tachycardia. The 0.87 second interval between the two tachycardia complexes that include the second VEB is shorter than two tachycardia cycle lengths (0.90 seconds), suggesting that an ectopic focus independent of other ventricular events is not likely to be responsible for the ventricular tachycardia.

The introduction of single, or pairs of, atrial or ventricular beats at specific coupling intervals to the tachycardia QRS complexes might have terminated the tachycardia but require sophisticated electronic equipment which was not available at this time.

Lidocaine might be administered in doses greater than those given during the first episode of ventricular tachycardia. DC cardioversion would terminate the rhythm as before.

After 150 mg intravenous lidocaine is administered without effect, this episode of ventricular tachycardia is converted to sinus bradycardia by DC cardioversion with 10 watt-seconds. The resulting ECG is identical to that in Fig. 41.2. Over the next several days, the patient continues to have marked sinus bradycardia at a rate of about 40/minute, and rhythms similar to that shown in Fig. 41.7. The first two beats are sinus. Following the second sinus beat is a wide bizarre QRS complex which is probably ventricular in origin, at a coupling interval of 0.77 seconds. Two more ventricular beats follow, at coupling intervals of 0.50 and 0.45 seconds, respectively. The P (p) waves appearing in the ST segments of the first and third ventricular beats are probably conducted in retrograde manner from the ventricles, as they bear no relationship to the sinus cycle length.

6. What further course of action might be taken at this time in this patient who is already taking quinidine sulfate in doses which achieve a therapeutic serum level?
   a) diphenylhydantoin administration
   b) procainamide administration
   c) ventricular pacing at rates aimed at suppressing ventricular ectopy
   d) cardiac catheterization with left ventricular and coronary angiography to evaluate the possibilities of myocardial revascularization and/or aneurysmectomy

ANSWER: (c, d) The very slow sinus rate suggests that increasing the heart rate with ventricular pacing is more likely to be successful in suppressing the arrhythmia than is additional antiarrhythmic medication such as diphenylhydantoin or procainamide. Cardiac catheterization and angiography would help to define more clearly a problem which might be amenable to surgical therapy, but in a 78-year-old man who is not symptomatic from angina or congestive failure, and who has an obvious left ventricular aneurysm, postponement of catheterization until all non-surgical therapeutic modalities

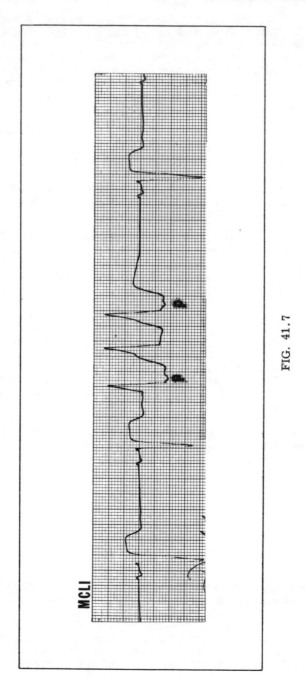

FIG. 41.7

have been attempted and found unsuccessful is a reasonable course
of action. Right ventricular pacing at rates varying from 70 to
110/minute is performed in an attempt to prevent recurrence of
the ventricular tachycardia. Fig. 41.8A shows a brief run of ventricular tachycardia during demand pacing at a rate of 79/minute;
Fig. 41.8B shows a long run of ventricular tachycardia during fixed
rate pacing at a rate of about 97/minute; pacemaker capture of the
ventricles is indicated by the dot (●). Following the pacemaker-
stimulated QRS complex, there is a less than complete compensatory pause, suggesting that a rapidly firing ectopic focus unaffected
by the paced beats is not the likely mechanism responsible for the
tachycardia. Although right ventricular pacing at a rate of about
80/minute is continued, the patient has numerous episodes of ventricular tachycardia, all requiring DC cardioversion, so procainamide and diphenylhydantoin, in addition to the quinidine sulfate,
are administered in doses which achieve therapeutic serum levels.
Ventricular tachycardia recurs despite the combination of medications, but can now occasionally be terminated by right ventricular pacing stimuli (Fig. 41.9).

In Fig. 41.9, wide QRS complexes occur with regularity at the
usual tachycardia rate of about 133/minute (RR interval about 0.44
seconds). At the first arrow, the pacemaker, which has been functioning in a demand mode and therefore does not pace during the
tachycardia, is converted to fixed rate mode in which it continuously
discharges at intervals of 0.76 seconds. The first pacing artifact
stimulates a QRS complex at a coupling interval of 0.38 seconds,
but does not terminate the tachycardia. A tachycardia QRS complex
follows the first paced beat at an interval (0.36 seconds) shorter than
the tachycardia cycle length (0.44 seconds) and the interval between
the tachycardia complexes which enclose the first paced beat is less
than twice the tachycardia cycle length (0.74 rather than 0.88
seconds), again suggesting that a rapidly firing ectopic focus is not
responsible for the ventricular tachycardia. The second paced beat,
occurring at a coupling interval of about 0.40 seconds, terminates
the ventricular tachycardia and the pacemaker rhythm continues.
At this point, with the patient taking several antiarrhythmic medications, the ventricular tachycardia, while not prevented, can intermittently be terminated by right ventricular pacing stimuli. This
indicates that the antiarrhythmic medications have altered the properties of the tissues responsible for the tachycardia sufficiently to
allow the pacing stimuli to interrupt the mechanism.

Cardiac catheterization and left ventricular and selective coronary
angiography are performed, revealing a large left ventricular aneurysm, a completely occluded left anterior descending coronary
artery, and insignificant stenoses of the left circumflex and right
coronary arteries. Cardiac surgery is performed, at which time
most of the large anterior wall aneurysm is removed, and a permanent demand ventricular pacemaker, set at a rate of 80 beats
per minute, is implanted. The patient has an uneventful postoperative course, and is discharged without medication. When seen

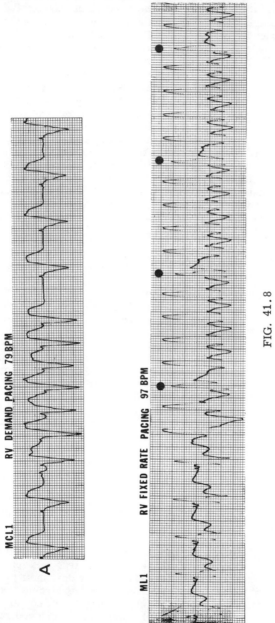

FIG. 41.8

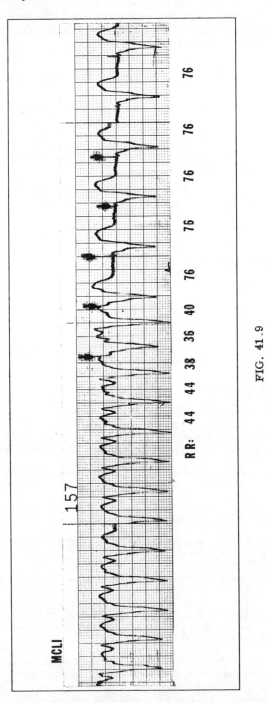

FIG. 41.9

twelve months after operation, he has had no further episodes of
ventricular tachycardia and feels well. His ventricular rhythm is
paced, and there is 1:1 VA conduction.

BIBLIOGRAPHY

Cohen HC, Arbel ER: Tachycardias and electrical pacing. Med
Clinics North Amer 60:II-343, 1976.

Cohn LJ, Donoso E, Friedberg CK: Ventricular tachycardia. Prog.
Cardiovasc Dis 9:29, 1966.

DeSanctis RW, Kastor JA: Rapid intracardiac pacing for treatment
of recurrent ventricular tachyarrhythmias in the absence of heart
block. Amer Heart J 76:168, 1968.

Haft JI: Treatment of arrhythmias by intracardiac electrical stimulation. Prog Cardiovasc Dis 6:539, 1974.

Han J, DeTraglia MD, Moe GK: Incidence of ectopic beats as a
function of basic rate in the ventricle. Amer Heart J 72:632, 1966.

Hellerstein HK, Levine B, Feil H: Electrocardiographic changes
following carotid sinus stimulation in paroxysmal supraventricular
tachycardia. J Lab & Clin Med 38:820, 1951.

Lown B, Levine S: The carotid sinus: Clinical value of its stimulation. Circulation 23:766, 1961.

Moe GK: Evidence for re-entry as a mechanism of cardiac arrhythmias. Rev Physiol Biochem Pharmacol 72:55, 1975.

Moss AJ, Aledort LM: Use of edrophonium (Tensilon) in the evaluation
of supraventricular tachycardias. Amer J Cardiol 17:58, 1966.

Wellens HJJ, Lie KI, Durrer D: Further observations on ventricular tachycardia as studied by electrical stimulation of the heart.
Chronic recurrent ventricular tachycardia and ventricular tachycardia during acute myocardial infarction. Circulation 49:647, 1974.

Wellens HJJ, Duren DR, Lie KI: Observations on mechanisms of
ventricular tachycardia in man. Circulation 54:237, 1976.

Wellens HJJ, et al.: Electrical stimulation of the heart in patients
with ventricular tachycardia. Circulation 46:216, 1972.

Wellens HJJ: Electrical stimulation of the heart in the study and treatment of tachycardias. University Park Press, Baltimore, 1971.

Willerson JT, Yurchak PM, DeSanctis RW: Ventricular tachycardia.
Cardiovasc Clinics 2:69, 1970.

Winkle RS, Alderman EL, Fitzgerald JW, Harrison DC:
Treatment of recurrent symptomatic ventricular tachycardia. Ann
Int Med 85:1-7, 1976.

Zipes DP: The contribution of artificial pacemaking to understanding
the pathogenesis of arrhythmias. Amer J Cardiol 28:211-222, 1971.

CASE 42: Rapid irregular cardiac action in a man with prior episodes of rapid regular heart action.

A 48-year-old man comes to the Emergency Room complaining of
rapid irregular heart action and a feeling of generalized weakness
which began three hours earlier while he was playing tennis. He
states that he has had three to four episodes of rapid heart action
yearly for the past 15 to 20 years, but that during these previous
episodes his heart rhythm has felt regular, and he has been able
to terminate the episodes within minutes by lying supine on the
floor with his legs elevated on a bed or table. This time, however,
this maneuver has had no effect, and the patient for the first time
feels weak. He has never had ischemic heart pain, and takes no
medications. Physical examination reveals a mildly anxious and
uncomfortable man, with pulses that are slightly weak and irregularly irregular at a rate of 140-150 beats per minute. Cardiac
examination suggests no valvular or myocardial disease. The
blood pressure is 110/70 in the recumbent position. The ECG is
shown in Fig. 42.1.

1. What is the rhythm?
    a) atrial flutter with variable AV conduction
    b) multifocal atrial tachycardia
    c) atrial fibrillation with rapid ventricular response

ANSWER: (c) The QRS complexes occur at irregularly irregular
intervals at an average rate of about 150/minute, and almost all of
the QRS complexes are narrow. P waves are not clearly identifiable.
The baseline seen during longer RR intervals is irregularly wavy,
suggesting that the atrial rhythm is fibrillation, which would explain
the irregular QRS rhythm. The absence of flutter waves in Leads
II, III, and aVF suggest that the rhythm is not atrial flutter. Multifocal atrial tachycardia is excluded by the absence of P waves.

2. How is the wide, bizarre contour of the second, predominantly
    upright beat in V2 explained?

ANSWER: In atrial fibrillation, when the majority of QRS complexes
that occur are narrow, QRS complexes that are wide and bizarre may
occur because of (1) ventricular ectopy or (2) aberrant intraventricular conduction of atrial fibrillatory impulses. Guidelines for the
differentiation between these two possibilities concern the contour
of the QRS complex in Lead V_1, and the relationships of the coupling
interval of the wide complex to the coupling interval of its preceding
narrow QRS complex.

3. What therapeutic interventions might reasonably be used at this
    time?
    a) digitalis administration   d) propranolol administration
    b) quinidine administration   e) DC cardioversion
    c) Tensilon® administration

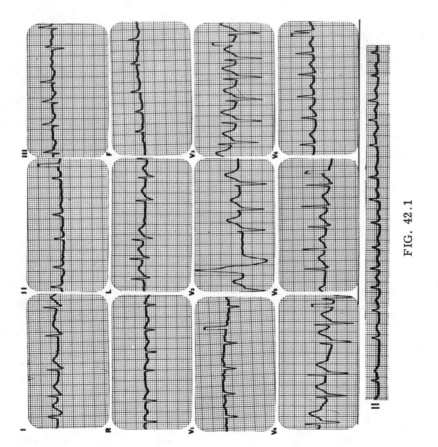

FIG. 42.1

ANSWER: (a, d, e) The management of atrial fibrillation in a patient who is hemodynamically stable involves administration of medication aimed at slowing the ventricular rate. Digoxin and/or propranolol would be expected to slow the ventricular rate. Quinidine preparations, given alone, might convert the atrial fibrillation to atrial flutter and then to sinus rhythm, but the rare possibility that 1:1 atrioventricular conduction will occur during atrial flutter makes its administration initially somewhat risky. While Tensilon®️ would increase atrioventricular nodal block and thereby slow the ventricular response, its effect is transient, lasting only seconds. DC cardioversion would be expected to be able to terminate the atrial fibrillation.

The patient is given Cedilanid®️ , 1.2 mg intravenously over a five minute period, and in the ensuing two hours the ventricular rate slows to about 120-130/minute. Another 0.4 mg of Cedilanid®️ is administered intravenously; and 30 minutes later sinus rhythm appears, at which time the 12-Lead ECG shown in Fig. 42.2 is recorded.

4. What are the abnormalities in this ECG and how are they explained?

ANSWER: The rhythm is sinus arrhythmia, at an average rate of about 60/minute. The P wave contour, axis, and duration are normal. The PR interval is normal at about 0.14 seconds. The QRS duration is about 0.11 seconds, and the slight slur on the upstroke of the R wave in Leads V1-4 suggests a delta wave. The QRS complex in Lead V_1 is completely upright. The frontal plane QRS axis is normal at about 0 degrees. The ST segments and T waves are normal. The suggestion of a small delta wave and the large R wave in V1 are abnormalities that could be due to initial excitation of the ventricles by an accessory atrioventricular conduction pathway. The normal PR interval suggests that either the accessory pathway lies at some distance from the sinus node such that at this time ventricular activation is attributable predominantly to impulses traversing the AV node-His-Purkinje system, and, to a lesser extent, to impulses traversing the accessory pathway; or, that the accessory pathway arises below the AV node in the area of the bundle of His (Mahaim fibers).

5. How and why does the QRS morphology during the episode of atrial fibrillation with rapid ventricular rate differ from that during sinus rhythm?

ANSWER: During atrial fibrillation, the frontal plane QRS axis is about +40 degrees. The QRS complexes in Leads V1-V4 are of shorter duration and have a more normal rS configuration than during sinus rhythm, suggesting that atrioventricular conduction during the episode of atrial fibrillation occurs virtually entirely through the normal AV node-His-Purkinje system, while during sinus rhythm ventricular tissue is activated at least partly via the anomalous pathway.

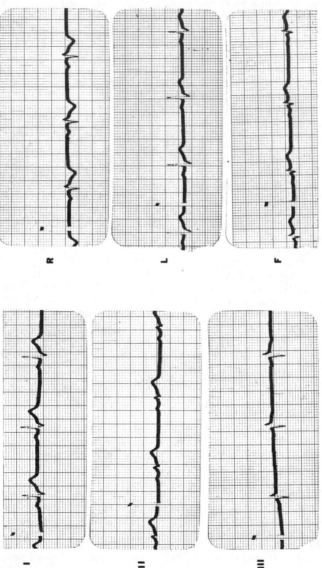

R   L   F

I   II   III

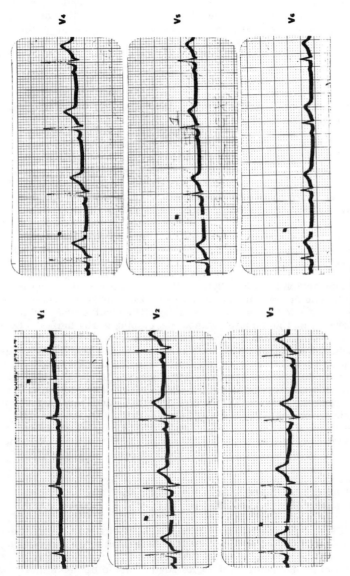

FIG. 42.2

6. How is the patient's propensity to episodes of rapid heart action explained in this clinical setting?

ANSWER: People with accessory atrioventricular conduction pathways have a predilection to develop atrial tachyarrhythmias. The development of paroxysmal supraventricular tachycardia in this clinical setting is readily understandable on the basis of the presence of two atrioventricular conduction pathways with different refractory periods and, probably, different conduction velocities. The onset of atrial fibrillation, which is more difficult to understand in that it probably does not require multiple atrioventricular conduction pathways, occurs much less commonly than paroxysmal supraventricular tachycardia.

This patient's episodes of rapid heart action that occurred with great frequency, during which he felt that the cardiac rhythm was regular, were probably paroxysmal supraventricular tachycardia. Their cessation within minutes of the patient performing his postural maneuver, thereby probably inducing a baroreceptor response, makes paroxysmal supraventricular tachycardia the likely arrhythmia in the previous episodes. It is not surprising that the present episode of rapid heart action did not respond to the postural maneuver, inasmuch as atrial fibrillation is unlikely to be terminated by baroreceptor responses.

After conversion to sinus rhythm, the patient feels well, and is sent home to resume his normal activities, taking digoxin, 0.25 mg daily. A few weeks later he performs a treadmill exercise test, achieving a heart rate of 160/minute, without developing arrhythmias, chest discomfort, or ST and T wave abnormalities. The PR interval throughout the exercise test is 0.16 seconds, and ventricular preexcitation does not occur. He does well for 14 months, while continuing to take digoxin. One day while ice-skating he has another episode of rapid irregular heart action which does not resolve on performing the previously effective postural maneuver, and which is again accompanied by a feeling of generalized weakness. He comes to the Emergency Room where his physical examination is essentially unchanged from that on his prior visit, except that the heart rate is slightly faster. The ECG is shown in Fig. 42.3.

7. What is the rhythm?
   a) atrial fibrillation with rapid ventricular rate
   b) ventricular tachycardia

ANSWER: (a) The irregularly irregular QRS rhythm occurs at a rate of about 180/minute and P waves are not identifiable, suggesting that once again the rhythm is atrial fibrillation with rapid ventricular rate. In ventricular tachycardia the QRS rhythm would be much more regular.

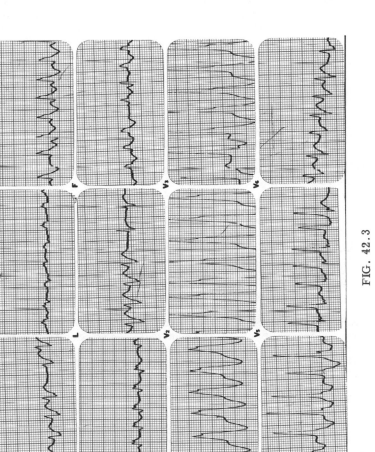

FIG. 42.3

8. How might the wide, bizarre QRS complexes be explained?
How might the two narrow QRS complexes at the end of Lead
aVL be explained?

ANSWER: The wide QRS complexes can be explained by aberrant
intraventricular conduction of the atrial fibrillatory impulses, and
the narrow QRS complexes by normal intraventricular conduction of
the atrial fibrillatory impulses. The coupling interval of the next to
last (narrow) QRS complex in Lead aVL is the longest coupling interval in the entire tracing, suggesting that rate-dependent aberrant
intraventricular conduction might explain the wide QRS complexes.
However, if the patient has an anomalous atrioventricular conduction pathway, it is possible that the "aberrant" intraventricular conduction is due to activation of the ventricles predominantly via this
accessory pathway.

The last two QRS complexes in Lead aVL in Fig. 42.3 are similar
to the QRS complexes seen in Lead aVL during sinus rhythm (Fig.
42.2), suggesting that these two QRS complexes are conducted predominantly over the AV node-His-Purkinje system pathway. The
QRS complexes in Lead V2 of Fig. 42.3 are very similar to the
second QRS complex in Lead V2 during the first episode of atrial
fibrillation (Fig. 42.1), suggesting that this latter beat could conceivably represent an atrial fibrillatory impulse that is conducted
to the ventricles via the accessory pathway.

9. What are possible explanations for the more rapid ventricular
rate and the aberrant intraventricular conduction in this second
episode of atrial fibrillation compared to the first episode?

ANSWER: The ventricular response to atrial fibrillation is determined by the ability of the atrioventricular conduction system to
transmit the fibrillatory impulses to ventricular tissue. When
atrioventricular conduction occurs only via the AV node-His-Purkinje system, the ventricular rate will be determined by conduction
through the AV node. Propagation of impulses through the AV node
is profoundly affected by autonomic stimuli as well as by pharmacologic agents, so the ventricular rate might be faster during the
second episode of atrial fibrillation than during the first episode because of a change in autonomic nervous system input. However,
the patient now takes digoxin which, by slowing conduction in the
AV node, would be expected to slow the ventricular response in atrial
fibrillation.

Atrioventricular conduction via an accessory pathway is also affected
by autonomic stimuli and pharmacologic agents. Some digitalis glycosides (ouabain and digoxin) have been shown to be able to improve
conduction in accessory pathways, probably by shortening the refractory period of the accessory pathway, and would therefore be
expected to increase the ventricular response to atrial fibrillation.

The most likely explanations for the more rapid ventricular response
and the aberrant intraventricular conduction now are that autonomic
stimuli and/or digoxin have shortened the refractory period of, and
perhaps have increased conduction velocity in, the accessory pathway, such that now it can conduct more fibrillatory impulses per
unit time than can the AV node, whose refractory period has probably been lengthened, and conduction velocity decreased, by digoxin.

The long rhythm strip seen in Fig. 42.4 shows that groups of QRS
complexes presumably conducted via the accessory pathway alternate
with groups of QRS complexes presumably conducted over the normal AV node-His-Purkinje system. The shortest coupling interval
between the wide QRS complexes (the 1st and 2nd, and 2nd and 3rd
beats in the top strip) is an estimate of the refractory period of the
accessory pathway (about 0.29 seconds). The shortest coupling interval between narrow QRS complexes (the 12th and 13th beats in the
bottom strip) is an estimate of the refractory period of the AV node-
His-Purkinje system (about 0.36 seconds). Thus, at this time, with
the patient taking digoxin, the refractory period of the accessory
pathway is shorter than that of the AV node-His-Purkinje system,
and atrial fibrillatory impulses might therefore be expected to be
conducted preferentially over the accessory pathway. However,
the accessory pathway, like the normal AV node-His-Purkinje system, may be bombarded with fibrillatory impulses in such rapid
succession that antegrade conduction through it is temporarily
blocked. Should this happen, fibrillatory impulses might then traverse the AV node-His-Purkinje system, resulting in the appearance
of normal QRS complexes. If the impulses that have been conducted
over the normal AV node-His-Purkinje system then penetrate the
accessory pathway retrogradely, antegrade accessory pathway conduction may be transiently blocked and only narrow QRS complexes
will be seen. Reappearance of wide QRS complexes could be explained by identical phenomena occurring during AV node-His-Purkinje system conduction: rapid bombardment of the AV node-His-
Purkinje system could result in transient failure of impulse conduction. Subsequent atrial fibrillatory impulses might traverse the
accessory pathway and enter the AV node-His-Purkinje system retrogradely, resulting in transient antegrade AV node-His-Purkinje
system block. Thus, concealed antegrade and retrograde conduction
of impulses into two pathways having different refractory periods
reasonably accounts for the alternation of groups of wide and narrow
QRS complexes.

The patient feels weak and anxious, but has a blood pressure of
110/70 in the recumbent position and there is no evidence of congestive heart failure. His cardiac output appears adequate.

10. Appropriate therapy at this time might include:
    a) lidocaine administration   e) sedation
    b) propranolol administration f) procainamide administration
    c) DC cardioversion   g) quinidine administration
    d) digoxin administration

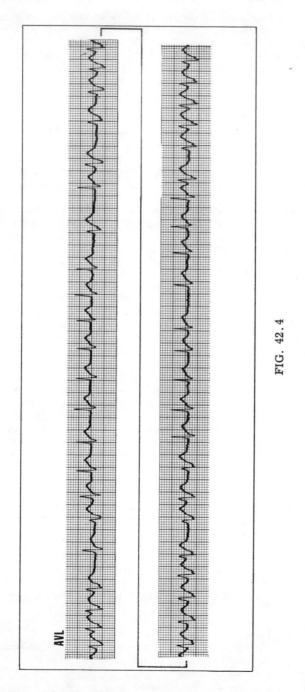

FIG. 42.4

ANSWER: (a, c, e, f, g) Lidocaine, procainamide, and quinidine
are likely to prolong the refractory period of the accessory pathway
and would be expected to slow the ventricular rate in this patient.
Quinidine might, in addition, convert the atrial fibrillation to atrial
flutter or to sinus rhythm, and, should DC cardioversion be required, might lessen the possibility of post-cardioversion arrhythmias. Propranolol is not likely to alter the refractory period of
the accessory pathway and would therefore probably not slow the
ventricular rate. Digoxin might shorten the refractory period
of the accessory pathway, and might thereby increase the ventricular rate. Both propranolol and digoxin would, however,
be expected to lengthen the refractory period of the atrioventricular node and thus slow the rate of impulse conduction that
occurs over the normal AV node-His-Purkinje system.

Sedation is not clearly established as an aid in slowing the ventricular response in atrial fibrillation, although this could conceivably
occur by diminishing catecholamine response to the stress of the
situation. DC cardioversion could be used to terminate the rhythm.

The patient is treated with 50 mg of lidocaine intravenously, and the
effect is shown in Fig. 42.5A. The shortest coupling interval between narrow QRS complexes is about 0.36 seconds (14th and 15th
QRS complexes), indicating that lidocaine has not measurably affected
the AV node-His-Purkinje system refractory period. However, the
wide QRS complexes now occur only rarely, even more rarely in
pairs (beats eight and nine), and the coupling intervals between the
wide complexes have lengthened dramatically to about 0.67 seconds,
indicating that lidocaine has effected either a marked depressant
effect on accessory pathway conduction velocity or a dramatic prolongation of accessory pathway refractory period. Fig. 42.5B is
recorded after another 50 mg intravenous lidocaine is administered.
There is again no measurable change in the shortest coupling interval between narrow QRS complexes (0.36 seconds, third and fourth
beats), but the wide QRS complexes have disappeared almost entirely.
Quinidine gluconate, 400 mg, is then administered intramuscularly,
in an attempt to aid conversion of the atrial fibrillation to sinus
rhythm, and in the event that DC cardioversion is required, to prevent post-conversion atrial premature beats which might initiate
atrial tachyarrhythmias. Ten mg Valium⊛ is given orally at the patient's request. Twenty-five minutes later the rhythm strip shown
in Fig. 42.5C is recorded, showing that the shortest coupling interval between narrow QRS complexes (eighth and ninth beats) is unchanged at about 0.36 seconds, and only a single wide QRS complex
is seen (second beat). The average ventricular rate has not changed
dramatically. One and one-half hours after administration of quinidine gluconate the patient states that he has felt a sudden thump in
his chest and that his rhythm is now normal. At this time the 12-
Lead ECG shown in Fig. 42.6 is recorded, showing a normal PR interval of 0.18 seconds, QRS duration of 0.10 seconds, an Rr' in
Lead V1, and no delta wave. Now the only suggestion of accessory
pathway conduction is the Rr' configuration in Lead V1.

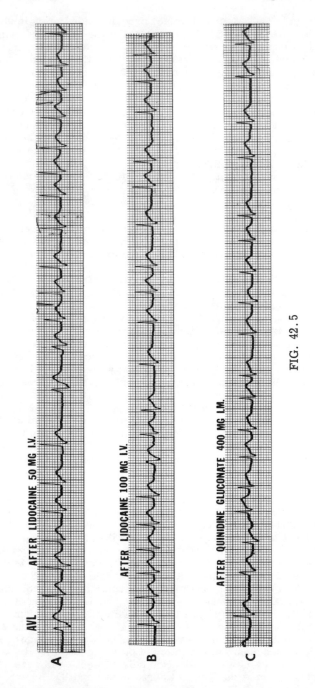

FIG. 42.5

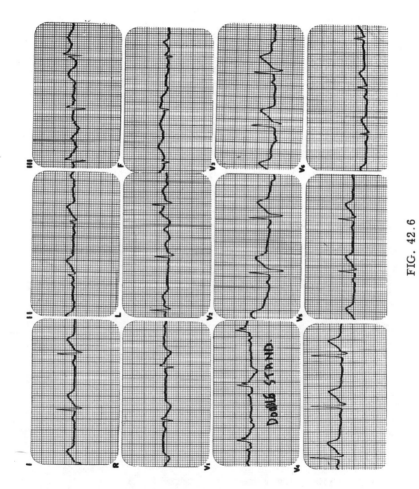

FIG. 42.6

The patient is discharged taking digoxin 0.25 mg daily, and is instructed to take quinidine sulfate, 400 mg by mouth, at the onset of another attack of rapid heart action. When last seen fourteen months later he reports that he has had no episodes of rapid heart action.

BIBLIOGRAPHY

Boineau JP, Moore EN, Spear JF, Sealy WC: Basis of static and dynamic electrocardiographic variations in Wolff-Parkinson-White syndrome. Amer J Cardiol 32:32, 1973.

Castellanos A Jr, Myerburg RJ, Craparo K, Befeler B, Agha AS: Factors regulating ventricular rates during atrial flutter and fibrillation in pre-excitation (Wolff-Parkinson-White) syndrome. Brit Heart J 35:811, 1973.

Chung KY, Walsh TJ, Massie E: Wolff-Parkinson-White syndrome. Amer Heart J 69:116, 1965.

Clifton J, Mandel WJ, Laks M, Hayakawa H: Effects of alterations in autonomic tone on AV conduction in the Wolff-Parkinson-White (WPW) syndrome. Circulation 50-51:II-109 (Abstr), 1972.

Denes P, Wu D, Dhingra RC, Chuquimia R, Rosen KM: Demonstration of dual A-V nodal pathways in patients with paroxysmal supraventricular tachycardia. Circulation 48:549, 1973.

Durrer D, Schuilenburg RM, Wellens HJJ: Pre-excitation revisited. Amer J Cardiol 25:690, 1970.

Gallagher JJ, Svenson RH, Sealy WC, Wallace AG: The Wolff-Parkinson-White syndrome and the pre-excitation dysrhythmias medical and surgical management. Med Clinics No Amer 60:I-101, 1976.

Gallagher JJ, Gilbert M, Svenson RH, Sealy WC, Kasell J, Wallace AG: Wolff-Parkinson-White syndrome. The problem, evaluation, and surgical correction. Circulation 51:767, 1975.

Mandel WJ, Laks MM, Obayashi K, Hayakawa H, Daley W: The Wolff-Parkinson-White syndrome: Pharmacologic effects of procainamide. Amer Heart J 90:744, 1975.

Narula OS: Wolff-Parkinson-White syndrome. A review. Circulation 47:872, 1973.

Neuss H, Schlepper M, Thormann J: Analysis of re-entry mechanisms in three patients with concealed Wolff-Parkinson-White syndrome. Circulation 51:75, 1975.

Rosen KM, Lopez-Arostegui F, Pouget JM: Pre-excitation with normal PR intervals. Chest 62:581, 1972.

Rosen KM, Barwolf C, Ehsani A, Rahimtoola SH: Effects of lidocaine and propranolol on the normal and anomalous pathways in patients with pre-excitation. Amer J Cardiol 30:801, 1972.

Spurrell RAJ, Krikler DM, Sowton E: Concealed bypasses of the atrioventricular node in patients with paroxysmal supraventricular tachycardia revealed by intracardiac electrical stimulation and Verapamil. Amer J Cardiol 33:590, 1974.

Wellens HJJ, Durrer D: The role of an accessory atrioventricular pathway in reciprocal tachycardia. Observations in patients with and without the Wolff-Parkinson-White syndrome. Circulation 52:58, 1975.

Wellens HJJ, Duren DR, Liem KL, Lie KI: Effect of digitalis in patients with paroxysmal atrioventricular nodal tachycardia. Circulation 52:779, 1975.

Wellens HJJ, Durrer D: Effect of procainamide, quinidine, and ajmaline in the Wolff-Parkinson-White syndrome. Circulation 50:114, 1974.

Wellens HJJ, Durrer D: Wolff-Parkinson-White syndrome and atrial fibrillation. Relation between refractory period of accessory pathway and ventricular rate during atrial fibrillation. Amer J Cardiol 34:777, 1974.

Wellens HJJ, Durrer D: Effect of digitalis on atrioventricular conduction and circus-movement tachycardias in patients with Wolff-Parkinson-White syndrome. Circulation 47:1229, 1973.

Zipes DP, DeJoseph RL, Rothbaum D: Unusual properties of accessory pathways. Circulation 49:1200, 1974.

CASE 43: Runs of wide QRS complexes in a man with extensive
         burns.

A 66-year-old man with no past history of cardiovascular disease
is hospitalized for treatment of extensive burns, which result in
substantial fluid and electrolyte losses, and necessitate endotracheal intubation. He is monitored in the Intensive Care Unit,
where the 12-Lead ECG shown in Fig. 43.1 is recorded. The
rhythm is sinus, at a rate of about 85/minute, with a normal PR
interval of about 0.18 seconds. Intraventricular conduction is normal. There are mild nondiagnostic ST and T wave abnormalities
and prominent U waves suggesting hypokalemia. Intermittently,
the cardiac rhythm seen on the oscilloscope shows wide, bizarre
QRS complexes, for which lidocaine, 100 mg, is given intravenously
without effect. In an attempt to define the rhythm more clearly the
tracings in Fig. 43.2 are recorded. Leads V1-V3 are recorded
simultaneously (Panel A) as are Leads V4-V6 (Panel B).

1. How are the wide QRS complexes best explained?
    a) ventricular premature beats
    b) atrial premature beats with aberrant intraventricular
       conduction
    c) junctional premature beats with aberrant intraventricular
       conduction

ANSWER: (b) In each Panel, the narrow QRS complexes are interrupted by two wide QRS complexes. These wide QRS complexes
have a left bundle branch block pattern, suggesting that during these
beats intraventricular conduction is occurring via the right bundle
branch. In Panel A, the narrow QRS complexes are preceded by P
waves at intervals of about 0.18 seconds, suggesting that they are
sinus beats with an intersinus interval of about 0.69 seconds. The
third and fourth QRS complexes are premature, having coupling
intervals of about 0.60 seconds and 0.54 seconds, respectively,
to their preceding QRS complexes. The U wave of the second
QRSTU complex has a slightly different contour from the U waves
of the first, fifth, and sixth QRSTU complexes, suggesting that a
superimposed P wave is deforming it. The downslope of the T
wave of the third QRS complex is deformed compared to that of the
fourth QRS complex, suggesting that a P wave is superimposed on
the T wave. These third and fourth P waves are both premature,
and the corresponding PR intervals are lengthened to about 0.19
seconds. The left bundle branch block pattern of the third and
fourth QRS complexes is therefore most likely due to aberrant intraventricular conduction of atrial premature beats. On the basis
of the events in Fig. 43.2, it is quite likely that the conduction delay in the left bundle branch is a rate-dependent phenomenon.

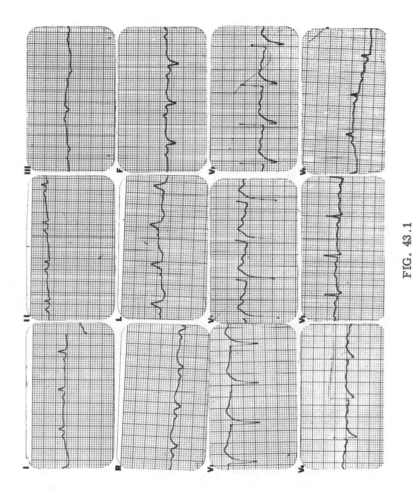

FIG. 43.1

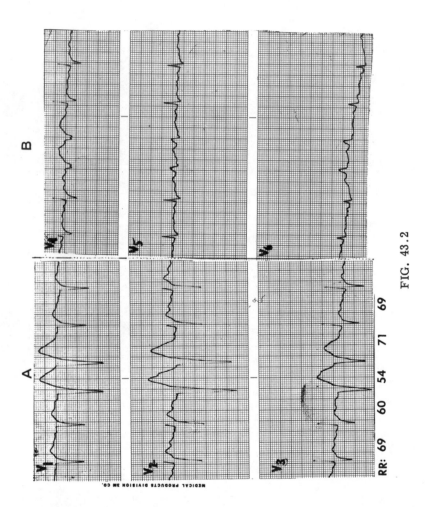

FIG. 43.2

Fig. 43.3 displays two continuous strips (Lead V1). Four sinus beats at intersinus intervals of 0.68 seconds are conducted with left bundle branch block pattern. They are followed by two atrial premature beats (●) also conducted with left bundle branch block pattern. After a pause of 0.72 seconds, sinus rhythm resumes at its previous rate, and intraventricular conduction is now normal. In the lower strip, sinus rhythm at intersinus intervals of 0.68-0.69 seconds with normal intraventricular conduction is interrupted by two atrial premature beats (↓), both of which are conducted with left bundle branch block pattern. This time however, the sinus cycle returns without a pause to its previous cycle length of about 0.68 seconds, and this first (X) and subsequent sinus beats are conducted with a left bundle branch block pattern. Thus, at RR intervals of 0.68-0.69 seconds, intraventricular conduction may be normal or may exhibit left bundle branch block.

2. How might the occurrence of normal and of left bundle branch block type of intraventricular conduction at identical RR intervals be explained?

ANSWER: It is possible that the refractory period of the left bundle branch may vary slightly from moment to moment such that at times it is 0.68 seconds and at other times it is slightly less than this. A more attractive explanation is that an atrial premature impulse is blocked antegradely in the left bundle branch but is conducted down the right bundle branch, spreads through the His-Purkinje system, and reenters the antegradely blocked left bundle branch from below, depolarizing it in a retrograde manner. The time required for an impulse which is blocked in one bundle branch to travel antegrade into ventricular tissue via the contralateral bundle branch, then retrograde into the antegradely blocked bundle branch has been estimated to be in the range of 0.04 to 0.08 seconds. In the present case, if the supraventricular (sinus or atrial) impulse following a left bundle branch block complex arrives at the left bundle branch at an interval less than the sum of the left bundle branch refractory period plus at most 0.08 seconds, it too will be conducted with a left bundle branch block pattern. In Fig. 43.2, Panel A, the RR interval following the second premature QRS complex is 0.71 seconds, and the QRS complex is normal. This indicates that the sum of the left bundle branch refractory period + 0.08 seconds has been exceeded, allowing recovery of the left bundle branch, and enabling it to conduct subsequent sinus impulses into the ventricles normally.

In estimating the refractory period of the left bundle branch in this patient at this time, the fact that normal intraventricular conduction appears at RR intervals as short as 0.68 seconds (Fig. 43.3) indicates that the refractory period of the left bundle branch is less than this. In the lower strip of Fig. 43.3, a QRS complex with left bundle branch block pattern stimulated by the first atrial premature beat (↓) occurs at an RR interval of 0.62 seconds, indicating that the

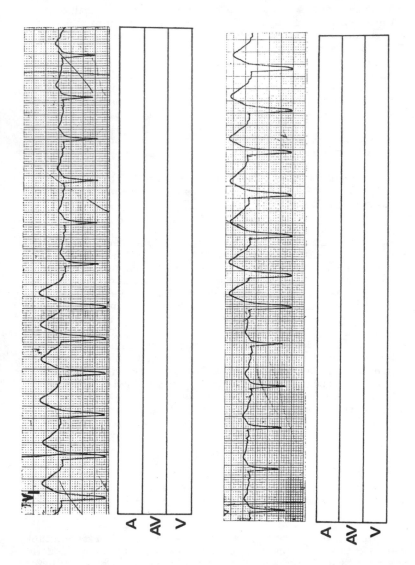

A   AV   V   A   AV   V

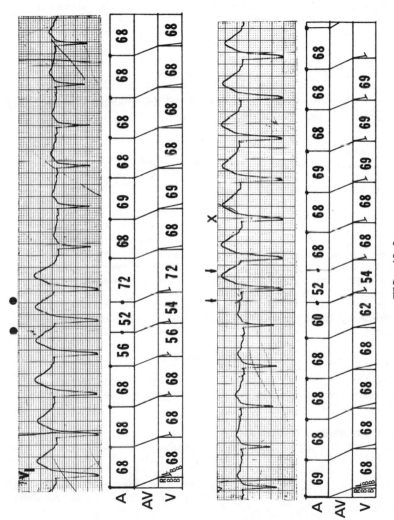

FIG. 43.3

refractory period of the left bundle branch is at least 0.62 seconds. Assuming that the left bundle branch refractory period is 0.62 seconds, and that during left bundle branch block retrograde activation of the left bundle branch occurs 0.08 seconds after the onset of the QRS complex, it would be expected that all QRS complexes which follow the left bundle branch block complexes by less than 0.70 seconds would be conducted with left bundle branch block, while all QRS complexes which follow the aberrantly conducted QRS complexes by 0.70 seconds or more would be conducted normally. This is indeed the case in Figs. 43.2 and 43.3, in which normal QRS complexes follow left bundle branch block complexes at intervals of 0.71 to 0.72 seconds, while left bundle branch block complexes follow other left bundle branch block complexes only by intervals of 0.69 seconds or less.

3. How might this patient's rhythm disturbance be managed at this point?
    a) correct fluid and electrolyte abnormalities
    b) administer digoxin
    c) administer propranolol
    d) maintain adequate arterial blood gases
    e) administer quinidine preparation

ANSWER: (a, d) Atrial premature beats, often a harbinger of sustained atrial tachyarrhythmias, are most likely related to this patient's respiratory and metabolic abnormalities resulting from the extensive burns. Attention should therefore be directed towards amelioration of these primary abnormalities rather than toward the arrhythmia itself. This patient died of sepsis and respiratory insufficiency; at no time did his arrhythmia play a major role in his illness.

BIBLIOGRAPHY

Katz AM, Pick A: Transseptal conduction time in the human heart: Evaluation of fusion beats in ventricular parasystole. Circulation 27:1061, 1963.

Moe GK, Mendez C, Han J: Aberrant A-V impulse propagation in the dog heart: A study of functional bundle branch block. Circulation Res 16:261, 1965.

Parameswaran R, Monheit R, Goldberg H: Aberrant conduction due to retrograde activation of the right bundle branch. J Electrocardiol 3:173, 1970.

Rosenbaum MB, Nau GJ, Levi RJ, Halpern MS, Elizari MV, Lazzari JO: Wenckebach periods in the bundle branches. Circulation 40:79, 1969.

Rosenbaum MB, Lepeschkin E: Bilateral bundle branch block. Amer Heart J 50:38, 1955.

CASE 44: Clinically insignificant arrhythmia prompting exhaustive discussion.

A 64-year-old man with chronic stable angina pectoris is admitted to the hospital for elective prostatectomy. A preoperative ECG is normal except for the rhythm disturbance shown in Fig. 44.1 (four continuous Lead V6 rhythm strips).

1. Which of the following is (are) present?
    a) exit block
    b) parasystolic rhythm
    c) sinus rhythm
    d) extrasystolic rhythm
    e) AV dissociation

ANSWER: (b, c, e) The predominant rhythm is sinus, indicated by the narrow qR complexes that are preceded by P waves at intervals of 0.14-0.15 seconds. Narrow QRS complexes with an RS contour are also present, but have no fixed temporal relationship to the P waves. Since the RS complexes are of similar duration to sinus-stimulated QRS complexes they probably originate in the His bundle or proximal portions of a fascicle, with the latter origin more likely because their contour differs from that of sinus beats. These ectopic beats follow the sinus-stimulated QRS complexes at intervals ranging from 0.54 to 1.14 seconds. The shortest interectopic interval is 1.58-1.59 seconds, and all other interectopic intervals are multiples of 1.50-1.55 seconds. The diagnosis of parasystolic rhythm is established by the variable coupling intervals of, and by identification of a common cycle length of the RS complexes. The absence of fusion beats is probably due to the proximal fascicle location from which the parasystolic impulse travels antegrade and retrograde so rapidly. For, were a fusion beat to occur, a sinus impulse would have to arrive at the fascicles in extremely close temporal relationship to the parasystolic focus, a phenomenon which might occur so rarely that it is not present in Fig. 44.1.

Occurrence of parasystolic beats at intervals that are multiples of the shortest observed interectopic interval might be due to the parasystolic focus discharging at a time when the surrounding tissue is in a refractory state. The refractory period of the tissue surrounding the parasystolic focus can be estimated from the shortest coupling interval of a parasystolic complex to a sinus-stimulated QRS complex. In Fig. 44.1, the refractory period of tissues surrounding the parasystolic focus is about 0.54 seconds, as measured in the last beat in the bottom strip. Impulses generated in, and about to exit from, the parasystolic focus earlier than 0.54 seconds after a QRS complex would therefore not be expected to stimulate a QRS complex. The failure of a parasystolic impulse to activate non-refractory surrounding tissue has been termed "exit block" because

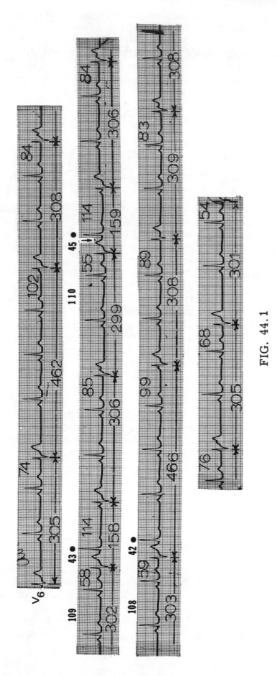

FIG. 44.1

the impulse presumably cannot leave the parasystolic focus. However, since at no time during the longer interectopic intervals in Fig. 44.1 are parasystolic beats expected to occur outside of the ventricular refractory period, exit block cannot be invoked to explain the longer interectopic intervals. It is always possible, however, that exit block is present at all times and that basic parasystolic cycle length is a fraction of the manifest cycle length of 1.58-1.59 seconds; but the presence of exit block can be established only by its transient disappearance, and since no parasystolic beats occur at intervals that are fractions of 1.58-1.59 seconds, there is no evidence that exit block is present here.

The parasystolic complexes occurring at coupling intervals of 1.02, 1.14, 1.14, and 0.99 seconds in Fig. 44.1 are preceded by P waves at intervals too short (0.10, 0.12, 0.13, and 0.08 seconds, respectively) to have stimulated them. At these times, then, there is AV dissociation, attributable to lack of opportunity for the sinus P wave to capture the ventricles in the brief time period before ventricular activation occurs via the parasystolic focus.

2. In Fig. 44.1, parasystolic beats which occur 0.55-0.59 seconds after a sinus-stimulated QRS complex are followed by normal QRS complexes at intervals of 0.42-0.45 seconds. What might explain the finding that the intervals between QRS complexes that enclose these parasystolic beats are shorter than those between two preceding sinus-stimulated QRS complexes that do not enclose one of the parasystolic beats?
   a) reentry
   b) echo phenomenon
   c) ventriculophasic sinus arrhythmia

ANSWER: (a, b, c) The earlier-than-expected appearance of a normal QRS complex following a parasystolic complex indicates that an impulse prematurely traversed the His-Purkinje system antegradely, activating ventricular tissue in the same manner as if it has been activated by a sinus impulse. The His-Purkinje system is able to be activated at very short cycle lengths (0.42-0.45 seconds) only because the preceding parasystolic beats occurred at relatively short cycle lengths (0.54-0.59 seconds). Possible explanations for the early appearance of these normal QRS complexes include ventriculophasic sinus arrhythmia, and AV nodal reentry of the parasystolic beat resulting in reactivation of the ventricles (i.e., a ventricular echo beat).

In the presence of intact AV conduction, ventriculophasic sinus arrhythmia is said to occur when the interval between two consecutive sinus P waves which enclose a premature QRS complex is shorter by up to 0.10 seconds than the interval between two consecutive sinus P waves that do not enclose one. Although ventriculophasic sinus arrhythmia most commonly occurs at slow heart rates and therefore may involve parasympathetic nervous system traffic, the exact mechanism is obscure. In Fig. 44.1, ventriculophasic sinus arrhythmia could conceivably be present, with early sinus P waves hidden in the T waves of the preceding parasystolic complexes.

The phenomenon in which an impulse originating in a particular portion of the heart activates that portion of the heart more than once
is called the "echo" phenomenon, and the resulting beat an "echo
beat". The mechanism of the echo beat is reentry. The early normal QRS complexes (●) in Fig. 44.1 could be echo beats caused by
AV nodal reentry of the parasystolic impulse. This would occur if
the parasystolic impulse, in addition to activating ventricular tissue,
has traveled retrograde into a portion of the AV node where it changes
direction (the "return level") and travels antegradely, activating the
His-Purkinje system in a normal manner and thus stimulating a normal QRS complex. If the retrogradely traveling parasystolic impulse
entered atrial tissue before the sinus node impulse entered it, retrograde atrial activation might occur, with the resulting P wave having
an axis opposite to that of the sinus P waves. If it entered atrial
tissue simultaneously with the sinus impulse, an atrial fusion beat
might occur. Whether retrograde atrial activation precedes, follows,
or occurs simultaneously with an early QRS complex will depend on
where in the AV node the parasystolic impulse turns around to travel
antegrade, and the relative conduction times of the impulse retrograde into atrial tissue and antegrade into ventricular tissue from
this return level.

In Fig. 44.2, recorded somewhat later, the first parasystolic beat
is followed by an unexpectedly early, normal QRS complex (●). The
ST segment and T wave of this first parasystolic beat is different
from that of the second parasystolic beat, suggesting that an inverted
P wave is superimposed on the T wave of the first parasystolic beat.
As sinus P waves are upright in Lead aVF, the inscription of an inverted P wave suggests that retrograde atrial activation by the parasystolic impulse has occurred. The similar interval from the retrograde P wave to the following QRS complex and the PR interval of
sinus beats suggests that the parasystolic impulse is reentering the
AV node in its upper portion, close to the atrium.

Fig. 44.3 shows two continuous Lead V1 rhythm strips recorded a
few minutes after Fig. 44.1.

3. Which of the following characterize(s) the third from last QRS
    complex in the bottom strip?
    a) echo beat with aberrant intraventricular conduction
    b) parasystolic beat, manifest because of transient disappearance
       of exit block
    c) fascicular premature beat
    d) sinus beat with aberrant intraventricular conduction

ANSWER: (a) Once again the rhythm is sinus, with fascicular parasystole. The third from last QRS complex in the bottom strip occurs
early. However, unlike the early QRS complexes in Figs. 44.1 and
44.2, this third from last QRS complex has a contour and duration
more like the parasystolic complexes than the sinus-stimulated QRS
complexes. This finding suggests that in this beat the ventricles

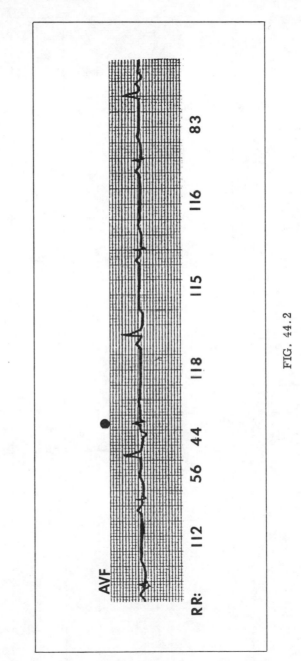

FIG. 44.2

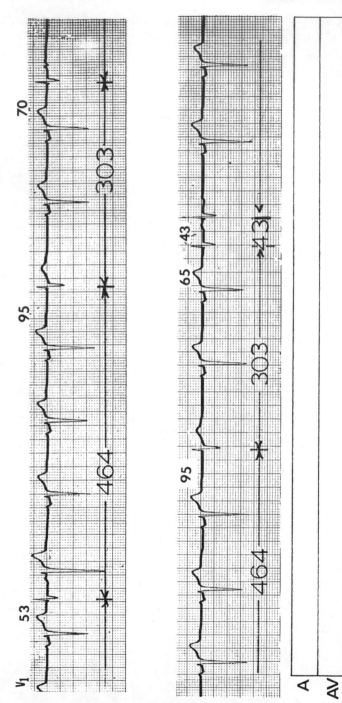

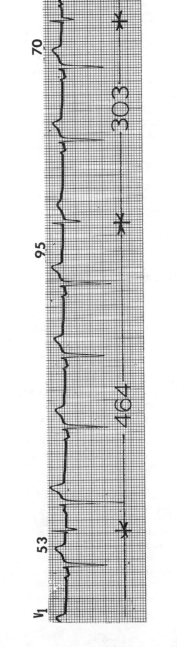

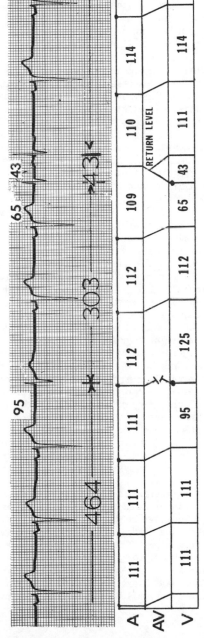

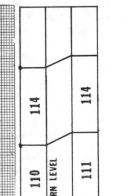

FIG. 44.3

are activated in a manner similar to that during activation by parasystolic beats. This complex is not likely to be a parasystolic beat
seen because of transient disappearance of exit block, as its coupling interval of 0.43 seconds to the preceding parasystolic beat
would mean that the basic parasystolic cycle length is 0.43 seconds,
of which the manifest cycle length of 1.50-1.59 is not a multiple.
It might be a sinus beat with aberrant intraventricular conduction
even though the time between it and the preceding sinus-stimulated
QRS complex is about 1.08 seconds, which is slightly shorter than
the preceding intersinus interval of about 1.12 seconds. Like other
early beats in these tracings, this beat is most likely an echo beat.
However, this echo beat following a parasystolic beat by 0.43
seconds is conducted into ventricular tissue aberrantly. As the
refractory period of the His-Purkinje system is determined on a
beat-by-beat basis and is shorter following QRS complexes which
occur at shorter cycle lengths, a parasystolic impulse reentering
the His-Purkinje system a fixed amount of time after the initiating
parasystolic impulse has activated ventricular tissue is more likely
to find the tissue refractory if the parasystolic beat followed the
preceding sinus beat by a longer interval than by a shorter one. In
Fig. 44.1, 44.2, and 44.3 the ventricular echo beats following parasystolic complexes that are coupled to sinus-stimulated QRS complexes by 0.53 - 0.59 seconds show normal intraventricular conduction,
while the last echo beat in Fig. 44.3, following a parasystolic beat
that follows a sinus-stimulated QRS complex by the longer interval
of 0.65 seconds, shows aberrant intraventricular conduction. This
aberrant intraventricular conduction indicates that the returning impulse initiates ventricular activation while a portion of the His-Purkinje system is in a refractory state. The contour of this echo beat,
similar to that of the parasystolic beats themselves, indicates that
the returning impulse activates ventricular tissue in a manner similar to activation by the parasystolic beat. This is not surprising in
view of the fact that later-activated portions of cardiac conduction
tissue will be refractory to a subsequent impulse at a time when
earlier-activated portions will be able to conduct the impulse. Thus,
an impulse reentering the His-Purkinje system shortly after a parasystolic beat will preferentially travel in tissue that has been activated earliest (and, presumably, has been repolarized earliest),
namely, in the area of the parasystolic focus itself. This time course
of activation will result in a QRS complex with a contour similar to
that of the parasystolic complex.

Electrophysiologic studies in animals and in man suggest that a His
bundle premature beat, a fascicular premature beat, or a ventricular premature beat will result in an echo beat only if the premature
beat occurs in a particular temporal relationship to the preceding
QRS complex. The time period following which a premature beat
can stimulate an echo beat is called an "echo zone". Table 44-1
shows the coupling intervals of the twenty-four parasystolic beats
of Figs. 44.1 through 44.3 to the preceding sinus-stimulated QRS
complexes, and categorizes them as to whether they are or are not

followed by ventricular echo beats. An echo zone exists from 0.53
to 0.65 seconds following a sinus-stimulated QRS complex. Experimental studies applied to this case indicate that in order for an echo
beat to occur, the retrogradely traveling parasystolic impulse must
arrive at the lower portion of the AV node at a time when some of
its fibers are capable of slow retrograde conduction while others,
still refractory, cannot conduct at all. When the slowly conducted
retrograde impulse reaches the upper portion of the AV node, it reenters the previously refractory - but now non-refractory - path-
way(s) and activates the ventricles via the His-Purkinje system. If
the parasystolic impulse arrives at the AV node later, when all AV
nodal pathways are capable of conducting impulses retrogradely,
the impulse will traverse the AV node and may cause retrograde
atrial activation but will not cause an echo beat to occur. In these
tracings there is no evidence that atrial activation is caused by VA
conduction of parasystolic beats that occur outside of the echo zone,
probably because the intersinus interval is shorter than the sum of
(1) the interval from the preceding sinus P wave to discharge of the
parasystolic focus, and (2) the time required for retrograde atrial
activation by parasystolic impulses occurring late, when all AV
nodal fibers are non-refractory.

TABLE 44-1

COUPLING INTERVALS OF PARASYSTOLIC BEATS TO PRECEDING SINUS-STIMULATED QRS COMPLEXES

Followed by echo beats	Not followed by echo beats
53	68
55	70, 70
56	74
58	76
59	83, 83
65	84, 84
	85
	89
	95, 95
	99
	102
	114, 114
	118

Fig. 44.4 shows a Lead V1 rhythm strip recorded a few days after
Figs. 44.1-3.

4. What best explains the finding that the interval between normal
   QRS complexes enclosing the parasystolic beat exceeds the interval between normal QRS complexes not enclosing a parasystolic beat?
   a) sinus arrhythmia
   b) concealed conduction of the parasystolic impulse into the AV
      node

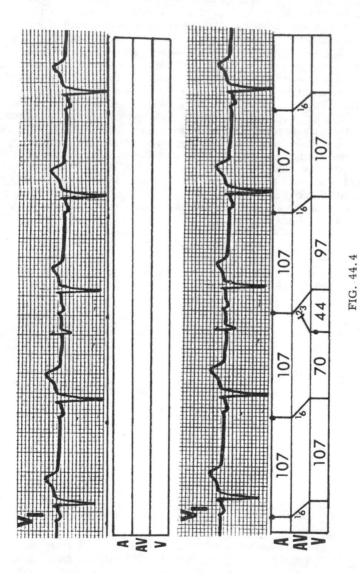

FIG. 44.4

c) reentry
d) echo beat

ANSWER: (b) P waves occur at regular intervals of about 1.07 seconds, excluding the diagnosis of sinus arrhythmia. The PR intervals of the first two and last two sinus beats are 0.16 seconds, while the PR interval of the sinus beat following the parasystolic beat is longer at about 0.23 seconds. The 0.07 second longer RR interval between the normal QRS complexes enclosing the parasystolic beat is thus attributable to the 0.07 second longer PR interval which follows the parasystolic beat. The sudden PR interval prolongation reflects slower conduction of the sinus impulse through the AV node-His-Purkinje system, which has shortly before been activated by the parasystolic beat. Although direct evidence of discharge of the AV node by the parasystolic impulse is not seen, its occurrence can be inferred by its effect on subsequent AV conduction. The phenomenon in which conduction of an impulse is manifested electrocardiographically only by its effect on conduction of and/or formation of subsequent impulses is called "concealed conduction". Reentry of the parasystolic impulse stimulating an echo beat would have resulted in a postparasystolic QRS complex that was either early or on time.

In contrast to the events in Fig. 44.4, in the top strip of Fig. 44.3, at similar sinus cycle length, a parasystolic beat following a sinus beat by the identical interval of 0.70 seconds is followed by a P wave which is on time but does not stimulate a QRS complex. This indicates that the AV nodal refractory period is longer at the time Fig. 44.3 was recorded than at the time Fig. 44.4 was recorded, and reflects the fact that the refractory period of the AV node is dependent upon factors other than merely the sinus rate.

This fascicular parasystole, by retrograde conduction into the AV node may result in (1) an echo beat which occurs early and which may show a normal or an aberrant intraventricular conduction pattern, (2) a delay in the AV nodal conduction causing the subsequent sinus-stimulated QRS complex to occur late, and (3) complete antegrade block of the subsequent sinus P wave. Which of these will occur depends on the temporal relationships of the parasystolic beat to the preceding sinus-stimulated QRS complex, the AV nodal refractory period at that time, and the intersinus interval.

This rhythm disturbance was without clinical significance in this patient, who underwent elective prostatectomy without problems. When last seen one year later he continued to have his chronic stable angina pectoris and his asymptomatic fascicular parasystole at essentially the same manifest rate.

BIBLIOGRAPHY

Chung EK: Parasystole. In: Principles of Cardiac Arrhythmias.
Williams and Wilkins Company, Baltimore, 1971.

Fisch C, Greenspan K, Anderson GJ: Exit block. Amer J Cardiol
28:402, 1971.

Kistin AD: Mechanisms determining reciprocal rhythm initiated by
ventricular premature systoles. Multiple pathways of conduction.
Amer J Cardiol 3:365, 1959.

Langendorf R, Pick A: Concealed conduction. Further evaluation
of a fundamental aspect of propagation of the cardiac impulse.
Circulation 13:381, 1956.

Moe GK, Mendez C: The physiologic basis of reciprocal rhythm.
Prog Cardiovasc Dis 8:461, 1966.

Moe GK, Mendez C, Han J: Some features of a dual A-V conduction
system. In: Mechanisms and Treatment of Cardiac Arrhythmias.
Dreifus LS and Likoff W, Eds. Grune and Stratton, New York, pp.
361-372, 1966.

Pick A: The electrophysiologic basis of parasystole and its variants.
In: The Conduction System of the Heart, Wellens HJJ, Lie KI, and
Janse MJ, Eds. Lea and Febiger, Philadelphia, 1976.

Schamroth L, Yoshonis KF: Mechanism in reciprocal rhythm.
Amer J Cardiol 24:224, 1969.

CASE 45: Intractable supraventricular tachycardia (SVT) in a
forty-two year-old woman.

A 42-year-old woman with no known cardiac disease is referred for
treatment of incapacitating paroxysmal supraventricular tachycardia
(SVT) which occurs three to four times daily and lasts up to six
hours, despite treatment with digoxin, maximally tolerated doses
of quinidine sulfate, and propranolol. Carotid sinus massage has
reportedly never converted an episode of SVT, and on the two occasions when intravenous Tensilon ⓡ was administered to terminate episodes, pauses of up to 15 seconds occurred following cessation of SVT. Therefore, prolonged episodes of tachycardia have
been treated with DC cardioversion on many occasions over the past
four years. The 12-Lead electrocardiograms during and after an
episode of SVT are shown in Fig. 45.1A and B.

1. Which of the following merit serious consideration at this time?
    a) increasing the doses of medication; advising the patient to
       try to tolerate their unpleasant side effects
    b) reviewing previous electrocardiograms for evidence of
       accessory AV conduction pathway(s)
    c) performing an electrophysiologic study to define the mech-
       anism and the effects of electrical stimulation on the SVT

ANSWER: (b, c) Since the patient has not been helped by those
medications effective in managing paroxysmal SVT in most patients,
electrophysiologic study of her atrioventricular conduction system
and mechanism of her SVT is in order. It does not seem reasonable
to ask her to suffer the side effects of increasing doses of medication when other therapies, albeit more risky, are available. As
a number of patients with paroxysmal SVT refractory to the usual
treatments have accessory AV conduction pathways, it is advisable
to review previous electrocardiograms for evidence of preexcitation.

2. Which of the following therapies might be expected to be useful
    in the management of paroxysmal SVT at this time in this patient?
    a) implantation of a carotid sinus nerve stimulator to terminate
       SVT
    b) surgical interruption of the AV node and/or His bundle to pre-
       vent SVT
    c) fixed-rate right ventricular pacing to terminate SVT
    d) rapid atrial pacing (200-300 beats per minute) to terminate
       SVT

ANSWER: (b, c, d) Initiation and perpetuation of SVT in most patients
in whom an accessory AV conduction pathway is not present involves
reentry within the AV node. Medications or autonomic nervous system maneuvers which alter conduction velocities and/or refractory

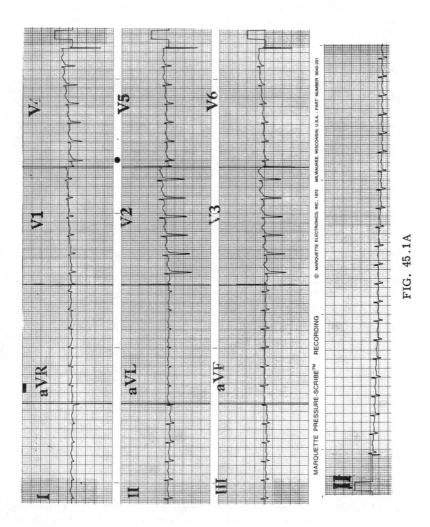

FIG. 45.1A

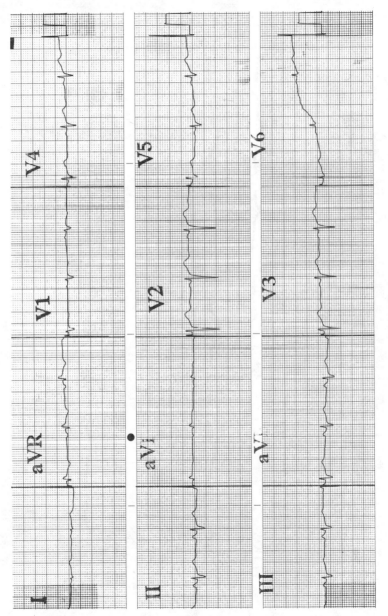

FIG. 45.1B

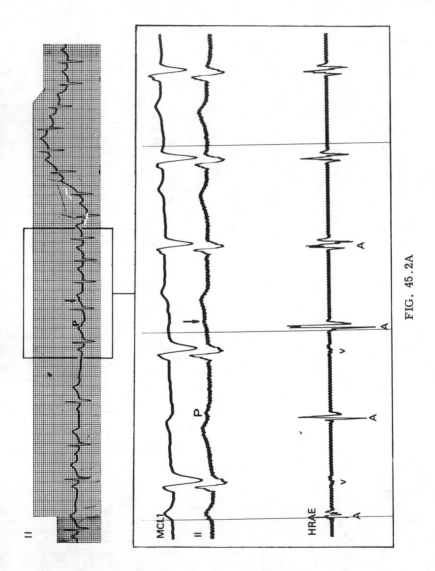

FIG. 45.2A

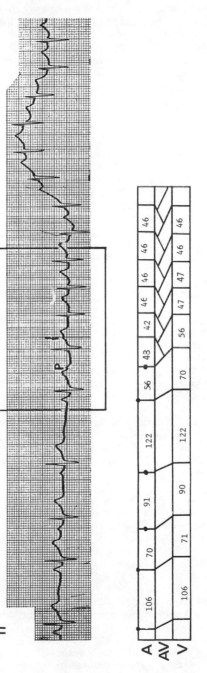

FIG. 45.2B

periods within the reentry circuit (AV node) may thus be useful in preventing the onset of, or in terminating, SVT. Electrical stimulation of the carotid sinus nerves, which causes withdrawl of sympathetic traffic from the AV node, has been used in terminating episodes of SVT refractory to pharmacologic treatment, but might not be effective in this patient whose SVT has never been terminated by carotid sinus massage. A disadvantage of this therapeutic modality is the necessity for bilateral dissections in the area of the carotid sinus nerves.

Fixed-rate right ventricular pacing stimuli might terminate SVT by retrograde depolarization of the His bundle and/or AV node, which may then be refractory when impulses that are traveling antegrade reach them. Pacing of the atrium at rates of 200-300 per minute would bombard the AV node with impulses, some of which would enter and depolarize the reentry circuit within seconds; retrogradely traveling impulses might then find the reentrant pathway refractory, and the tachycardia would terminate.

Surgical section of the AV node and/or His bundle would prevent the onset of SVT by causing complete atrioventricular block, in which case maintenance of adequate heart rate would depend on the normal function of an implanted ventricular pacemaker.

The patient undergoes electrophysiologic study, which reveals (1) no antegrade or retrograde accessory AV conduction pathway, (2) failure of premature ventricular impulses to initiate SVT, and (3) reproducible initiation of SVT by electrically and mechanically (catheter) induced atrial premature impulses. Fig. 45.2A and B show the onset of an episode of catheter-induced SVT. Fig. 45.2A, top, displays a Lead II rhythm strip recorded on a standard ECG machine, and Fig. 45.2A, bottom, displays surface Leads MCL$_1$ and II, and a high right atrial electrogram (HRAE) recorded on photographic paper simultaneously with the enclosed portion of the top strip. Fig. 45.2B shows the Lead II rhythm strip from Fig. 45.2A, with a corresponding ladder diagram based on the intracardiac recordings.

In Fig. 45.2A and B, two sinus impulses are followed by two atrial premature beats, after which there is a pause in atrial rhythm of about 1.22 seconds, terminated by a sinus impulse. The following atrial impulse (P) occurs at very short cycle length (i.e., is premature), is conducted with a PR interval much longer than that of sinus-stimulated QRS complexes (0.30 vs. 0.15 seconds), and the QRS complex stimulated by it has a P wave (arrow) deforming its ST segment. The QRS cycle length then abruptly shortens to about 0.46 seconds (rate about 130 per minute), the P waves disappear from Lead II, and a regular tachycardia is established. Although the sharp contours of the T waves during tachycardia suggest that P waves are superimposed, the right atrial electrogram of Fig. 45.2A (HRAE) shows that the P waves actually occur within the QRS complexes, and confirms a 1:1 relationship between atrial and ventricular activity.

The effect of fixed-rate high right atrial pacing stimuli at an interval of about 0.80 seconds (rate about 75/minute) on the SVT is shown in Fig. 45.3A and B.   Fig. 45.3A, top, displays a Lead II rhythm strip and Fig. 45.3A, bottom, displays surface Leads MCL$_1$ and II, and high and low right atrial electrograms (HRAE, LRAE) recorded in the same manner as Fig. 45.2A.   Fig. 45.3B shows the Lead II rhythm strip from Fig. 45.3A and a corresponding ladder diagram based on the intracardiac recordings.

3. Termination of the SVT involves which of the following?
    a) electrically stimulated atrial premature impulse
    b) ventricular capture by an electrically stimulated atrial premature impulse
    c) concealed conduction of electrically stimulated atrial premature impulse into the AV node

ANSWER: (a, c) In Fig. 45.3A, pacing artifacts (S) occur at intervals of 0.80 seconds. The third, the eighth through twelfth (and probably the fifth although this is not well-seen) pacing artifacts stimulate P waves, while the others do not, as they presumably fall within the atrial refractory period. The time interval from the onset of a QRS complex to the earliest pacing artifact which stimulates a P wave is an estimate of atrial refractory period at this cycle length.   In Fig. 45.3A, pacing artifacts occurring at QRS-to-stimulus (QRS-S) intervals of 0.35 seconds or greater stimulate P waves, while those occurring at intervals of 0.28 seconds or less do not, indicating that the atrial refractory period lies between 0.29 and 0.34 seconds. (Measurements from longer strips indicate an atrial refractory period of about 0.34 seconds.)

The final QRS complex of the SVT (V) follows by 0.15 seconds a P wave that is stimulated by a pacing artifact occurring about 0.35 seconds after a QRS complex. As this last QRS complex of the SVT is on time (i.e., occurs at the SVT cycle length of about 0.50 seconds), and follows a P wave by an interval shorter than that of paced atrial beats on termination of SVT (0.15 seconds vs. 0.24 seconds, despite the longer atrial cycle length after termination), the final QRS complex of the SVT is not stimulated by the preceding paced atrial impulse. Therefore, the SVT must somehow be terminated by this paced premature P wave even though it itself fails to capture the ventricles. It is likely that this paced premature atrial impulse, which reaches the low right atrium about 0.05-0.06 seconds before the onset of ventricular activation (Fig. 45.3A), enters the AV node and depolarizes a part of it. When the reentrant impulse traveling retrograde in the AV node reaches this recently activated - and now refractory - part of the AV node, it cannot traverse it to reenter the AV conduction pathway antegradely, or to activate the atrium. The penetration of the paced premature atrial impulse into the AV node is electrocardiographically silent, but is inferred on the basis of subsequent events. Thus, it is an example of concealed conduction of an impulse into the AV node.

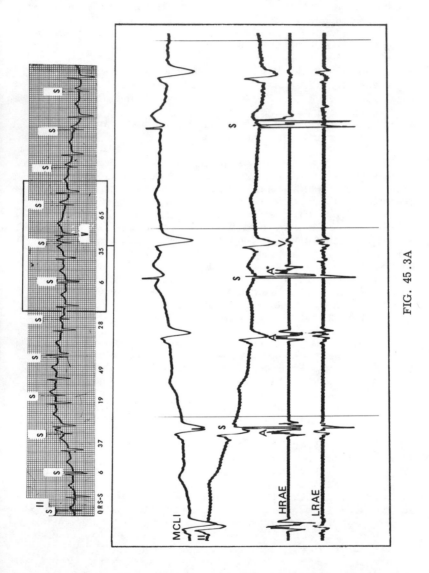

FIG. 45.3A

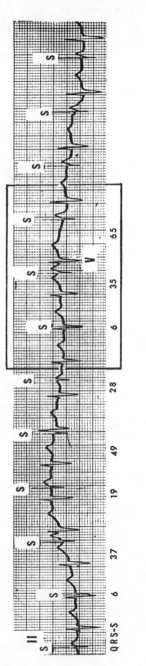

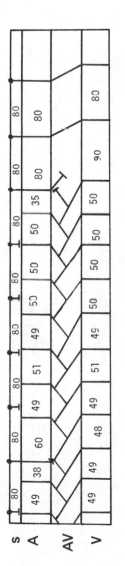

FIG. 45.3B

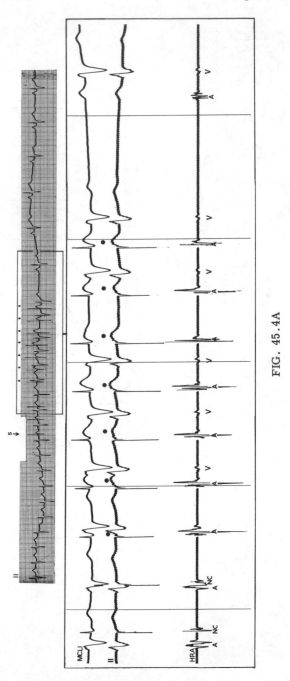

FIG. 45.4A

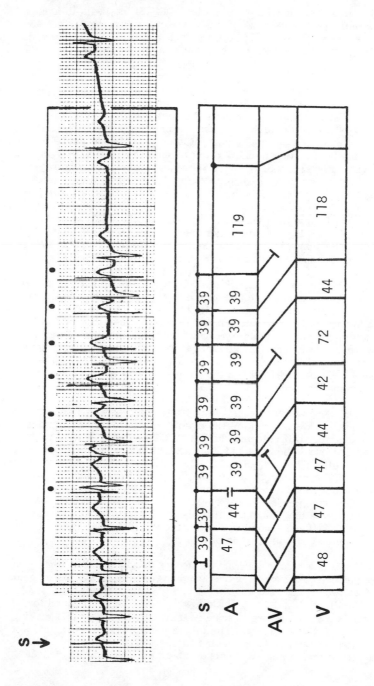

FIG. 45.4B

Measurements of the QRS-to-stimulus (QRS-S) intervals in longer
strips indicate that whereas pacing artifacts occurring 0.35-0.49
seconds after a QRS complex stimulate P waves, SVT is terminated
only by a stimulated P wave occurring at a QRS-S interval of 0.35
seconds.

There is thus a very narrow time frame within which a premature
impulse stimulated high in the right atrium can terminate SVT.
This limited time interval reflects the fact that the sum of the refractory period of the high right atrium plus the conduction time
from the high right atrium to that point in the AV node where the
retrogradely traveling impulse turns around to travel antegradely
(the "return level") approximates the time interval after retrograde
atrial activation when the reentrant impulse turns to travel antegradely.

The effect of rapid high right atrial pacing on the SVT is shown in
Fig. 45.4A and B, at a time when the pacing interval is about 0.39
seconds (rate about 154/minute), and the cycle length of the SVT is
about 0.47 seconds (rate about 128/minute). The arrow indicates
the onset of a four second period of high right atrial stimulation.
The first four of the eleven stimuli follow QRS complexes (and therefore atrial complexes which occur virtually simultaneously with the
QRS complexes, as seen in Fig. 45.2A) at intervals of up to 0.24
seconds, and fail to activate the atria (NC) because they fall within
the high right atrial refractory period. The fifth stimulus artifact,
following a QRS complex by about 0.44 seconds, and the remaining
six stimulus artifacts, following atrial activity by about 0.36 seconds,
stimulate P waves (●). When the pacing stimuli are discontinued,
sinus rhythm resumes.

The rapid burst of paced atrial impulses, some of which capture the
ventricles, makes analysis of the events surrounding cessation of
SVT much more difficult than during atrial pacing at slower rates.
However, it would be expected that the last QRS complex of the SVT
would be followed by a QRS complex at cycle length shorter or longer
than the SVT cycle length, depending on the rate of the paced atrial
beats and on the time relationships of these paced beats to the tachycardia QRS complexes. In the enclosure, the fifth QRS complex
occurs at cycle length shorter than the SVT cycle length (0.44 seconds vs. 0.47-0.48 seconds), suggesting that the fourth QRS complex is the last in this episode of SVT.

Fig. 45.4B is a ladder diagram of the events surrounding termination of SVT based on the intracardiac recordings. In this diagram,
the first two pacing artifacts do not capture the atrium; the third
pacing artifact stimulates a P wave which may be contributed to,
at least in part, by the retrogradely traveling impulse, this making
it an atrial fusion complex. The fourth pacing artifact stimulates a
P wave which activates ventricular tissue with a markedly long AV
conduction time; it must have depolarized the AV node in advance

of the arrival of the retrogradely traveling impulse, which is therefore blocked. Block of the retrogradely traveling impulse by earlier
depolarization of the AV conduction pathway by the paced atrial impulse interrupts the circus movement and the tachycardia terminates. The ladder diagram suggests that the P waves stimulated
by the fourth, fifth, and sixth, and by the seventh, eighth, and ninth
pacing artifacts are conducted to the ventricles with Wenckebach
type 3:2 second degree AV block.

An operation is performed in which two pacing electrodes are sewn
onto the right atrial appendage and connected to a subcutaneously
implanted pacing device which can be activated by externally applied
radiofrequency stimuli. A few days after surgery, the patient has
a spontaneous episode of SVT at cycle length of about 0.43 seconds
(rate about 140/minute), during which Fig. 45.5 is recorded. At
"S" the patient turns on the external pacing unit for a period of about
2.1 seconds, during which pacing stimuli (●) occur at intervals of
about 0.30 seconds (rate about 200 per minute). All stimulus artifacts appear to stimulate P waves but not all P waves stimulate
QRS complexes. The last tachycardia QRS complex probably occurs
between the second and third pacing artifacts, as that following the
third artifact occurs at a shorter cycle length than that of the SVT
(0.37 vs. 0.43 seconds).

The patient is taught how to use the device, and is discharged from
the hospital with instructions to take propranolol, 20 mg, and quinidine sulfate, 200 mg, four times daily. When last seen one month
later, she was having rare attacks and was able to terminate them
within seconds on the first, second, or third attempt, each attempt
lasting four seconds, with the pacing rate set at about 200/minute.

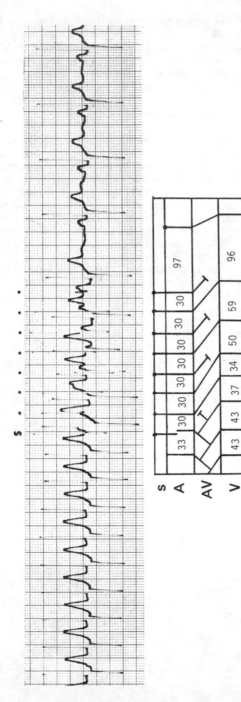

FIG. 45.5

BIBLIOGRAPHY

Braunwald E, Sobel BE, Braunwald NS: Treatment of paroxysmal supraventricular tachycardia by electrical stimulation of the carotid-sinus nerves. New Engl J Med 281:885, 1969.

Davidson RM, Wallace AG, Sealy WC, Gordon MS: Electrically induced atrial tachycardia with block. A therapeutic application of permanent radiofrequency atrial pacing. Circulation 44:1014, 1971.

Denes P, Wu D, Dhingra R, Pietras RJ, Rosen KM: The effects of cycle length on cardiac refractory periods in man. Circulation 49:32, 1974.

Fruehan CT, Meyer JA, Klie JH, Johnson LW, Obeid AI, Smulyan H, Eich RH: Refractory paroxysmal supraventricular tachycardia. Amer Heart J 87:229, 1974.

Goyal SL, Lichstein E, Gupta PK, Chadda KD: Refractory reentrant atrial tachycardia. Successful treatment with a permanent radiofrequency triggered atrial pacemaker. Amer J Med 58:586, 1975.

Iwa T, Wada J: Treatment of tachycardia by atrial pacing. Jap Circulation J 38:82, 1974.

Massumi RA, Kistin AD, Tawakkol AA: Termination of reciprocating tachycardia by atrial stimulation. Circulation 36:637, 1967.

Pick A, Langendorf R: Recent advances in the differential diagnosis of A-V junctional arrhythmias. Amer Heart J 76:553, 1968.

Pittman DE, Makar JS, Kooros KS, Joyner CR: Rapid atrial stimulation: successful method of conversion of atrial flutter and atrial tachycardia. Amer J Cardiol 32:700, 1973.

Vergara GS, Hildner FJ, Schoenfeld CB, Javier RP, Cohen LS, Samet P: Conversion of supraventricular tachycardias with rapid atrial stimulation. Circulation 46:788, 1972.

Zeft HJ, McGowan RL: Termination of paroxysmal junctional tachycardia by right ventricular stimulation. Circulation 40:919, 1969.

CASE 46:   Tachycardia following emergency aortic valve replacement in a young woman with acute severe aortic
regurgitation.

A 26-year-old woman with no previous history of symptoms of
cardiac disease is admitted to the hospital with acute severe
shortness of breath of two hours duration.   Physical examination
indicates cyanosis, hypotension (BP of 80/60), low cardiac output, pulmonary edema, peripheral vasoconstriction, and severe
aortic regurgitation.   Despite treatment with supplemental inspired oxygen, several doses of intravenous Lasix (R) and intravenous digoxin 1.5 mg over 12 hours, she becomes obtunded and
anuric.   Cardiac catheterization and cineangiography reveal a
profoundly depressed cardiac index of 1.1 L/min/m^2, aneurysmal
dilatation of the ascending aorta, severe aortic regurgitation, and
markedly elevated intracardiac pressures, with the left ventricular pressure in mid to late diastole exceeding the pulmonary
artery wedge pressure.   She is taken from the catheterization
laboratory to the operating room where a prosthetic aortic valve
is implanted and a graft interposed between the aortic sinuses
and the upper portion of the ascending aorta.   When cardiopulmonary bypass is discontinued hemodynamic measurements show
minimal change in the cardiac index, a high mean left atrial pressure of 30 mmHg, and an intraarterial pressure of 90/70.   Therefore, digoxin 0.5 mg, and isoproterenol 2 μg/min are administered
intravenously and the operation completed.   The patient is moved to
the Intensive Care Unit, where the cardiac rhythm shown in Fig.
46.1 (two continuous Lead MCL$_1$ strips) is recorded.

1. Which terms might characterize this rhythm?
    a) group beating
    b) ventricular ectopic beats
    c) AV dissociation
    d) capture beats
    e) accelerated junctional rhythm (junctional tachycardia) with
       retrograde block
    f) sinus tachycardia with junctional tachycardia
    g) aberrant intraventricular conduction
    h) complete AV block
    i) ventricular echo beats
    j) double tachycardia

ANSWER: (a, b, c, d, e, f, g, i) There is group beating, a wide
bizarre QRS complex following eight narrow QRS complexes.   The
normal MCL$_1$ contour of the narrow QRS complexes suggest that the
ventricles are activated in a normal manner via the His-Purkinje
system.   The six narrow QRS complexes preceding the wide QRS
complexes occur at regular intervals of 0.45 seconds (corresponding
rate about 133/minute), while the narrow complexes immediately
following the wide QRS complexes occur earlier (coupling interval
of 0.39-0.40 seconds).

While P waves are not identifiable at all times, they are clearly seen preceding the second through fifth narrow QRS complexes of a group, and they are barely visible in the initial portion of the ST segment of the eighth narrow QRS complex of the group. The P waves, occurring at regular intervals of about 0.49 seconds (corresponding rate about 122/minute), and having a normal contour for Lead MCL_1, are probably sinus in origin.

The simultaneous occurrence of regular atrial and regular ventricular rhythms at different rates indicates that the two rhythms are independent, that is, there is AV dissociation. The marked variability in PR intervals reflects the different atrial and ventricular rates. The regular QRS rhythm, composed of complexes of normal contour and duration, is likely to be junctional in origin, and its rapid rate establishes the diagnosis of accelerated junctional rhythm, or junctional tachycardia. Junctional tachycardia is seen most commonly in the settings of digitalis intoxication and following open heart surgery.

As the interval between the two narrow QRS complexes enclosing a wide, bizarre complex (0.28 + 0.40 = 0.68) is less than twice the interval between narrow QRS complexes occurring consecutively, the wide QRS complex somehow affected the narrow QRS rhythm. The differential diagnosis of the wide bizarre QRS complexes includes sinus capture beats with aberrant intraventricular conduction and ventricular ectopic beats.

If the wide bizarre QRS complexes were ventricular ectopic beats, they would be expected to travel retrograde into the AV junctional area. If they arrived there before the junctional pacemaker discharged, they would probably depolarize it. The junctional focus would then have to repolarize and the subsequent junctional impulse would not occur before 0.45 seconds after the wide bizarre QRS complex; the junctional complex following the wide bizarre QRS complex in fact, however, occurs much earlier (0.39-0.40 vs. 0.45 seconds). The early narrow QRS complex could be a ventricular echo beat stimulated by the hypothesized ventricular premature impulse. If so, the ventricular premature beat would have had to travel retrogradely in the His-Purkinje system and into the AV node in which it changed direction and re-entered the His-Purkinje system, activating it antegradely in a normal fashion to stimulate a normal QRS complex. The second narrow QRS complex following the wide bizarre QRS complex could be a sinus-stimulated beat, or a junctional beat which occurs at cycle length slightly in excess of the subsequent junctional cycle length (0.48 vs. 0.45 seconds) because of transient depression of automaticity caused by premature discharge of the junctional pacemaker by the hypothesized ventricular premature beat.

Alternatively, the wide bizarre QRS complexes could be aberrantly conducted sinus impulses. The P wave preceding these wide bizarre

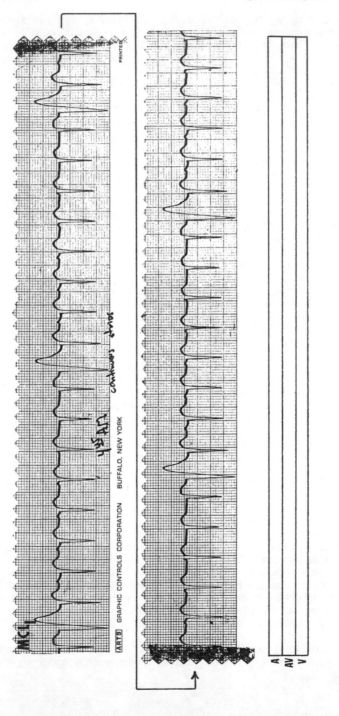

MCl₁

[ART B] GRAPHIC CONTROLS CORPORATION   BUFFALO, NEW YORK

Continuous strips

A
AV
V

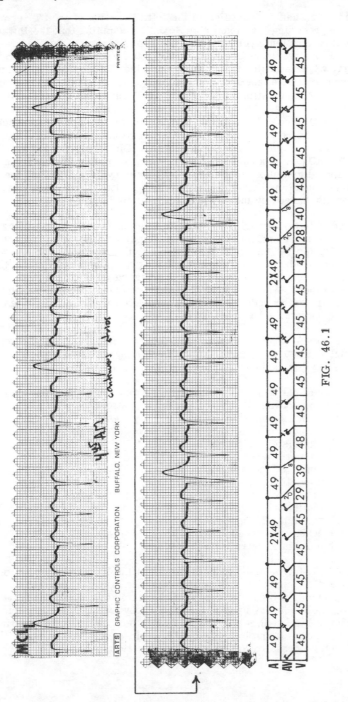

FIG. 46.1

complexes can be identified in the initial portion of the ST segment of the preceding junctional complexes. Assuming that the P waves occur at constant cycle lengths, the wide bizarre beats are preceded by P waves at intervals of about 0.20 seconds. The first narrow QRS complex that follows the wide QRS complex, occurring at shorter cycle length than the subsequent junctional rhythm, is also likely to be stimulated by a sinus P wave, but at a PR interval of 0.18 seconds. The normal contour and duration of this first narrow QRS complex indicate that the cycle length at which it occurs exceeds the refractory periods of all portions of the intraventricular conduction system. The second narrow QRS complex following the wide QRS complex could also be a sinus-stimulated beat, or, a junctional complex which occurs at longer cycle length than the subsequent junctional rhythm because the junctional pacemaker has been discharged by the two preceding sinus impulses.

If the wide bizarre QRS complex and the subsequent narrow one (or two) are indeed stimulated by sinus impulses, they would be termed sinus "capture" beats. The AV dissociation in these tracings would then be attributable to intermittent lack of opportunity for the sinus P wave to capture the ventricles, and there would be no evidence of AV block. Whereas antegrade atrioventricular conduction appears to occur, retrograde block of the junctional impulses is suggested by the undisturbed P wave rhythm.

Double tachycardia refers to the simultaneous presence of ectopic atrial and ectopic QRS rhythms. In this patient, the presence of sinus rhythm excludes the diagnosis of double tachycardia.

2. How might this rhythm disturbance reasonably be managed in this hemodynamically compromised patient?
   a) maintain adequate arterial blood gases
   b) maintain normal serum potassium level
   c) administer additional digoxin
   d) discontinue digoxin
   e) continue isoproterenol
   f) discontinue isoproterenol
   g) administer intravenous diphenylhydantoin
   h) administer intravenous atropine
   i) watchful waiting
   j) DC cardioversion
   k) administer intravenous lidocaine

ANSWER: (a, b, d, e, f, g, i) At this time the patient is hemodynamically compromised probably because of underlying heart muscle disease, myocardial depression related to the prolonged period of cardiopulmonary bypass, and the arrhythmia. The deleterious effect of this rhythm is likely to be due both to the rapid ventricular rate and also to the loss of atrial contribution to ventricular filling. Therefore, restoration of 1:1 AV conduction is desirable.

Maintenance of adequate arterial blood gases and normal serum
potassium level are cardinal aspects of the treatment of all arrhythmias. Since the junctional tachycardia could be due to the previously administered digoxin, it is essential at this time to withhold this medication; its further administration might cause even
more dangerous arrhythmias.

Isoproterenol is unlikely to be a primary cause of the junctional
rhythm, but it might be contributing to its rapid rate. It might
also be causing the ventricular ectopy if this is indeed what the
wide QRS complexes represent. However, since isoproterenol is
an extremely useful medication in treating postoperative low cardiac output states, its continued use may be life-saving.

Diphenylhydantoin has been documented to suppress ventricular
arrhythmias induced by digitalis glycosides; its use in suppressing
digitalis-induced junctional tachycardia is less well-documented.
The most serious problem encountered with intravenous administration of diphenylhydantoin is hypotension.

In this patient who has a sinus rate of about 122/minute and a low
cardiac index, significant parasympathetic input to the sinus node
is not likely to be present. Thus, atropine administration will probably not increase the sinus rate to the degree required for complete
ventricular capture. In addition, atropine will not be expected to
effect the junctional rate per se.

Watchful waiting, while continuing the intravenous isoproterenol, is
also reasonable management since the rapid junctional rate, whether
due to digoxin and/or the effects of cardiac surgery, will likely be
transient.

Since the junctional rhythm is intermittent, being terminated every
three to four seconds by sinus P waves, DC cardioversion of the
junctional rhythm to sinus will offer no beneficial effect. Intravenous
lidocaine might be effective in suppressing the wide bizarre QRS
complexes if indeed they are ventricular ectopic beats. There is
little if any documentation of the effects of lidocaine on junctional
tachycardia.

The patient is given intravenous lidocaine in two 50 mg boluses two
minutes apart, without effect on the rates or rhythms. Diphenylhydantoin, 150 mg, is administered intravenously over a six minute
period of time, resulting in a transient fall in blood pressure from
90 to 80 mmHg systolic, at which time the rhythm strip shown in
Fig. 46.2 is recorded. The group beating continues, but now consists of four, rather than eight, narrow QRS complexes separated
by wide bizarre ones. The cycle length of the junctional pacemaker
has lengthened from 0.45 seconds (corresponding rate about 133/
minute) to 0.51 to 0.52 seconds (corresponding rate 115-118/min-
ute), the sinus cycle length from 0.49 (rate about 122/minute) to

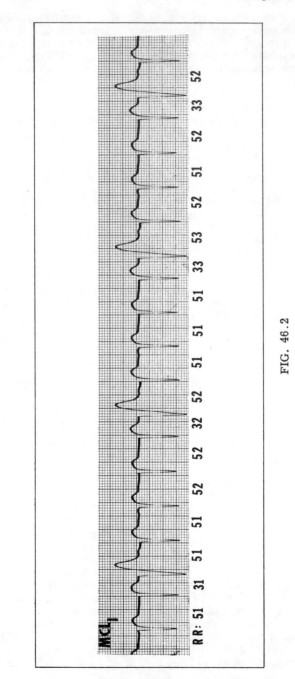

FIG. 46.2

about 0.60 seconds (rate about 100/minute), and the interval between the wide bizarre QRS complex and its preceding narrow complex has increased from about 0.29 to 0.31-0.33 seconds. Over
the next 60 minutes the patient's blood pressure rises somewhat
and the urine output increases. In the next thirty minutes the wide
bizarre beats disappear, but on occasion, narrow QRS complexes
occur at short cycle length, illustrated in Fig. 46.3. The sensitivity of the monitoring equipment has been increased to facilitate
accurate identification of P waves.

All the QRS complexes are narrow, indicating that the ventricles
are being stimulated in a normal manner via the His-Purkinje system. There is minor variation in RR intervals from about 0.50 to
about 0.53 seconds, except for the very short cycle lengths of 0.35
and 0.40 seconds in the bottom strip. P waves are clearly seen in
the top strip, in the initial portion of the middle strip, and in most
of the bottom strip. The PP intervals vary only slightly and are
of about the same cycle length as the QRS complexes. The PR intervals of the first three QRS complexes in the top strip, and of the
last 12 QRS complexes in the bottom strip, are equal at about 0.16
seconds, suggesting that they are stimulated by sinus impulses.
Following the three sinus beats in the top strip, the QRS cycle length
shortens, probably because the junctional pacemaker discharges.
This junctional beat initiates a long run of AV dissociation which
occurs because of lack of opportunity for the P wave to capture the
junctional pacemaker.

3. What might explain the appearance of the two QRS complexes at
the unexpectedly short cycle lengths of 0.35 and 0.40 seconds
in the bottom strip?
a) junctional premature beat followed by a ventricular echo beat
b) sinus capture beats
c) atrial premature beats

ANSWER: (b) The normal contour and duration of these two QRS
complexes indicate that the impulses which stimulate them have
activated the ventricles in a normal manner. Since the P wave rate
is essentially constant throughout the tracing, atrial premature beats
are not present. It is conceivable that the first of these two QRS
complexes is a premature junctional beat which is conducted retrogradely into the AV node, whence it turns antegradely and reenters
the His-Purkinje system, stimulating the second QRS complex.
More likely, however, these early QRS complexes are stimulated
by on-time sinus P waves which arrive in the AV junction before
the junctional pacemaker is scheduled to discharge. In Figs. 46.1,
46.2, and 46.3, pairs of QRS complexes at short but differing cycle
lengths follow a junctional complex which has a P wave early in its
ST segment. Presumably, the mechanism in all tracings is the
same. The P waves most likely stimulate the subsequent QRS complexes and therefore represent sinus capture beats. When sinus
capture beats occur at very short cycle lengths (0.28-0.29 seconds
in Fig. 46.1, and 0.31-0.33 seconds in Fig. 46.2), intraventricular

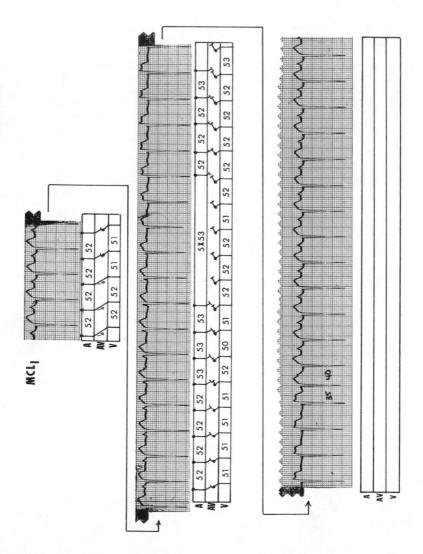

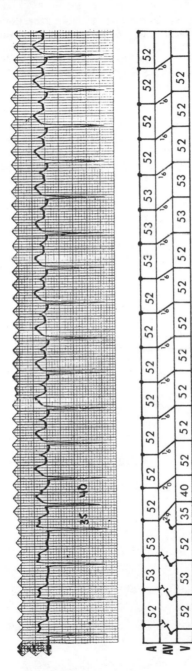

FIG. 46.3

conduction is aberrant, and when it occurs at the longer cycle
length (0.35 seconds in Fig. 46.3), intraventricular conduction
is normal. Junctional complexes follow the pairs of beats in
Fig. 46.1 and 46.2 because the junctional cycle length is
shorter than the sinus cycle length, whereas sinus rhythm continues following the pair of beats in Fig. 46.3 because the junctional
and sinus cycle lengths are about equal.

If the pairs of QRS complexes in these tracings were all due to the
mechanism of premature beats followed by ventricular echo beats,
the occurrence of a normal early QRS complex in Fig. 46.3 would
indicate that the wide bizarre QRS complexes in Figs. 46.1 and
46.2 would have had to be aberrantly conducted junctional premature
beats. It would be most unlikely if, over a period of about one hour,
a junctional premature beat followed by a ventricular echo beat always followed and only followed QRS complexes which had P waves
in their ST segments. Over a period of two hours the junctional
complexes disappear, sinus rhythm at a rate of about 100/minute
persists, and the patient's hemodynamic state improves. Isoproterenol is gradually discontinued, with no noticeable change in the
hemodynamic state. The remainder of the hospital course is uneventful and the patient is discharged. Over a four-week period at
home she begins to have symptoms of congestive heart failure with
paroxysmal nocturnal dyspnea and orthopnea, despite diuretic and
digoxin administration. She is readmitted to the hospital with acute
pulmonary edema which responds to the usual therapies. Repeat
cardiac catheterization and angiography at this time indicate markedly elevated intracardiac pressures, moderately reduced cardiac
output, severe left ventricular dysfunction, and a normally functioning prosthetic valve. It was felt that irreversible ventricular dysfunction was present. The patient continued to have symptoms of
congestive heart failure over the next few weeks, and died suddenly
at home.

BIBLIOGRAPHY

Bigger JT Jr, Schmidt DH, Kutt H: Relationship between the plasma
level of diphenylhydantoin sodium and its cardiac antiarrhythmic
effects. Circulation 38:363, 1968.

Dreifus LS, Bartolucci G, Likoff W: Nodal tachycardia. Etiology
and treatment. Circulation 22:741, 1960.

Igarashi M: Electrocardiogram in potassium depletion. II. Atrial
and nodal tachycardia in digitalis intoxication. Jap Circulat J
27:476, 1963.

Moore EN, Knoebel SB, Spear JF: Concealed conduction. Amer J
Cardiol 28:406, 1971.

Pick A, Langendorf R: The dual function of the A-V junction. Amer
Heart J 88:790, 1974.

Pick A, Dominguez P: Non-paroxysmal A-V nodal tachycardia. Circulation 16:1022, 1957.

Resnekov L: Prevalence, diagnosis, and treatment of digitalis-induced dysrhythmias. In: Symposium on Cardiac Arrhythmias. Sande E, Flenstead-Jensen E, Olesen KH, Eds. A.B. Astra, Sodertalje, Sweden, pp. 573-599, 1970.

Schott A: Various arrhythmias due to digitalis intoxication recorded in the same patient in the course of one month. Dis Chest 38:560, 1960.

Ayres SM, Grace WJ: Inappropriate ventilation and hypoxemia as causes of cardiac arrhythmias. Amer J Med 46:495, 1969.

Rose MR, Glassman E, Spencer FC: Arrhythmias following cardiac surgery: relation to serum digoxin levels. Amer Heart J 89:288, 1975.

Pick A, Langendorf R: Recent advances in the differential diagnosis of A-V junctional arrhythmias. Amer Heart J 76:553, 1968.

CASE 47: Twenty year history of paroxysmal tachycardia, some of
which have wide, and some narrow, QRS complexes.

A 57-year-old woman is hospitalized with acute appendicitis. She
has been taking digoxin 0.25 mg daily and quinidine sulfate 200 mg
four times daily for about eight years in an attempt to prevent episodes of rapid heart action which she has had for about 20 years.
The episodes of rapid heart action begin and end abruptly, and last
minutes to hours. They had occurred almost monthly until she began taking the medications; they now occur only once or twice yearly.
She has been told that her electrocardiogram indicated that she had
had a "heart attack" at some time in the past, but she has never experienced chest discomfort suggestive of myocardial ischemia and
she has never had syncope. The admission ECG is shown in Fig.
47.1.

1. This tracing is most suggestive of:
   a) old inferior myocardial infarction
   b) left ventricular hypertrophy with septal hypertrophy
   c) ventricular preexcitation
   d) accessory atrioventricular (AV) pathway conduction

ANSWER: (c, d) The rhythm is sinus at a rate of about 83/minute.
The P waves are normal, and the PR interval is normal at 0.14
seconds. The QRS duration is normal at 0.10 seconds, the mean
frontal plane QRS axis is normal at about +15 degrees, there are
prominent "Q" waves in Leads II, III, and aVF, and there are delta
waves best appreciated in Leads I, V4, and V5. There are non-
diagnostic ST segment and T wave abnormalities.

The delta wave indicates that initial ventricular activation occurs
via an accessory AV conduction pathway. The prominent "Q" waves
in the inferior Leads represent inverted delta waves and almost certainly do not represent myocardial infarction. Ventricular pre-
excitation, defined as activation of ventricular tissue prior to the
time when it is activated via the normal AV node-His-Purkinje system, may be occurring even when the PR interval is normal. Ventricular preexcitation with a normal PR interval suggests that the
accessory pathway is located somewhat distant from the sinus node,
and/or its conduction velocity is only slightly faster than that of normal nodal tissue.

The patient undergoes an appendectomy which she tolerates well.
After operation, a nasogastric tube is in place, so digoxin and quinidine sulfate are not administered. She does well until about 48 hours
postoperatively when she reports that she is having her typical rapid
heart action. The ECG recorded at this time is shown in Fig. 47.2.

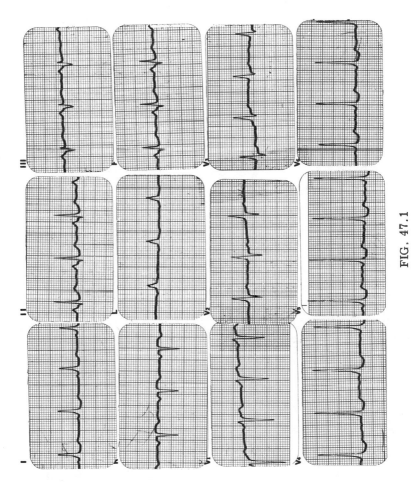

FIG. 47.1

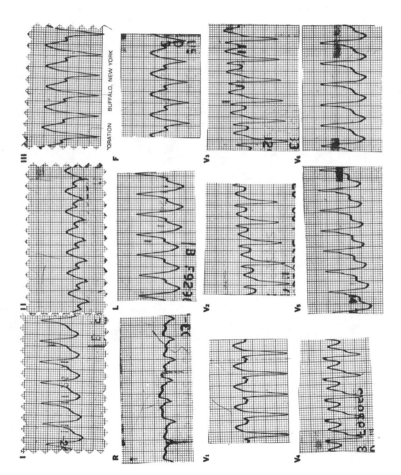

FIG. 47.2

2. What is this rhythm likely to be in this patient?
   a) ventricular tachycardia
   b) supraventricular tachycardia (SVT)
   c) atrial flutter with 2:1 AV conduction

ANSWER: (b) Wide bizarre QRS complexes occur at regular intervals of about 167/minute. Atrial activity probably accounts for the
upright deflections preceding each QRS complex by about 0.12 seconds in Lead aVR, and for the downward deflections in Lead V1.
There is a fixed temporal relationship between atrial and ventricular activity. The rhythm could therefore be SVT, ventricular tachycardia with 1:1 ventriculoatrial conduction, or atrial flutter with
2:1 AV conduction. Whether or not there is a 1:1 or a 2:1 relationship between atrial and ventricular activity cannot be established
with certainty, but if atrial flutter with a 2:1 AV relationship is present, the atrial rate would have to be about 334/minute, which would
be unusually rapid. In this patient with numerous prior episodes of
tachycardia and an accessory AV conduction pathway, the most likely
diagnosis is SVT.

The blood pressure is 150/105 mmHg, there is no evidence of congestive heart failure, and the patient has no chest discomfort. Carotid sinus massage is performed without effect. Edrophonium (Tensi-
lon®) administration and the performance of the Valsalva maneuver
are felt to be ill-advised in view of the recent abdominal surgery.
Quinidine gluconate, 300 mg, is administered intramuscularly without effect on rate or rhythm, and repeat carotid sinus massage 30
minutes later is again ineffective. Intravenous lidocaine, 100 mg,
is administered, and DC cardioversion is then attempted with a 10
watt-second discharge after intravenous Valium © administration.
The pre- and post-cardioversion Lead I rhythm strips are shown in Fig.
47.3A, B, and C.

3. Which of the following characterize the post-cardioversion
   rhythm in the top three strips (Fig. 47.3A and B)?
   a) sinus rhythm
   b) atrial arrest
   c) atrial fibrillation
   d) ventricular tachycardia
   e) accessory AV pathway conduction
   f) normal AV node-His-Purkinje system conduction
   g) ventricular premature beats
   h) aberrant intraventricular conduction

ANSWER: (c, e, f, h) A 10 watt-second discharge at the arrow in
the top strip is followed by a 1.2 second period during which the
ECG machine is not recording. The QRS complexes which emerge
occur at variable RR intervals and are of two types: (1) wide, bizarre,
and essentially identical to those occurring prior to the electrical
discharge, and (2) narrow, and of normal contour. The irregular
baseline suggests that the atrial rhythm is fibrillation rather than

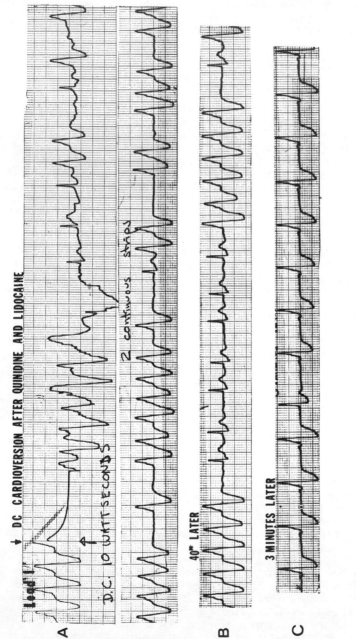

FIG. 47. 3

sinus or atrial arrest; the marked variability in RR intervals of both
the wide and narrow QRS complexes suggests that all the QRS complexes are stimulated by the fibrillatory impulses. The narrow,
normal QRS complexes indicate ventricular activation via the normal AV node-His-Purkinje system pathway, while the wide bizarre
beats with prominent delta waves indicate ventricular activation via
an accessory AV conduction pathway. The wide bizarre QRS complexes could conceivably be ventricular ectopic beats and bursts of
ventricular tachycardia, but the irregularly irregular intervals at
which they occur would not be expected in ventricular tachycardia.

In Fig. 47.3B, recorded about 40 seconds after the top strip, groups
of wide bizarre QRS complexes are separated by a group of seven
narrow QRS complexes. The RR intervals are variable, suggesting
that the QRS complexes are stimulated by fibrillatory impulses. The
shortest coupling interval between wide QRS complexes (3rd and 4th,
16th and 17th, and 18th and 19th beats in the lower strip of Fig. 47.3A)
is a measure of the refractory period of the accessory AV conduction
pathway (about 0.30 seconds). The shortest coupling interval between
narrow QRS complexes (6th and 7th, 8th and 9th, and 10th and 11th
beats in Fig. 47.3B) is an estimate of the refractory period of the
AV node-His-Purkinje system (about 0.46 seconds). At this time,
then, the refractory period of the AV node-His-Purkinje system exceeds that of the accessory pathway, and fibrillatory impulses are
therefore expected to be conducted into the ventricles preferentially
via the accessory pathway. In atrial fibrillation, however, the
accessory pathway, like the normal AV node-His-Purkinje system,
may be bombarded with fibrillatory impulses in such rapid succession
that antegrade conduction through it is temporarily blocked. If this
occurs, fibrillatory impulses might then traverse the AV node-His-
Purkinje system, resulting in the appearance of normal QRS complexes. If the impulses that have been conducted via the normal AV
node-His-Purkinje system then penetrate the accessory pathway,
retrogradely, antegrade conduction via the accessory pathway may
be transiently blocked and only narrow QRS complexes will be seen.
Reappearance of wide QRS complexes could be explained by identical
phenomena occurring during normal AV node-His-Purkinje system
conduction, in which rapid bombardment of the AV node-His-Purkinje
system by fibrillatory impulses could result in transient failure of
impulse conduction. Subsequent impulses might then traverse the
accessory pathway and enter the AV node-His-Purkinje system retrogradely, resulting in transient block in the AV node-His-Purkinje system. The alternation of groups of wide and narrow QRS complexes is
thus accounted for by concealed antegrade and retrograde conduction of
impulses via two conduction pathways with differing refractory periods.

At this point, another 50 mg of lidocaine is administered intravenously,
and three minutes later (four minutes after the electrical discharge)
sinus rhythm at a rate of about 82/minute appears (Fig. 47.3C). The
PR interval is short (0.11 seconds), the QRS duration prolonged (0.13
seconds), and the delta wave more prominent, suggesting that AV
conduction is occurring via the accessory pathway to a greater extent
than previously (Fig. 47.1). The fifth beat is an atrial premature
beat, which is conducted with a normal PR interval, normal QRS

duration, and no delta wave, suggesting that AV conduction of the
atrial premature impulse occurs via the normal AV node-His-Purkinje system. The atrial premature beat might be conducted with
normal QRS duration and contour because (1) the additional lidocaine administration has caused the refractory period of the accessory pathway to exceed that of the AV node-His-Purkinje system,
and (2) the atrial premature beat originated closer to the AV node
and distant from the atrial portion of the accessory pathway, thereby preferentially entering the AV node. Preexcitation of the ventricles by sinus impulses suggests that conduction velocity in the
accessory pathway exceeds that in the AV node-His-Purkinje system. A 12-Lead ECG performed shortly after restoration of sinus
rhythm is shown in Fig. 47.4. Compared with the preoperative
tracing (Fig. 47.1), the PR interval has shortened from 0.15 seconds to about 0.14 seconds, the QRS duration has increased from
about 0.10 seconds to 0.13 seconds, the QRS axis has shifted from
about +15 degrees to -45 degrees, the delta wave has become more
prominent, and the ST segment and T wave abnormalities are more
marked. These changes can be attributed to ventricular activation
via the accessory pathway now occurring relatively earlier than via
the AV node-His-Purkinje system. Marked variability in PR interval and in QRS contour, duration and axis is commonly seen in patients with accessory AV conduction pathways.

4. Assuming the tachycardia in Fig. 47.2 is SVT, what char-
   acterizes the tachycardia circuit?
   a) antegrade conduction via the AV node-His-Purkinje system,
      with aberrant intraventricular conduction
   b) antegrade accessory pathway conduction
   c) retrograde accessory pathway conduction
   d) retrograde conduction via the AV node
   e) AV nodal reentry

ANSWER: (b, d) The wide QRS complexes during tachycardia (Fig.
47.2) have the same contour and axis as do the sinus beats in the
post-cardioversion tracing (Fig. 47.3), suggesting that during this
tachycardia antegrade conduction occurs via the accessory pathway,
and retrograde conduction occurs presumably via the AV node-His-
Purkinje system. It is possible, however, that retrograde ventriculoatrial conduction is occurring over a second accessory pathway.
AV nodal reentry, while probably a mechanism of SVT in a small per-
centage of patients with accessory pathways and SVT, is excluded
as the mechanism in this tachycardia in which antegrade AV conduction is occurring via the accessory pathway.

The electrical conversion of the tachycardia to atrial fibrillation is
not surprising in view of the low (10 watt-second) electrical energy
discharge that was delivered. Although there is little reported experience in the electrical conversion of SVT to sinus rhythm, it is
known that a sizable number of patients undergoing DC cardioversion
of atrial flutter will be converted to atrial fibrillation if the discharge
energy is low (less than 75 watt-seconds). In such patients, atrial

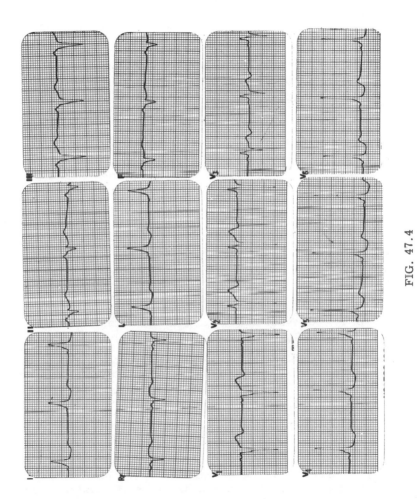

FIG. 47.4

fibrillation may spontaneously convert to sinus within minutes, as happened in this patient. If spontaneous conversion to sinus rhythm does not occur, repeat DC cardioversion with higher energy levels (greater than 100 watt-seconds) will usually restore sinus rhythm.

The patient recovers from her operation and returns home taking digoxin 0.25 mg daily and quinidine sulfate 200 mg four times daily. She has only rare episodes of rapid heart action, all of which are brief. Upon admission to the hospital two and one-half years later for gynecologic surgery, her medications are continued in the same dosages but are administered parenterally during the early post-operative period. On the tenth postoperative day she complains of the abrupt onset of rapid heart action, at which time the 12-Lead ECG shown in Fig. 47.5 is recorded.

5. What is the rhythm?
   a) SVT
   b) atrial flutter with 1:1 AV conduction
   c) atrial flutter with 2:1 AV conduction

ANSWER: (a) Narrow QRS complexes occur at regular intervals at a rate of 200/minute. Atrial activity, identifiable in the ST segments preceding each QRS complex by about 0.17-0.18 seconds, has a 1:1 relationship to the QRS complexes. The isoelectric segments in the inferior leads exclude the presence of flutter waves. The rhythm is thus SVT. At this time, antegrade conduction occurs via the AV node-His-Purkinje system, and retrograde conduction occurs presumably via the accessory pathway. This pattern of impulse transmission in SVT in patients with accessory pathways is more common than that which occurred during the tachycardia in Fig. 47.2. The longer PR interval in this narrow-QRS tachycardia (about 0.17-0.18 seconds) compared to the episode of SVT with wide-QRS complexes (about 0.12 seconds) probably reflects antegrade AV node-His-Purkinje system conduction that is slower than antegrade accessory pathway conduction. The faster QRS rate in the narrow-QRS tachycardia compared with the wide-QRS tachycardia might be due to the ability of the AV node to conduct impulses more rapidly in an antegrade than in a retrograde direction. While AV nodal reentry cannot be excluded as the mechanism of SVT at this time, it appears to be a much less common mechanism of SVT in patients with accessory AV pathways.

Right carotid massage results in termination of SVT and return of sinus rhythm. The post-conversion ECG (Fig. 47.6) indicates that accessory pathway conduction is occurring. Since the patient had been able to conduct antegradely in a normal manner via the AV node-His-Purkinje system at a rate of 200/minute and therefore has an AV node-His-Purkinje system refractory period less than 300 milliseconds, conduction via the accessory pathway at this slower rate can best be explained by greater conduction velocity via the accessory pathway than via the AV node-His-Purkinje system.

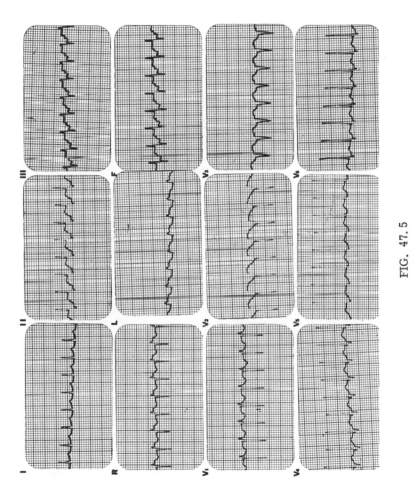

FIG. 47. 5

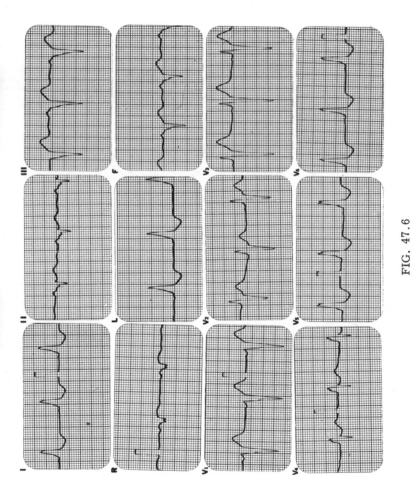

FIG. 47.6

The patient recovers from her surgery and is discharged on digoxin 0.25 mg daily and quinidine sulfate 200 mg four times daily. When last seen two years after this episode she has had only one episode of tachycardia which she terminated with a brisk cough.

BIBLIOGRAPHY

Castellanos A Jr, Lemberg L, Gosselin A, Fonseca EJ: Evaluation of countershock treatment of atrial flutter. Arch Int Med 115:426, 1965.

Guiney TE, Lown B: Electrical conversion of atrial flutter to atrial fibrillation. Brit Heart J 34:1215, 1972.

Lown B: Electrical reversion of cardiac arrhythmias. Brit Heart J 29:469, 1967.

Neuss H, Schlepper M, Thormann J: Analysis of reentry mechanisms in three patients with concealed Wolff-Parkinson-White syndrome. Circulation 51:75, 1975.

Wellens HJJ, Durrer D: The role of an accessory atrioventricular pathway in reciprocal tachycardia. Circulation 52:58, 1975.

Rosen KM: A-V nodal reentrance. An unexpected mechanism of paroxysmal tachycardia in a patient with preexcitation. Circulation 47:1267, 1973.

Wellens HJJ, Durrer D: Patterns of ventriculoatrial conduction in the Wolff-Parkinson-White syndrome. Circulation 49:22, 1974.

Wellens HJJ, Durrer D: Pathway of tachycardia in Wolff-Parkinson-White syndrome. Circulation 49-50 (III-58), 1974.

Rosen KM, Lopez-Arostegui F, Pouget JM: Preexcitation with normal PR intervals. A case secondary to slow Kent bundle conduction. Chest 62:581, 1972.

CASE 48:   Onset of tachycardias four years after aortocoronary
           bypass graft surgery in a man with chronic obstructive
           pulmonary disease and congestive heart failure.

A 56-year-old man with chronic obstructive pulmonary disease had
saphenous vein aortocoronary bypass grafts placed in the left
anterior descending and right coronary arteries for severe angina
pectoris. Over the next four years he had only occasional anginal
pain, but began to experience very bothersome episodes of rapid
heart action that caused a feeling of breathlessness and chest discomfort and lasted minutes to hours. Since they only rarely terminated spontaneously and reportedly were unaffected by carotid
sinus massage, they were terminated with DC cardioversion. When
daily administration of digoxin and quinidine sulfate did not prevent
the episodes, the patient was hospitalized for electrophysiologic
study of the mechanism of his tachycardia. Physical examination
revealed normal blood pressure, signs of moderately severe obstructive pulmonary disease, mild jugular venous distension, right
ventricular hypertrophy, mild pulmonary hypertension, and scattered
rales. The 12-Lead ECG is shown in Fig. 48.1.

1. Which of the following terms describe the rhythm?
    a) sinus rhythm   d) atrial fibrillation
    b) ventricular premature beats   e) AV dissociation
    c) junctional beats   f) fusion beats

ANSWER: (a, b, c, e, f) The second QRS complexes in the first panel
(simultaneously recorded Leads I, II, and III), being narrow and preceded by normal-appearing P waves at intervals of about 0.15 seconds
are probably sinus stimulated. All other narrow QRS complexes are
probably junctional in origin as the preceding P waves occur at intervals too short (≤ 0.11 seconds) to be stimulating them. At such times,
therefore, AV dissociation is present. The wide, bizarre QRS complexes, occurring at short coupling interval (≤ 0.53 seconds) are
premature ventricular impulses, and the sharp deflections in the ST
segments of some of them may be antegrade or retrograde P waves.
The first complexes in the first panel are P waves in the middle of
which occur QRS complexes which have contour similar, but not
identical, to the ventricular premature impulses which are the final
complexes in these Leads. The initial QRS complexes are therefore
probably fusion complexes in which the ventricles are activated by
both sinus and ventricular impulses.   The presence of discrete P
waves excludes the diagnosis of atrial fibrillation.

2. In view of the patient's history of coronary artery disease and
    obstructive lung disease, and the ECG in Fig. 48.1, which
    rhythm disturbance is most likely to be causing his symptoms
    of breathlessness and chest discomfort?
    a) ventricular tachycardia
    b) supraventricular tachycardia
    c) multifocal atrial tachycardia

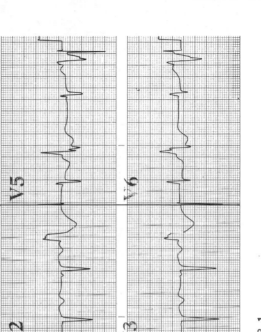

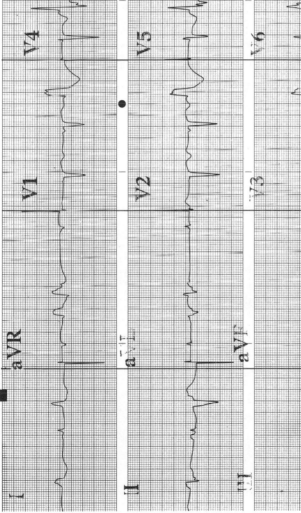

FIG. 48.1

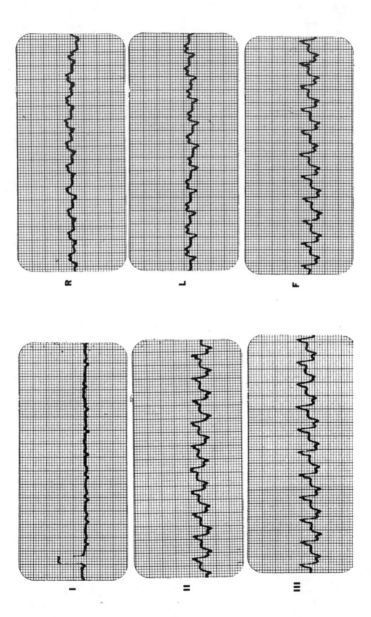

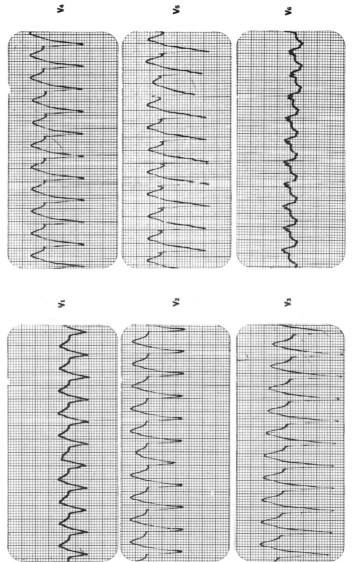

FIG. 48.2

ANSWER: (a) Episodes of rapid heart action occurring in a patient with symptomatic coronary artery disease and frequent premature ventricular beats are more likely to be ventricular tachycardia than supraventricular tachycardia (SVT). Multifocal atrial tachycardia, a common rhythm disturbance in patients with chronic obstructive pulmonary disease and with congestive heart failure, is unlikely to occur in the absence of acute exacerbations of respiratory or cardiac failure.

A 12-Lead ECG recorded during an episode of rapid heart action is shown in Fig. 48.2.

3. What is the rhythm likely to be?
   a) SVT with aberrant intraventricular conduction
   b) ventricular tachycardia with 1:1 retrograde atrial activation
   c) atrial flutter with 2:1 AV conduction and aberrant intraventricular conduction
   d) nonparoxysmal junctional tachycardia with aberrant intraventricular conduction

ANSWER: (a, b) Wide QRS complexes occur with regularity at intervals of about 0.34 seconds (rate about 176/minute). The abnormally rightward frontal plane QRS axis and the left bundle branch block pattern of the QRS complexes appreciated in the precordial Leads suggest that ventricular activation occurs via the right bundle branch and anterior fascicle of the left bundle branch. Atrial activity, most apparent in the limb Leads, has a fixed 1:1 relationship to the QRS complexes, but whether the P wave axis is directed superiorly or inferiorly cannot be stated with certainty. Thus, the rhythm could be either ventricular tachycardia with 1:1 ventriculoatrial conduction or SVT with aberrant intraventricular conduction. The 1:1 relationship between atrial and ventricular activity at this rate, and the absence of flutter waves in Leads II, III, and aVF exclude the diagnosis of atrial flutter. Nonparoxysmal junctional tachycardia, an accelerated junctional rhythm occurring most commonly in the first several hours following cardiac surgery and in the setting of digitalis intoxication, may have rates as high as 130 beats per minute and usually occurs in the presence of an independent atrial rhythm; the paroxysmal occurrence of this patient's tachycardias, the rapid rate, and constant 1:1 relationship between atrial and ventricular activity excludes the diagnosis of nonparoxysmal junctional tachycardia.

Fig. 48.3 shows two continuous Lead MCL$_1$ rhythm strips recorded while the patient was lying in bed. In the top strip there is a run of bigeminal rhythm, in which a sinus-stimulated QRS complex is followed by a ventricular premature beat. The seventh QRS complex, similar but not identical in contour to the preceding ventricular premature beat, and occurring at cycle length shorter than the coupling interval of the preceding ventricular premature beat (0.33 seconds vs. 0.42 seconds), initiates a run of regular tachycardia (cycle length about 0.36 seconds, corresponding rate about 167/minute) in which the contours of the QRS complexes are very different

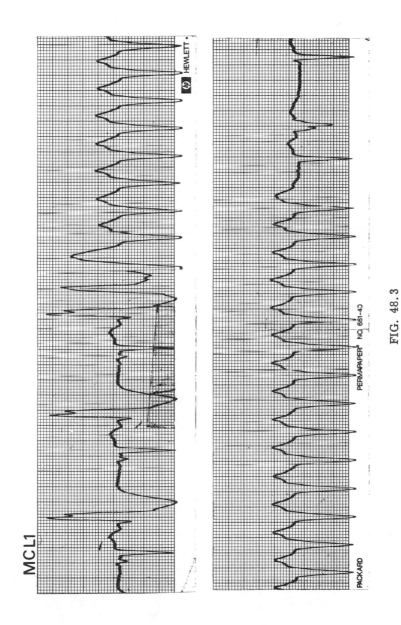

FIG. 48.3

from those of the ventricular premature beat, but are identical to
those during the episode of tachycardia seen in Lead V_1 of Fig.
48.2.   The peaked T waves of the tachycardia complexes suggest
a superimposed P wave.   The lower strip shows the spontaneous
termination of the tachycardia about seven seconds later.

4. Does the initiation of tachycardia by the ventricular premature
    beat establish the diagnosis of ventricular tachycardia?
    a) yes
    b) no

ANSWER: (b) Ventricular premature beats have been documented to
initiate both ventricular and supraventricular tachycardias.   A
premature ventricular impulse initiates ventricular tachycardia by
establishing a reentry circuit usually in Purkinje fibers within the
ventricular myocardium, while it initiates supraventricular tachycardia by establishing a reentry circuit usually in the AV node. The
initiation of AV nodal reentry by a ventricular premature beat may
be explained by hypothesizing that the AV node consists of two
longitudinally dissociated pathways which differ with respect to
their individual refractory periods, conduction velocities, excit-
abilities, and abilities to transmit impulses in a particular direction.
In order for AV nodal reentry to occur, the ventricular premature
impulse must reach the AV node when there is undirectional block
(allowing conduction to occur in only one direction) in one of these
pathways, and slow conduction in the other.

Fig. 48.4 diagrams the hypothesized initiation of a run of SVT by a
single ventricular premature beat.   In Fig. 48.4A two sinus beats
are followed by a premature ventricular beat which, traveling retrogradely, reaches the lower portion of the AV node which has not
fully repolarized.   The ventricular impulse is therefore blocked in
one pathway and conducted more slowly than usual in the other; when
the slowly conducted impulse reaches the upper portion of the AV
node it continues to travel retrograde to activate the atrium resulting in a retrograde P wave (P) but also enters the upper portion of
the previously refractory pathway in which it turns antegrade to
travel into the lower portion of the AV node, and then into the His-
Purkinje system to stimulate a second QRS complex which is a ventricular echo beat (E).   If, when the impulse reaches the lower
portion of the AV node, it also turns around to travel retrograde,
another reentrant cycle may occur.   By this mechanism of repeated
reentry, SVT can be established and sustained, as shown in Fig.
48.4B.   The hypothesized locations in the AV node where an impulse changes direction are called "return levels".

In view of the inability to differentiate between SVT with aberrant
intraventricular conduction and ventricular tachycardia with 1:1
ventriculoatrial conduction, the patient is taken to the cardiac
catheterization laboratory where the mechanism of onset and termination of tachycardia is studied.   Electrophysiologic study reveals

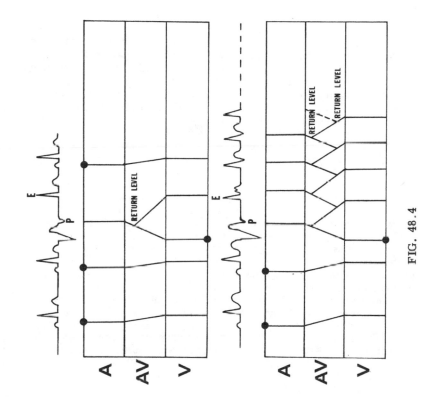

FIG. 48.4

that (1) the spontaneously occurring tachycardia can reproducibly be initiated by atrial premature beats, (2) during tachycardia atrial activity is seen to occur in the T waves of each QRS complex, and (3) during tachycardia a His bundle deflection precedes each ventricular complex by an interval identical to that during sinus rhythm. These findings establish the diagnosis of SVT, with the prolonged QRS duration being due to aberrant intraventricular conduction.

Fig. 48.5 shows simultaneously recorded Lead MCL_1, Lead II, a His bundle electrogram, and a ladder diagram based on these events during induction of tachycardia. Two sinus beats occurring at cycle length of about 0.93 seconds (rate about 65/minute) are followed by two consecutive electrically stimulated (S) premature atrial impulses at coupling intervals of about 0.86 and 0.40 seconds. The second stimulated premature atrial impulse, conducted to the ventricles much more slowly than preceding beats (PR interval about 0.21 seconds vs. 0.14 seconds), initiates a run of tachycardia that is identical in contour and rate to that shown in Lead V_1 and Lead II of Fig. 48.2. The second atrial premature impulse probably reached the AV node at a time when it could enter and travel antegrade in one of the two AV nodal pathways, albeit more slowly than usual, but was blocked in the other. When the slowly conducted impulse reached the lower portion of the AV node, it (1) turned to travel retrograde in the previously refractory pathway and (2) traveled antegrade into the His-Purkinje system to stimulate a QRS complex. The stimulated QRS complex is wide because the impulse reached the His-Purkinje system when it was partially refractory, so that intraventricular conduction is aberrant. The retrogradely traveling impulse, on reaching the upper portion of the AV node (1) activated the atria and (2) turned antegrade to reexcite the ventricles. Thus, as illustrated by the ladder diagram in Fig. 48.5, SVT is initiated by a premature atrial impulse, and sustained by AV nodal reentry.

Having established that the tachycardia is supraventricular, the mechanism of onset of SVT by the pair of ventricular premature beats (Fig. 48.3) may be hypothesized. In Fig. 48.6, the top strip is the same as the top strip in Fig. 48.3, and a ladder diagram of the hypothesized events is shown below it. During the period of ventricular bigeminy, sinus impulses fall within the premature QRS complexes such that the sinus and ventricular impulses probably collide with each other in the AV node. The seventh QRS complex, occurring at cycle length shorter than the preceding ventricular premature beats (0.33 vs. 0.42 seconds) reaches the lower portion of the AV node when it is not yet fully repolarized (thus meeting one of the conditions required for initiation of reentry), and well before the next sinus impulse is expected to occur. Continued retrograde conduction of the impulse into the upper portion of the AV node is followed by retrograde atrial activation and return of the impulse into the His-Purkinje system, resulting in a ventricular echo beat. The tachycardia is established because the AV nodal reentry is sustained.

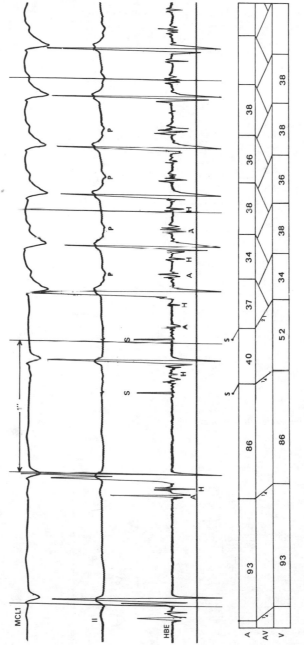

FIG. 48.5

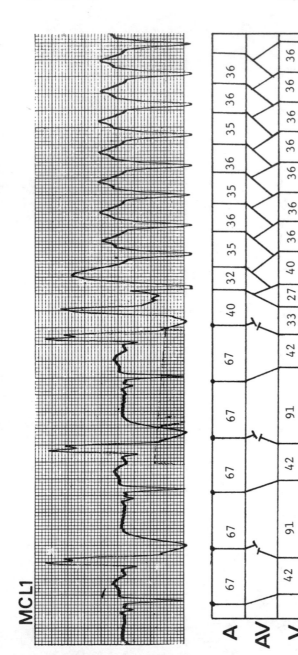

FIG. 48.6

The effect of fixed-rate right ventricular apical endocardial pacing on the episode of SVT is shown in Fig. 48.7. The strip begins with the tachycardia complexes occurring at intervals of about 0.38 seconds (rate about 158/minute). At the arrow, the pacemaker is turned on and stimulus artifacts (●) are barely seen to occur at intervals of about 0.72 seconds (rate about 83/minute). The first five stimulus artifacts fail to capture the ventricles because they fall within the refractory period of ventricular tissue. The sixth pacing artifact probably activates a portion of the ventricles for it falls in the early portion of a QRS complex (F) which, as seen in Lead II, is of somewhat lower amplitude than the preceding QRS complexes, and is probably a fusion beat. The seventh pacing arti- fact stimulates a QRS complex (C_1) which is followed by a non-paced QRS complex. The interval between the two QRS complexes enclos- ing this paced QRS complex (0.33 seconds + 0.43 seconds) is exactly twice the tachycardia cycle length, indicating that this paced QRS complex did not effect the reentry rhythm. The tachycardia QRS complex (X) that follows this paced beat is of shorter (actually nor- mal) duration than preceding tachycardia QRS complexes, probably because the slight pause in QRS rhythm (0.43 seconds) occasioned by the paced beat allowed the His-Purkinje system to repolarize completely by the time the antegradely traveling reentrant impulse reentered it. This narrow QRS complex (X) is followed by a paced QRS complex (C_2) which, followed by no atrial activity and only by paced QRS complexes, has terminated the tachycardia. The termi- nation of the tachycardia by the second, but not by the first, paced QRS complex probably relates to the shorter coupling interval of the second compared to the first paced QRS complex (0.29 seconds vs. 0.33 seconds). The first paced QRS complex (C_1) must have pene- trated into the AV node only after the antegradely traveling impulse had turned to travel retrogradely, while the second paced impulse (C_2), occurring at shorter cycle length, must have reached the re- turn level in the AV node and depolarized it in advance of the ante- gradely traveling impulse, which was blocked because the reentry circuit was interrupted. This explanation would account for the pre- sence of retrograde P waves (P) at the expected times after the first paced beat and the subsequent (narrow) QRS complex (X), and its absence after the second paced QRS complex (C_2).

5: How might this patient be reasonably managed at this time?
   a) optimize therapy of his pulmonary disease
   b) optimize therapy of his congestive heart failure
   c) measure serum digoxin level
   d) increase his dose of quinidine sulfate
   e) administer procainamide
   f) administer propranolol
   g) implant a permanent right ventricular endocardial pacemaker

ANSWER: (a, b, c, d, e) Since the SVT can be initiated by spontan- eously occurring ventricular premature beats and by electrically in- duced atrial premature beats, prevention of both ventricular and atrial

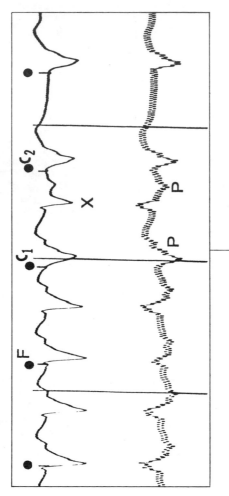

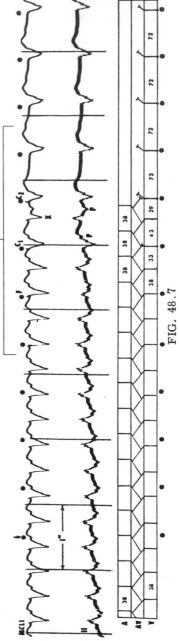

FIG. 48.7

ectopic activity is in order. Treatment achieving maximal improvement in the pulmonary disease and in the congestive heart failure
should be tried first, as it may result in disappearance of ectopic
beats. The serum digoxin level should be measured to assess the
possibility that digoxin is causing the ventricular premature beats.
Increasing the dose of quinidine sulfate to achieve higher(but non-
toxic) serum levels, or administering procainamide in place of
quinidine sulfate may also suppress ectopic beats. Propranolol,
often useful in preventing atrial and ventricular premature beats
and in terminating SVT, may have the detrimental effects of depressing cardiac performance and increasing bronchospasm in this
patient with coronary artery disease and chronic obstructive pulmonary disease. It does not seem reasonable to implant a right
ventricular endocardial pacemaker for use in terminating SVT until
all measures aimed at prevention of SVT have been found to be unsuccessful.

Over the next few days vigorous treatment of the congestive heart
failure and chronic obstructive pulmonary disease is undertaken,
digoxin is continued when the serum digoxin level is found to be
within the normal range, quinidine sulfate is discontinued and procainamide is administered orally every three hours in doses which
achieve therapeutic serum levels. The ventricular premature beats
now occur only rarely, atrial premature beats are never seen, and
SVT does not occur, but the patient continues to have a moderate degree of congestive heart failure. He returns home and has no symptomatic episodes of SVT. Two months later, following several
hours of ischemic heart pain, he dies suddenly, presumably from
ventricular fibrillation.

BIBLIOGRAPHY

Barold SS, Coumel P: Mechanisms of atrioventricular junctional
tachycardia. Role of reentry and concealed accessory bypass tracts.
Amer J Cardiol 39:97, 1977.

Bigger JT Jr, Goldreyer BN: The mechanism of supraventricular
tachycardia. Circulation 42:673, 1970.

Damato AN, Lau SH, Bobb GA: Studies on ventriculo-atrial conduction and the reentry phenomenon. Circulation 41:423, 1970.

Denes P, Wu D, Dhingra RC, Chuquimia R, Rosen KM: Demonstration of dual A-V nodal pathways in patients with paroxysmal
supraventricular tachycardia. Circulation 43:549, 1973.

Goldreyer BN, Bigger JT Jr: Site of reentry in paroxysmal supraventricular tachycardia in man. Circulation 43:15, 1971.

Goldreyer BN, Damato AN: The essential role of atrioventricular
conduction delay in the initiation of paroxysmal supraventricular
tachycardia. Circulation 43:679, 1971.

Kitchen JG III, Goldreyer BN: Demand pacemaker for refractory paroxysmal supraventricular tachycardia. New Engl J Med 287:596, 1972.

Knoebel SB, Fisch C: Accelerated junctional escape. A clinical and electrocardiographic study. Circulation 50:151, 1974.

Schamroth L, Yoshonis KF: Mechanisms in reciprocal rhythm. Amer J Cardiol 24:224, 1969.

Wu D, Denes P: Mechanisms of paroxysmal supraventricular tachycardia. Arch Int Med 135:437, 1975.

Wu D, Amat-y-Leon F, Denes P, Dhingra RC, Pietras RJ, Rosen KM: Demonstration of sustained sinus and atrial reentry as a mechanism of paroxysmal supraventricular tachycardia. Circulation 51:234, 1975.

Wu D, Denes P, Wyndham C, Amat-y-Leon F, Dhingra RC, Rosen KM: Demonstration of dual atrioventricular nodal pathways utilizing a ventricular extrastimulus in patients with atrioventricular nodal reentrant paroxysmal supraventricular tachycardia. Circulation 52:789, 1975.

CASE 49: Onset of tachycardia one day after aortocoronary bypass
graft surgery.

A 50-year-old furniture salesman with angina pectoris is referred
for evaluation when propranolol and sublingual nitrate therapy fails
to enable him to perform his work. The physical examination,
chest x-ray, and 12-Lead ECG are within normal limits. Cardiac
catheterization with left ventricular and selective coronary cine-
angiography are performed, revealing normal ventricular function
and a high-grade proximal stenosis in the right coronary artery.
A saphenous vein bypass graft is interposed between the aorta and
the right coronary artery and the patient is transferred to the Intensive Care Unit where he has sinus rhythm at a rate of about 100/
minute and is judged to be hemodynamically stable. Eighteen hours
postoperatively, when arterial blood gases and 12-Lead ECG are
within normal limits, the endotracheal tube is removed and the patient says he feels well except for incisional pain. Two hours later
the heart rate is observed to abruptly increase from 100/minute to
about 150/minute, at which time the rhythm strip shown in Fig. 49.1
is recorded. The Lead is a modified Lead II, in which the negative
electrode is located near the right shoulder, the positive electrode
just below the usual V6 electrode position, and the ground electrode
near the left shoulder.

1. Which of the following is (are) likely to be present in Fig. 49.1?
    a) sinus tachycardia
    b) supraventricular tachycardia (SVT)
    c) atrial flutter with 2:1 AV conduction
    d) atrial fibrillation
    e) ventricular tachycardia with 1:1 ventriculoatrial conduction

ANSWER: (c) The normal duration and contour of all QRS complexes
indicate that ventricular activation is occurring normally via the AV
junction-His-Purkinje system, and excludes the diagnosis of ventricular tachycardia. The regular QRS rhythm at a rate of 148-150/
minute (RR intervals about 0.40-0.41 seconds) could be present with
sinus tachycardia, SVT, and atrial flutter with 2:1 AV conduction.
A regular ventricular rhythm would not, however, be expected to
occur in atrial fibrillation, in which variable depths of penetration
of the irregularly occurring atrial impulses into the AV node results
in variable RR intervals. The absence of an isoelectric period in
the baseline could result from the presence of atrial flutter waves,
but might also occur with sinus rhythm or SVT if T and U wave abnormalities were present. The abrupt increase in heart rate is not
likely to occur in sinus rhythm, in which the atrial rate usually rises
gradually. As atrial flutter is a much more common rhythm than
SVT in this setting, and as the absence of an isoelectric period in
the baseline is more easily explained by atrial flutter waves than by

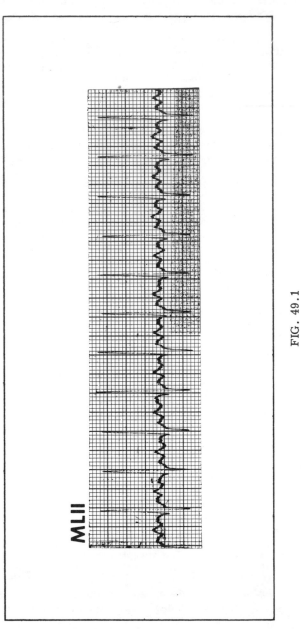

FIG. 49.1

SVT with T and U wave abnormalities, the rhythm in Fig. 49.1 is most likely atrial flutter with 2:1 AV conduction. Since flutter waves are best seen in Leads II, III, and aVF, a 12-Lead ECG should be performed for accurate diagnosis of the atrial rhythm. Fig. 49.2A displays a Lead II rhythm strip, recorded shortly after Fig. 49.1, in which flutter waves are clearly demonstrated.

Physical examination at this time reveals minimal change in blood pressure and in signs of peripheral perfusion. The chest is clear and a loud pericardial friction rub is present. An arterial blood gas determination is within normal limits.

2. How might this rhythm be reasonably managed in this patient at this time?
   a) DC cardioversion
   b) administration of digoxin
   c) administration of propranolol
   d) administration of a quinidine preparation
   e) administration of procainamide

ANSWER: (b, c) Atrial flutter occurring within the first few days following cardiac surgery is attributable both to intraoperative trauma to the sinus node and atrial tissue and to postoperative pericarditis. The atrial flutter is usually transient, lasting minutes to days, but may recur over a period of days. Since this patient is having no discernible hemodynamic problem as a consequence of the atrial flutter, and since the atrial flutter may recur even if sinus rhythm is restored, it does not seem reasonable to subject him at this time to the possible risks of anesthesia and/or rhythm disturbances associated with DC cardioversion. If, however, this rhythm had caused hemodynamic deterioration, DC cardioversion would be the most rapid and effective means of restoring sinus rhythm. Slowing the ventricular rate to a hemodynamically more favorable rate is reasonable since 150/minute is too rapid for optimum ventricular performance. The medication most commonly used to diminish AV nodal conduction velocity, and thereby decrease the ventricular response to atrial flutter has been digoxin. However, propranolol can also slow ventricular response and it does so more rapidly than digoxin, and may be used safely so long as left ventricular dysfunction is not present. Quinidine preparations and procainamide may slow the ventricular rate by slowing the atrial rate, and may even convert the flutter to sinus rhythm, but since these medications do not dramatically alter AV conduction, they do not significantly slow the ventricular rate. Furthermore, they may slow the flutter rate to a range in which 1:1 AV conduction can occur, resulting in a dramatic increase, rather than a decrease, in ventricular rate. Therefore, administration of quinidine preparations or procainamide in an attempt to convert atrial flutter to sinus rhythm is best undertaken after digoxin and/or propranolol have achieved a depressant effect on AV conduction.

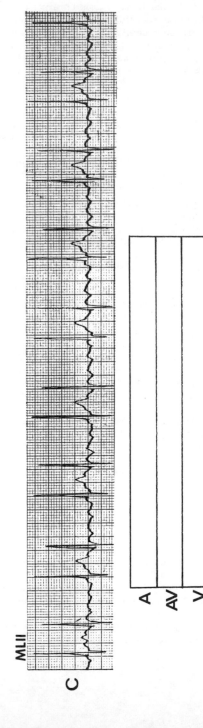

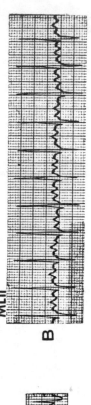

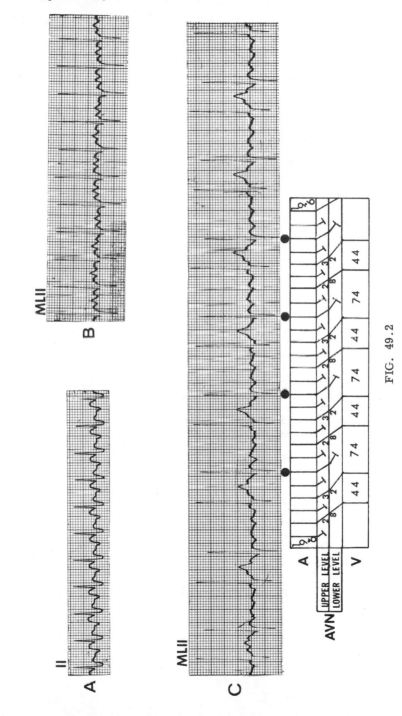

FIG. 49.2

At this time the patient is given intravenous digoxin 0.5 mg, but as
AV conduction is unaltered, additional 0.25 mg doses are administered twice in the next four hours. Five hours after the initial
digoxin administration, the tracing shown in Fig. 49.2C is recorded
from a modified Lead II. Fig. 49.2B, identical to Fig. 49.1, is
included for comparison.

3. Which of the following terms describe the rhythm in Fig. 49.2C?
   a) group beating
   b) bigeminal rhythm
   c) AV Wenckebach periods
   d) 3:1 AV conduction
   e) different depths of penetration of atrial flutter impulses into
      the AV node

ANSWER: (a, b, c, e) All QRS complexes are of similar contour
and narrow, indicating that ventricular activation occurs via the
AV junction-His-Purkinje system. There is group beating in a
bigeminal pattern with RR intervals alternating between 0.74 and
0.44 seconds, the average RR interval (0.44 + 0.74)/2 = 0.59
seconds corresponding to a ventricular rate of about 102/minute.
The atrial rhythm consists of flutter waves occurring with reasonable regularity at intervals averaging 0.196 seconds (corresponding
rate about 306/minute). The constant temporal relationship of the
QRS complexes occurring at longer cycle length to preceding flutter
waves indicates that the flutter impulses stimulate the ventricular
rhythm. Although the flutter rate of 306/minute is three times the
average ventricular rate of 102/minute, the bigeminal rhythm indicates that AV conduction is not occurring in a simple 3:1 relationship. Rather, there appears to be alternating 2:1 and 4:1 AV conduction of flutter impulses. However, as the shorter RR intervals
(0.44 seconds) are about 0.05 seconds longer than twice the flutter
wave intervals (2 X 0.196 = 0.39 seconds), and the longer RR intervals (0.74 seconds) are about 0.04 seconds less than four times the
flutter wave intervals (4 X 0.196 = 0.78 seconds), it appears that
AV conduction time ("FR interval") during 2:1 AV conduction is
longer than during 4:1 AV conduction. * The pattern of apparent alternating 2:1 and 4:1 AV conduction, and the longer FR interval of
the QRS complex occurring at shorter cycle length can be explained
by hypothesizing two regions of impedance to impulse transmission
in the AV node, one located above the other. Conduction properties
of the uppermost level are such that at this flutter rate only every
other flutter impulse can be conducted so it is this upper region which
is responsible for the 2:1 AV conduction in Fig. 49.1 and 49.2A and
B. The alternate flutter waves which manage to traverse the upper

* As the actual onset of a flutter wave cannot be determined, exact
FR intervals cannot be accurately measured, but any portion of a
flutter wave may be used to compare FR intervals so long as this
portion is used consistently.

region encounter a second, lower region of impedance to conduction, which also is not capable of conducting all impulses reaching it. Second degree block may occur in this lower region, with one of every two, two of every three, three of every four, etc. impulses traversing it to stimulate the ventricles. In Fig. 49.2C the apparent alternating 2:1 and 4:1 AV conduction pattern can be explained by 2:1 conduction of the flutter impulses through the upper level, and 3:2 conduction of those impulses traversing the upper level through the lower level and into the ventricles. In the ladder diagram of Fig. 49.2C, the FR intervals of the QRS complexes occurring at short cycle length are greater than those occurring at longer cycle length, due to progressive conduction delay in the lower portion of the AV node; the flutter impulses denoted by the solid circles (●) are blocked within this lower portion of the AV node. The effect of digoxin in this patient has therefore been to slow the ventricular rate by causing Wenckebach type of 3:2 second degree block within the lower region of the AV node.

About one hour after the recording of Fig. 49.2C, another 0.25 mg intravenous digoxin is administered, and thirty minutes later the monitor strip shown in Fig. 49.3 is recorded. Except for the seventh QRS complex (●) which occurs at short cycle length (0.44 seconds), and the eighth QRS complex which occurs 0.71 seconds later, the QRS complexes occur with reasonable regularity at intervals of 0.74-0.78 seconds (corresponding rate about 77-81/minute). The interval between flutter waves appears to be about 0.19 seconds (corresponding rate about 316/minute), or about one-fourth the longer RR intervals, suggesting that during longer RR intervals only every fourth flutter impulse traverses the AV conduction system. In the framework of two levels of impedance to conduction within the AV node, at this time there is 2:1 conduction of flutter impulses through the upper level of the AV node, and, as only alternate impulses reaching the lower level of the AV node traverse it to activate the ventricles, there is 2:1 second degree block in the lower level of the AV node; whereas prior to this last dose of digoxin, 3:2 second degree block existed in this region. The QRS complex (●) occurring at cycle length about 0.06 seconds greater than twice the flutter interval probably represents transient 3:2 second degree block within the lower level of the AV node. The interval from the QRS complex preceding to that following the early QRS complex (●) (0.44 + 0.71 = 1.15 seconds) is almost exactly six times the flutter interval (6 X 0.19 = 1.14 seconds), and supports this hypothesized mechanism of AV conduction of the flutter impulses. The digoxin has thus effected a further delay in conduction through the lower level of the AV node, either by directly depressing conduction in this area and/or by increasing the rate of the atrial flutter (from about 302 to about 316 per minute), which in itself will slow AV conduction. About one hour after recording the tracing in Fig. 49.3, the rhythm abruptly changes from atrial flutter with predominantly 4:1 AV conduction to sinus at a rate of about 84/minute. Digoxin, continued for two weeks during which only sinus rhythm is

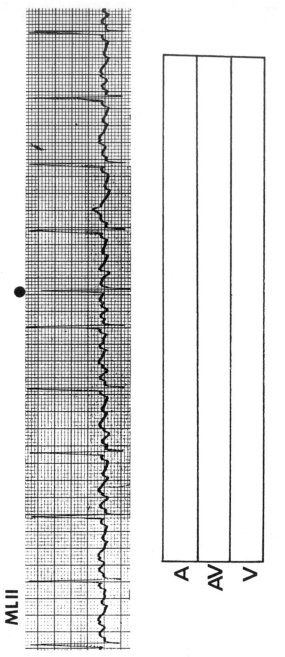

MLII

A

AV

V

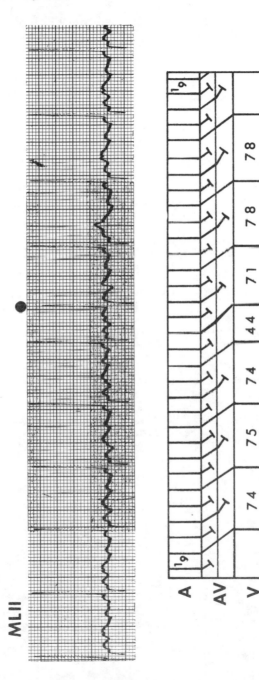

FIG. 49.3

present, is not prescribed upon discharge. When last seen ten months postoperatively, the patient was feeling well, having no angina, and no arrhythmias.

BIBLIOGRAPHY

Berkowitz WD, Wit AL, Lau SH, Steiner C, Damato AN: The effects of propranolol on cardiac conduction. Circulation 40:855, 1969.

Fisch C, Greenspan K, Knoebel S, Feigenbaum H: Effects of digitalis on conduction of the heart. Prog Cardiovasc Dis 6:343, 1964.

Katz LN, Pick A: Clinical Electrocardiography. Part I. The Arrhythmias. Lea and Febiger, Philadelphia, pp. 382-502, 1956.

Kayden HJ: The current status of procainamide in the management of cardiac arrhythmias. Prog Cardiovasc Dis 3:331, 1961.

Kosowsky BE, Haft JI, Lau SH, Stein E, Damato AN: The effects of digitalis on atrioventricular conduction in man. Amer Heart J 75:736, 1968.

Pick A: Digitalis and the electrocardiogram. Circulation 15:603, 1957.

Przybyla AC, Paulay KL, Stein E, Damato AN: Effects of digoxin on atrioventricular conduction patterns in man. Amer J Cardiol 33:344, 1974.

Rabbino MD, Dreifus WL, Likoff W: Cardiac arrhythmias following intracardiac surgery. Amer J Cardiol 7:681, 1961.

CASE 50: Fatigue and paroxysmal lightheadedness in an elderly
          man with bradycardia.

A 72-year-old previously healthy man complains of feeling fatigued
and intermittently lightheaded for the past three weeks. His
physical examination is remarkable only in that the apical pulse is
36/minute. The 12-Lead ECG shows abnormally leftward mean
frontal plane QRS axis of -40 degrees, probably due to left anterior
fascicle block. A Lead V_1 rhythm strip is shown in Fig. 50.1.

1. Which of the following terms describe the rhythm?
    a) sinus rhythm
    b) junctional escape beat
    c) first degree AV block
    d) second degree AV block, Type I (Wenckebach)
    e) second degree AV block, Type II
    f) second degree AV block, type uncertain
    g) AV dissociation
    h) ventriculophasic sinus arrhythmia

ANSWER: (a, c, f) The QRS complexes, occurring at regular intervals of about 1.76 seconds (corresponding rate 34/minute) are narrow and of normal contour, indicating that ventricular activation
occurs normally via the AV junction-His-Purkinje system. Normal-
appearing P waves, occurring at intervals of about 0.88 seconds
(corresponding rate about 68/minute) are probably sinus in origin,
and P waves precede each QRS complex by a constant interval. The
QRS complexes are stimulated by the P waves preceding them, but
the slightly prolonged PR interval of about 0.21 seconds indicates
abnormally slow conduction through the AV conduction system (first
degree AV block). The presence of sinus P waves that follow each
QRS complex but do not themselves stimulate QRS complexes indicates that second degree AV block is also present. The presence
of 2:1 AV conduction does not allow differentiation between Type I
(Wenckebach type) and Type II second degree AV block. Autonomic
nervous system maneuvers and/or administration of pharmacologic
agents may allow more accurate diagnosis to be made by altering
sinus rate and/or AV conduction system velocity or refractory
period.

Carotid sinus massage, for example, by withdrawal of sympathetic
traffic from, and enhancement of parasympathetic traffic into, the sinus
and AV nodes, will slow both sinus rate and AV nodal conduction velocity
but would not be likely to affect impulse conduction velocity through
the more distal His-Purkinje system. As the conduction abnormality
in Type I AV block is almost invariably located within the AV node,
carotid sinus massage would be expected to worsen (prolong) AV
conduction if sinus rate did not slow. As the conduction abnormality

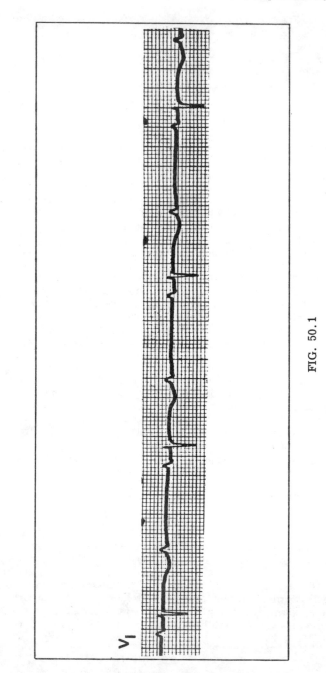

FIG. 50.1

in Type II AV block is almost invariably located within the His
bundle and/or proximal bundle branches, carotid sinus massage,
by slowing sinus rate, would allow the His-Purkinje system more
time to repolarize and thus improve AV conduction. Atropine, a
parasympatholytic agent, would be expected to improve AV conduction in Type II AV block so long as the increase in sinus rate was
not excessive. However, should atropine cause marked acceleration
in sinus rate, AV conduction might worsen. Since atropine has no
effect on conduction within the His-Purkinje system, it would not
be expected to improve AV conduction in Type II AV block. On the
contrary, atropine-induced increase in sinus rate, by increasing
the frequency with which impulses reach the His-Purkinje system,
usually worsens AV conduction in Type II AV block.

Since all QRS complexes in Fig. 50.1 are stimulated by P waves,
neither AV dissociation nor junctional escape beats are present.
The failure of junctional escape beats to occur during a pause as
long as 1.76 seconds could be due to (1) depressed AV junctional
automaticity or (2) conduction of the blocked sinus impulses into,
and depolarization of, a subsidiary AV junctional pacemaker which,
shortly thereafter, might otherwise have stimulated a QRS complex.
Conduction of this sinus impulse into, and depolarization of, a
latent AV junctional pacemaker is electrocardiographically silent.
It is inferred on the basis of subsequent events and is thus an example of concealed conduction of an impulse into the AV junction,
resulting in concealed discharge of a subsidiary pacemaker. Since
the PP intervals are constant, ventriculophasic sinus arrhythmia
is not present.

The patient is admitted to the hospital in order to establish the
severity of conduction system abnormalities, and whether or not
they are of recent onset and therefore possibly reversible. As a
diagnostic maneuver he is given atropine, 1.2 mg intravenously,
and the MCL_1 rhythm strip shown in Fig. 50.2 is recorded about
five minutes later.

2. Which of the following terms describe the rhythm?
    a) sinus rhythm
    b) junctional escape beats
    c) second degree AV block, Type I
    d) second degree AV block, Type II
    e) second degree AV block, type uncertain
    f) AV dissociation
    g) first degree AV block
    h) escape-capture bigeminy
    i) atrial premature beats

ANSWER: (a, b, c, f, h, i) All QRS complexes are narrow and of
normal appearance, indicating that ventricular activation occurs normally via the AV junction-His-Purkinje system. The QRS rhythm
occurs in a bigeminal pattern. Those QRS complexes occurring at

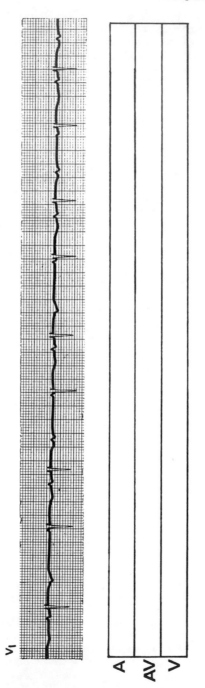

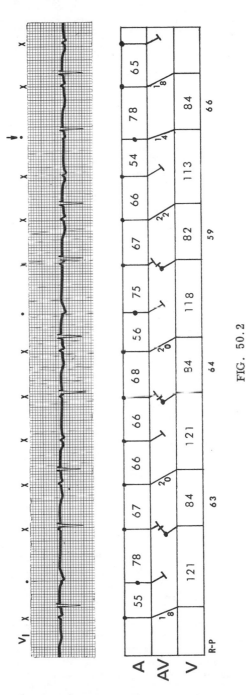

FIG. 50.2

shorter cycle length (0. 82-0. 84 seconds) are preceded by P waves
at intervals of 0.18-0.22 seconds, and are probably stimulated by
these P waves. The QRS complexes occurring at longer cycle
length (1. 18-1.24 seconds) are preceded by P waves at intervals
too short ($\leq$ 0.08 seconds) to be stimulated by them and are therefore junctional escape beats. The rhythm is thus AV dissociation
with capture. The next-to-last QRS complex, occurring at cycle
length of about 1.13 seconds, is likely to have been stimulated by
the preceding P wave occurring about 0.14 seconds earlier (vide
infra). The longer PR intervals following shorter RP intervals
during AV dissociation with capture supports the probability that
the AV conduction abnormality is Type I, for it reflects the phenomenon that conduction velocity of impulses through the AV conduction
system is slower shortly after depolarization when the AV node is
more refractory than it is later on. P waves labeled "X", occurring at cycle lengths of 0.65-0.68 seconds, are sinus impulses. The
remaining P waves (●), occurring at shorter cycle lengths of 0.55,
0.56, and 0.54 seconds, are most likely atrial premature beats, a
possibility supported by the clearly seen twelfth P wave (arrow),
which has a contour somewhat different from sinus beats. The P
waves following the premature P waves by 0.78, 0.75, and 0.78
seconds are probably sinus P waves because they follow the preceding sinus beat by an interval about twice the sinus cycle length
(i.e., there is a complete compensatory pause). Since not all consecutive sinus P waves are conducted, there is second degree AV
block. As the last two QRS complexes in the strip are stimulated
by two consecutive atrial impulses occurring 0.78 seconds apart,
the refractory period of the AV conduction system must be at most
0.78 seconds at this time, whereas prior to the administration of
atropine, it must have exceeded the intersinus interval present at
that time, about 0: 88 seconds. Shortening of the refractory period
of the AV conduction system by atropine suggests that AV block is
occurring in the area of the AV node, and supports the inference
that the second degree AV block may well be Type I (Wenckebach).

The observed effects of atropine in this patient have been to (1) increase the sinus rate from about 68/minute to 91/minute, (2) shorten the PR intervals of the conducted sinus beats despite shorter
RP intervals, (3) not measurably change the degree of AV block,
and (4) facilitate the appearance of junctional escape beats. The
appearance of the junctional escape beats following atropine could
be due to (1) shortening of the escape interval of the junctional pacemaker by parasympatholysis, and/or (2) a change (decrease) in the
depth of penetration of the blocked sinus impulse into the AV node
so that the impulse does not reach and discharge the junctional escape pacemaker as readily as it had previously (Fig. 50.1).

The bigeminal rhythm in Fig. 50.2, consisting of junctional escape
beats followed by sinus beats is termed "escape-capture bigeminy".
This rhythm occurs because the escape interval of the AV junctional
pacemaker is shorter than the reasonably constant intervals between
consecutive atrial impulses reaching the AV junctional pacemaker.

When the final atrial premature beat in Fig. 50.2 (arrow) makes the interval between two consecutive atrial impulses reaching the AV junction shorter than the escape interval of the AV junctional pacemaker, there is transient interruption of the escape-capture bigeminy.

3. How might this patient be reasonably managed at this time?
   a) implantation of a permanent transvenous demand ventricular pacemaker
   b) close observation to determine the reversibility of the conduction abnormality
   c) administration of parasympatholytic medication
   d) reassurance that the patient will feel better with time and that he needs no treatment at this time

ANSWER: (a, b) The patient's fatigue and lightheadedness are most likely related to the slower than optimum ventricular rate occasioned by the AV block. Since these symptoms have been present, though stable, for about three weeks, and there are no symptoms or electrocardiographic evidence of recent myocardial ischemia or other potentially reversible processes, it is unlikely that the conduction abnormality is reversible; it is nevertheless reasonable to monitor the cardiac rhythm in an attempt to document that this is the case. It is unlikely that the patient's symptoms will abate spontaneously unless AV conduction improves, and treatment with parasympatholytic agents almost always causes unpleasant side effects and only rarely produces significant improvement in AV conduction. Permanent ventricular demand pacing is currently the only reliable treatment for bradycardia-related symptoms in this clinical setting.

The patient's cardiac rhythm is monitored for 48 hours while serial electrocardiograms and serum creatine kinase and lactic dehydrogenase determinations are performed. There is no change in AV conduction and no evidence of recent myocardial necrosis, so a permanent demand right ventricular apical pacemaker is implanted. Within one week the patient feels normal and when last seen four years later was continuing to feel well.

BIBLIOGRAPHY

Damato AN, Lau SH: Concealed and supernormal atrioventricular conduction. Circulation 43:967, 1971.

Dreifus LS, Watanabe Y, Haiat R, Kimbiris D: Atrioventricular block. Amer J Cardiol 28:371, 1971.

Bradley SM, Marriott HJL: Escape-capture bigeminy. Amer J Cardiol 1:640, 1958.

Narula OS, Cohen LS, Samet P, Lister JW, Scherlag B, Hildner FJ: Localization of A-V conduction defects in man by recording of the His bundle electrogram. Amer J Cardiol 25:228, 1970.

Narula OS, Scherlag BJ, Samet P, Javier RP: Atrioventricular
block. Amer J Med 50:146, 1971.

Langendorf R, Cohen H, Gozo EG: Observations on second degree
atrioventricular block, including new criteria for the differential
diagnosis between Type I and Type II block. Amer J Cardiol
29:111, 1972.

Langendorf R, Pick A: Concealed conduction. Further evaluation
of a fundamental aspect of propagation of the cardiac impulse.
Circulation 13:381, 1956.

Pick A, Langendorf R: The dual function of the A-V junction. Amer
Heart J 88:790, 1974.

Schamroth L, Dubb A: Escape-capture bigeminy. Mechanisms in
S-A block, A-V block, and reversed reciprocal rhythm. Brit Heart
J 27:667, 1965.

Schamroth L: Principles governing 2:1 AV block with interference
dissociation. Brit Heart J 31:780, 1969.

INDEX

433